Human Ecology and Public Health

Edited by

Edwin D. Kilbourne, M.D.

Professor and Chairman, Department of Microbiology,
Mount Sinai School of Medicine of The City University of
New York, New York. Formerly, Professor of Public Health,
Cornell University Medical College, New York

Wilson G. Smillie,
            M.D., D.P.H., Sc.D. (Hon.)

Professor Emeritus of Public Health and Preventive Medicine,
Cornell University Medical College, New York

THE MACMILLAN COMPANY
COLLIER-MACMILLAN LIMITED, LONDON

Human Ecology and Public Health

FOURTH EDITION

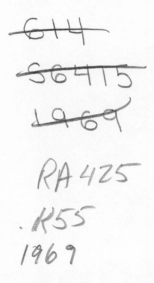

To the student,
with the hope that he will be
provoked to learn,
persuaded to agree,
encouraged to dissent,
and led to teach.

PREFACE
to the Fourth Edition

Human Ecology and Public Health is a direct lineal descendant of the third edition of *Preventive Medicine and Public Health*, but it is almost wholly a new book. The spirit and purpose of the present volume (and the editorship) remain the same. However, the increasing complexity of the subject, reflected in the title and content of *Human Ecology and Public Health*, has dictated a change to multiple authorship. The editors have undertaken this change with some reluctance because the intent of the present book, like that of earlier editions of *Preventive Medicine and Public Health*, has been to present an integrated and cohesive discussion of the concepts that underlie man's approach to the prevention of disease and the preservation of health. Yet a subject that encompasses demography, human and microbial genetics, epidemiology, clinical medicine, systems analysis, and health services administration is presently beyond the scope of one or two men and demands the insight and depth of the expert. The answer to the dilemma has been to recruit fifteen experts of like philosophy (from five different academic institutions and representing six academic disciplines) and to invite discussion of assigned topics in their areas of special competence. During the preparation of manuscript many contributors shared their thoughts with other contributors by permitting the editors to circulate tentative outlines of their chapters. This tactic has largely prevented duplication of material and sometimes has had a catalytic effect—certainly upon the editors!

There was good reason to believe that the seemingly disparate elements of this text could be blended into a coherent educational experience. Certain of the contributors, including Drs. Bearn, McDermott, Schulman, and one of the editors (E. D. K.) had collaborated earlier in the design and presentation of a lecture series for third-year medical students in the Department of Public Health at Cornell University Medical College. These lectures embraced much of the content and philosophy of Part One ("Human Ecology and Human Disease") of the present book. Drs. McCarroll and Cassell are former members of this department, while Dr. Johnson has joined the department recently. Dr. Lynn heads a department on the Ithaca campus of Cornell which has had frequent interchange with the medical college. Among this group, there has been no lack of strong-minded (but friendly) dissension, but more often there has been agreement on the general goals and concepts of the vast subject called "public health." In any event, an integration of the thoughts and scholarship of these independent and creative investigators has been essayed here. The success of this effort must be judged by the reader.

The editors are especially indebted to Mrs. Wilhelmina Jacquet for her invaluable assistance in the preparation of the manuscript and also to Miss Marie Magnani for her efficient and untiring stenographic aid.

E. D. K.
W. G. S.

CONTRIBUTORS

Barondess, Jeremiah A., M.D.

Associate Professor of Clinical Medicine, Cornell University Medical College, New York.

Bearn, Alexander G., M.D.

Professor and Chairman, Department of Medicine, Cornell University Medical College, New York.

Béhar, Moises, M.D.

Director, Institute of Nutrition of Central America and Panama, Guatemala City, Guatemala.

Cassell, Eric J., M.D.

Associate Clinical Professor of Community Medicine, Mount Sinai School of Medicine of The City University of New York, New York.

Johnson, Kenneth G., M.D.

Associate Professor of Public Health and Director, Division of Epidemiology, Cornell University Medical College, New York.

Kilbourne, Edwin D., M.D.

Professor and Chairman, Department of Microbiology, Mount Sinai School of Medicine of The City University of New York, New York.

Lynn, Walter R., Ph.D.

Professor of Environmental Systems Engineering, Director, Center for Environmental Quality Management, Cornell University, Ithaca.

McCarroll, James, M.D.

Professor of Preventive Medicine and Director, Environmental Health Division, University of Washington, Seattle.

McDermott, Walsh, M.D.

Livingston Farrand Professor of Public Health and Chairman, Department of Public Health, Cornell University Medical College, New York.

Mountain, Isabel M., Ph.D.

Research Associate, Department of Public Health, Cornell University Medical College, New York.

Reader, George G., M.D.

Professor of Medicine, Cornell University Medical College, New York.

Schulman, Jerome L., M.D.

Associate Professor of Microbiology, Mount Sinai School of Medicine of The City University of New York, New York.

Scrimshaw, Nevin S., Ph.D., M.D.

Professor and Chairman, Department of Nutrition and Food Science, Massachusetts Institute of Technology, Cambridge.

Smillie, Wilson G., M.D., D.P.H., Sc.D. (Hon.)

Professor Emeritus of Public Health and Preventive Medicine, Cornell University Medical College, New York.

Yerby, Alonzo S., M.D.

Professor and Head, Department of Health Services Administration, Harvard University School of Public Health, Boston.

CONTENTS

Section II
The Methods and Techniques of Public Health

Section III
Specific Problems of Public Health and Their Containment

Part Three
The Administration of Health Services

INDEX

Human Ecology and Public Health

Introduction

Human Ecology, Public Health, and Preventive Medicine

Edwin D. Kilbourne

The semantic distinctions and connotations of the terms *human ecology*, *public health*, and *preventive medicine* could easily occupy the few pages set aside for this introduction—but they will not. The denotations of these terms, when they are removed from their common context as labels of medical school departments, are remarkably explicit. *Ecology*, an "in" word these days (and used here therefore with some trepidation), denotes the study of the "mutual relations among organisms and between them and their environment." The prefatory adjective "human" indicates that one of the organisms in question is man. *Public health* concerns the health of the public. Although the term sometimes implies public responsibility in the control of disease and surveillance of health, in current usage it implies equally that the recipient of this responsibility and concern is the public (individuals collectively as they live together). Indeed, benefits *for* the public are generally administered *by* the public (or more precisely, by its elected or selected representatives). As stressed by several contributors to this book (especially in Chapters 13 and 14), the functions of public health are no longer limited to the prevention of disease but are increasingly concerned with medical care. *Preventive medicine*—as emphasized in the predecessor of this book (Smillie and Kilbourne, *Preventive Medicine and Public Health*, 3rd ed.)—is an integral part of the practice of medicine as carried out by the individual practitioner for the individual patient. Thus, preventive medicine is not a medical subspeciality but a viewpoint that permeates all medical specialties and a stratagem employed by the physician in the battle against disease. It should be clear that the prevention of disease is by no means solely the province of preventive medicine and just as clear that preventive medicine as a narrower and restricted discipline has, by definition, no other role to fill. Indeed, it is the increasing importance of a wide variety of nonmedical factors in both the genesis and control of human diseases that suggests that the total ecology of man must be evaluated in any consideration of human health.

It is hardly revolutionary to propose that the causation of disease is multifactorial. The probable contribution of the "poor environment" or of deficient genetic endowment to the expression even of disease related to extrinsic agents has always been appreciated intuitively by the physician. But ecology implies *interaction* and the importance of this interaction is not yet fully understood. Modern man interacts with his environment and with other organisms in ways that have no biologic precedent. In this interaction man is more than a 150-pound animal who intermittently drains oxygen from the atmosphere, replaces it with carbon dioxide, and finally contributes his meager share of nitrogen to the soil upon his demise. Almost alone among organisms, man has acquired the power to manipulate his environment, other organisms, and himself. His contributions to the atmosphere now include a frightening array of products of the combustion processes required for his present-day survival. Even the least toxic of these (CO_2) has increased to an amount that may alter the heat balance of the earth (See Chapter 4). This effect is less dramatic perhaps than the raw mutagenic power of an atomic bomb, but it is the more awesome because it derives directly and inevitably from our established contemporary patterns of daily existence.

The development of powerful antimicrobial drugs has given the physician control over life and death that he never had in the past, (see Chapter 1), but this same dramatic innovation also has provided a sharp reminder of the genetic plasticity of microorganisms, as we have learned about microbial persistence and drug resistance (see Chapters 3 and 10) and the unlikelihood of total eradication of microbial species. These are ecologic problems. The interaction of man and microbe has been influenced and the effects extend beyond the outcome of disease in the individual patient into the world into which his mutated pathogens emerge.

And, of course, man himself is mutable. His self-imposed increased exposure to ionizing radiation, whether diagnostic or bellicose in origin, has undoubtedly changed the frequency of neoplastic disease in association with effects on his somatic cells. The ultimate effect on his genes is less readily ascertained. But not only radiation and mutation are involved in man's manipulation of himself—or more properly of his personal and genetic endowment. The great advances in genetics in the past decade provide the startling suggestion that at least some genetic diseases are correctable—that the genetic cripple can be rehabilitated by biochemical alteration of his phenotype (see Chapter 2). In simpler but less general terms, a genetically determined enzyme deficiency can be corrected for by appropriate control of the diet. But in the opposite direction, man's battle to control infectious diseases by the use of vaccines has introduced grim and quite unsuspected hazards in the form of alien nucleic acids with carcinogenic potential (see Chapter 3). And even if vaccines have not yet been proved to induce human genetic change, they do alter human phenotype (immunity) as they alter resistance to disease. We have never seriously questioned the principle of artificial immunization, but to the extent that it may affect unfavorably the patterns of disease it now must be cautiously scrutinized. Immunization that only postpones infection until a more vulnerable age or that sensitizes the recipient to a viral antigen is worse than meddlesome (see Chapter 10).

What this all means is that as the complexity of human existence increases and man becomes more powerful in his actions, even his actions for good may have exaggerated consequences for evil. The twin factors of power and complexity also dictate that now less than ever can health and medicine be isolated and considered apart from the society in which they exist without regard for the total of human ecology. When it is appreciated that the greatest public health problem in the world is too many people, then it can be seen why public health considerations must enter the bedroom, the church, and the legislature—although perhaps in disguise. If poverty contributes (as it does) to the risk of disease, then the remedies for certain ills are socioeconomic and political, not medical.

Malnutrition is a deficiency disease and the deficiency—food—cannot be supplied by the best-equipped and best-intentioned physicians or by paramedical personnel. But the nature and extent of the problem and approaches to a solution can be and have been defined by medical science and epidemiologic methods (see Chapter 11). Within both domestic and international health agencies there is an increasing emphasis on research in all fields of public health as a judicious investment of the limited funds available for the solution of vast problems. A large section of the present text (see Chapters 6, 7, 8, 9) is devoted to methods and techniques used in primary research in public health and also in the more efficient utilization of the resources of public health.

As societies evolve they do not become free of disease but they substitute new diseases for old (see Chapter 12), or a technological "advance" in packaging may revive an old disease such as botulism (see Chapter 10) languishing from earlier technologic improvements. This dynamism and change in disease patterns is reflected in the administration of health services (see Chapters 13, 14, 15). The administration of these services is now undergoing a genuine revolution with the quite recent recognition that medical care and services are not merely a commodity in the market place but are the right of every human being.

PART ONE

Human Ecology and Human Disease

1

Demography, Culture, and Economics and the Evolutionary Stages of Medicine

Walsh McDermott

Health, like happiness, cannot be defined in exact measurable terms because its presence is so largely a matter of subjective judgment. About as precise as one can get is that health is a relative affair that represents the degree to which an individual can operate with effectiveness within the particular circumstances of his heredity and his physical and cultural environment. Definitions that embrace the concept of "the absence of disease" in reality are rather misleading. For all living things are diseased—our crops, our lawns, our household pets, and ourselves. Even our microbes are themselves diseased with still smaller microbes—the bacteriophages.

As a concept, therefore, a disease-free society would be biologically unreal, and hence something hardly to be set as a goal. But what is a realizable goal is to modify significantly the pattern of disease within a society; and certain disease patterns are clearly preferable to certain others. For disease *is* measurable, and to a surprising extent in any society the particular disease pattern that is present is a reflection of the over-all forces we set up or tolerate. The relation of disease patterns to such forces and the institutions developed for their management form the basis for this chapter. By using disease rather than health as an indicator, it is possible to obtain objective data for comparison among different societies or in the same society at different points in history.

7

THE EVOLUTIONARY STAGES OF MEDICINE

In approaching this question it has been helpful to consider both the historic sequence of disease patterns and the different systems for using medical knowledge as a single stepwise evolutionary process punctuated by certain stages from the primitive or traditional to the modern. The resulting conceptual model is crude; it by no means describes the way things have always occurred throughout history. But it does serve to sift out certain forces and effects in a way that permits their easier study. The model as presented here represents a modified version of what has been presented in earlier publications (McDermott, 1964; June 1966) and is an obvious borrowing from the concept of the stages of economic growth of Rostow and Millikan.

In broad outline the *first stage of biomedical growth* in the change away from the most primitive society (and perhaps the most effective single step of all) *is the introduction of impersonal measures that are not customarily regarded as being related to disease at all*. In this Stage I, the initial steps consist of such things as the innovation of eating off a table instead of from a dirt floor. Along with this come the beginnings of the economic infrastructure—the footpaths, roads, and bridges, and ultimately the dams and communications systems. The capability of spanning 300 miles by telephone to find out what to do about a local outbreak of disease can make a considerable difference in the health of a community.

Stage II of growth is similarly nonpersonal. It consists of purposeful attempts to affect disease by introducing a change in the nonpersonal environment. Examples of this are the provision of a safe water supply and the spraying of residual insecticides for the control of malaria. In this stage too, the effect on the disease pattern may obviously be considerable, and this stage marks the start of medical institutions as we have created them.

In Stage III, the system becomes personal but the personal relationship is *noncontinuing*. In this stage, the program involves such actions as immunization programs every two or three years for remotely situated villages, or for school children if schools exist. Such a program is a "one-shot" affair and the deliverers of the technology pull out after only one or two days with a clear understanding that their return is not to be expected for another year or so.

These three stages all consist of programs that are essentially nonpersonal. The application of the biomedical sciences to the problems of an individual is indirect rather than by the direct method exemplified in the classic physician-patient relationship.

Between these three stages and the fourth is the great divide—once this is crossed, forces are set in motion that in effect are chain reactions, with each creating a need for still additional innovations. For *in Stage IV, the society assumes the responsibility for the provision of services on a continuing basis—the regular delivery of medical services to each person as an individual*. In other words, some form of the classic physician-patient relationship is present.

Each stage is grafted on to its predecessors; it does not supplant them. Thus, introduction of Stage IV (continued personalized services) is in addition to Stage III and what went before. But each of these two stages represents a quite different system for the application of biomedical science and technology for man's benefit, and the earlier stages also represent forms that conceivably might be exploited as delivery systems. In a historic sense, what characterizes the individual stages or delivery systems is the extent to which each stage or system had a decisive technology. By this is meant the capability to perform acts based on science—acts with predictable consequences that are decisive in altering the status of disease.

Using decisive influence on disease as the yardstick, the presently modernized world remained in Stage III well into this century. To be sure, in the preceding two or three centuries there had gradually developed an institutional form recognizable as the forerunner of today's personal physician. These rather haphazardly trained and educated men and women provided great human comfort, but in retrospect, it is clear that they had virtually no power to alter the course of a disease in a predictable and decisive fashion. With a few notable exceptions, the only real capability to influence disease *decisively*, really as late as the mid-nineteen-twenties, was through the noncontinuing, group approach of Stage III. From the mid-twenties on, however, there was a relatively rapid development of a decisive technology. Yet this technologic decisiveness was engrafted on to the ongoing system that had lacked any such capability. As a consequence, it is not altogether easy to distinguish how much of what we apply today represents the modern decisive technology and how much is the carry-over of practices of dubious value from a prescientific past. Without question, an appreciable portion of what the public voices as the medical services they need and should have is not really this decisive portion of our medicine at all, but practices that have survived from a day when we could not act decisively.

THE DELIVERY OF MEDICAL TECHNOLOGY

Let us examine modern medicine and its delivery systems from this standpoint, i.e., their degree of decisiveness with respect to demographic/disease patterns of quite different kinds. Before doing this, however, it is worth making the point that the decisive technology is only one part of the total medical influence. For medicine is not a science but a learned profession deeply rooted in a number of sciences and charged with the obligation to apply them for man's benefit. As we have noted, the actual applying is done by two quite different sorts of physicians: those who care for one patient at a time and those who deal with people as groups. Both kinds of physician exercise compassion. In the one, compassion takes the form of a cultivated instinct to lend support and comfort to a particular fellow human being; in the other, it is necessarily what I call "statistical compassion," namely that imaginative compassion for people one never knows about except as dots on a graph. But the technology of modern medicine—its capability to take decisive acts—is separable from this humanitarian component with its long and honorable tradition, and it is on this technologic component that the present discussion is focused.

As indicated before, the respective stages are, in effect, delivery systems, categorizable on the basis of the persons by whom the biomedical knowledge gets applied for the public good. There are three such categories. There is the kind of biomedical knowledge that can be applied by an individual physician to manage the problems of an individual patient. I call this *the clinical or personal physician delivery system*. There is the kind of biomedical knowledge that can be applied to people in groups. I call this *the nonclinical or public physician* delivery system*. In large measure it is the conventional public health program but it is considerably more than that. And there is the kind of knowledge developed in other walks of science, including biology, that can be applied in such a way that it has a beneficial impact on health. I call this *the nonphysician delivery system*.

The respective contributions of the individual systems to change in the disease/demographic pattern of the United States may be seen by comparing two eras; the period from 1900 to 1935 and from 1935 to the present. The year 1935 is chosen as the historic watershed because it was in that year that sulfonamide was first introduced into clinical practice. In a strict historic sense one could choose either 1910, when arsphenamine was introduced, or 1921, the year of the announcement of insulin, as representing the great change-over to the present period in which science and technology put decisive weapons in the hands of the personal physician. Following the introduction of insulin there were a number of other developments, such as liver extract and vitamin D. But the widespread impact of this modern technologically based medicine was not perceptible until 1935, a year that conveniently and evenly divides the seven decades of this century.

In looking at the earlier era (1900–35) in terms of its most important diseases, a fruitful approach is to analyze the infant mortality, which is conventionally expressed as the total of deaths occurring during the first year of life per each 1,000 infants who were born alive. One frequently hears that there is "a lot" of this or that disease in a particular locality, but it is far from easy to obtain any very clear idea of what people actually have in mind when they use the term "a lot." It is even more difficult to find observed data on disease frequency. Obviously, what one has to have is quantitative information on how much of one disease is present in comparison with all the others. Surprisingly enough, the data on diseases of adults are seldom presented in these terms, yet without looking at such disease inventories we are simply not looking at the problem. Fortunately, the disease pattern for infants is more often characterized in this way as may be seen in Figure 1-1, which represents the infant deaths from all causes in New York City during the first 30 years of this century.

The first striking feature of the graph is that it is important as an indication that diseases readily recognizable by name—and they include such well-known entities as tuberculosis, diphtheria, and the streptococcal diseases—make up only a small portion of the total causes of infant deaths. As one may see, this group of "name" diseases forms a relatively thin band compared with the two diseases above them in the graph. The great killer—and it accounted for approximately one half the total deaths—is the pneumonia-diarrhea complex.

Diarrhea is a manifestation rather than a disease, and even when considered broadly it is not as easy either to identify or define as one might think. Nevertheless, when large numbers of cases are examined, there is a clustering within a 12-month period

---

* The term "managerial physician" formerly used by this writer to describe the public physician has been abandoned because it is also used to describe the managerial role of the personal physician in working with subprofessionals.

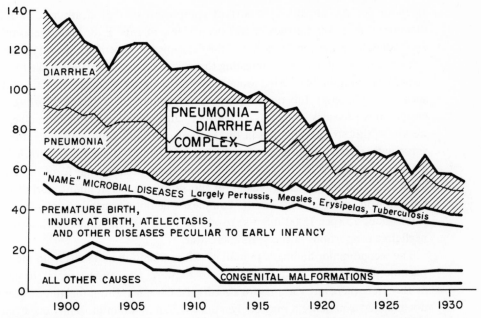

FIGURE 1-1. Infant mortality by prominent causes in New York City (rates per 1,000 births). (Modified from *Weekly Reports of the Department of Health, New York City.* 21: 396, 1932.)

from the sixth to the eighteenth month of age. Gordon and his associates (Gordon *et. al.*, 1963) call this "weanling diarrhea," and the term is a useful one. Weanling diarrhea has an important linkage to protein-calorie malnutrition (see Chapter 11), but it can also occur in high incidence, although it is probably far less lethal, in societies with an abundance of high-quality protein.

The pneumonia part of the diarrhea-pneumonia complex is not the sharply distinguishable group of pneumonias we can so readily define and diagnose in adults. Instead it is a syndrome in an infant or young child characterized by clinical or radiographic evidence of lower respiratory tract disease. It is this pneumonia and diarrhea, occurring either individually or together, that represents the great killer in any society before it is modernized. In 1900, in New York City, the annual fatality rate from diarrhea (exclusive of the pneumonia) was more than 5,000 per 100,000 infants. In the late-nineteen-fifties we observed similar rates in our Navajo studies. Assuming that in both societies at these two different points in time, the infants represented about 4 per cent of the population (the actual Navajo rate was 3.7), this diarrhea rate alone, not counting the pneumonia, would yield a death rate of over 200 per 100,000 population. This is higher than the present annual United States mortality from all forms of cancer. Here we have one definition of "a lot," and it includes only the infants; if the preschool children were also included, the diarrhea death rate would be considerably higher.

Now let us compare these diarrhea deaths with deaths from all the other diseases and then examine how our biomedical science and technology were applied to manage this pneumonia-diarrhea complex in New York. Throughout the nineteenth century, the birth rate in New York City stayed around 55 per 1,000 and the death rate continued at about 30. An obviously important component of that death rate in 1900 was the more than 5,000 diarrhea deaths per 100,000 infants. Four highly relevant points are evident from the consideration of the three-decade experience shown in Figure 1-1.

As mentioned above, it is interesting to note what a small portion of the total deaths at the beginning of the period were contributed by the "name" infectious diseases, such as diphtheria, tuberculosis, or the streptococcal diseases. Throughout the ensuing three decades, there was a steady straight-line fall in deaths from all causes. As we know, this straight-line fall in total infant mortality continued thereafter until in subsequent decades it leveled off at 24 instead of the 140 per 1,000 recorded in 1898 and seen on the left of the graph. But in the three decades that form the graph it is quite clear that the principal reason for this gratifying fall in infant mortality was the reduction in just that one disease complex, pneumonia-diarrhea, which had fallen from about 75 (per 1,000 infants) to about 17 in 1930.* And, it dwindled away to negligible proportions in the years thereafter.

The second major finding is that all of this marked fall in deaths from the diarrhea-pneumonia complex occurred before there were any antimicrobial drugs at all; neither were there any vaccines for this disease complex. From this three-decade, well-documented experience it may be seen that the fall in infant mortality occurred during a time in which biomedical science and technology could put no specific, decisive therapies or preventives into the hands of our clinical or personal physicians.

The third major finding is that, if we could put no decisive tools into the hands of our physicians then, the fact is that we are only very slightly better off now.

Unlike the situation among adults, probably 90 per cent, at least, of these pneumonias of infancy are viral in origin (Coriell 1967). One must say "probably" because, strange as it may seem, our biomedical science has not yet produced a systematic study of the question employing both bacteriologic and virologic technics. Thus the 90 per cent can be no more than an estimate. Whatever the precise distribution may turn out to be, it is virtually certain we will find that no more than one or two in five, and perhaps even fewer, of the infants with this pneumonia-croup-lower-respiratory-tract disease would be significantly benefited by the administration of an antimicrobial drug. This is in full agreement with the clinical impressions of those who have used such drugs in the treatment of these pneumonias.

The situation with the diarrhea is even worse from the standpoint of decisive therapies available to be put into the hands of the personal physician. As is well known, the diarrhea is thought to have both a microbial and a nutritional component. Careful studies, made in localities scattered all over the world, have all shown the same thing— there is no microbe, neither a virus nor a bacterium, that can be convincingly implicated as *the* cause of the microbial part of the disorder. Moreover, most clinicians with experience with the disease would agree that antimicrobial therapy per se is not a decisive therapy for this disease.

At the present time, the concept is once again gaining acceptance, largely from studies by the Army Medical College and at the Institute for Nutrition of Central America and Panama (INCAP), that the microbial component of weanling diarrhea is

* The birth rate in 1926–30 was 18.7 per 1,000 population.

one or more of the microbes that become a part of the intestinal flora of us all (Gordon *et al.*, *Bull WHO*, 1964.) This concept was originally developed in 1902 as the result of of the work of Park and Holt. In this respect, the diarrheas appear to resemble the steadily increasing endogenous microbial disease we are seeing on our adult wards today, in which commonplace microbes, generally harmless for most people, are nevertheless capable of producing serious disease. In any case, it is clear that except for the occasional infant with shigellosis, and the small portion of those with pneumonia in whom the pneumonia is bacterial in origin, we have today no decisive treatments or preventives that we can put into the hands of a clinical physician confronted with an infant with the diarrhea-pneumonia complex.

The fourth major point is that not only was the job done without there being decisive tools in the hands of the clinical or personal physicians, it is not possible to identify the impact of individual decisive measures introduced through the nonclinical system. Thus the chlorination of the central water supply and the uniform pasteurization of milk—both representing major applications of biomedical science and technology—cannot be shown to have affected the rate of the falling mortality in New York. Whatever was done that produced the result was many things not just one or two. This gives rise to the questions of what were the essential elements in the package of developments and how much of what was done is transferable elsewhere.

It would not be useful to dwell long on these questions because we lack truly meaningful information on the subject. We do know that the first part of this period was one of lively social reform movement aimed at ameliorating the conditions in the New York slums. There were milk kitchens, visiting nurses, and the beginnings of well-baby clinics; there was the growth of pediatrics with Jacobi and Holt and the work of Park and of Lillian Wald. There were major campaigns against illiteracy and a big push in primary school education. There was a substantial fall in the birth rate (from 35 in 1900 to 18.7 in the late-nineteen-twenties), so there were not quite so many infants and young children in the society. In short, it was a period of intense community development in which many people, including some of the leading physicians, played a big role. It was also a period of considerable increase in the standard of living. Thus the experience of the first of the two eras represents more of a broad social triumph in which medicine and public health played some part rather than a result largely attributable to modern medicine as such. Nevertheless, the impact on changing the length of life expectancy from the time of birth was obviously very great. When the era started in 1900, a 70-year old man had a greater chance of surviving a year than had an infant and the life expectancy at the time of birth was 47.3 for whites and 33.0 for nonwhites.

It is when one looks at what happened in the second era that the impact of modern decisive medicine delivered through the personal physician system becomes clear. The observations in Figure 1-2 also start in 1900 and show the age-adjusted death rate for the United States as a whole. (An age-adjusted death rate is one in which the data are corrected to ensure that the populations being compared each year contain comparable numbers of young people and old people.) As may be seen, except for the influenza epidemic of 1918, the curve of the death rate shows a steady fall from year to year until 1937, close to the dividing point (1935) between our two eras.

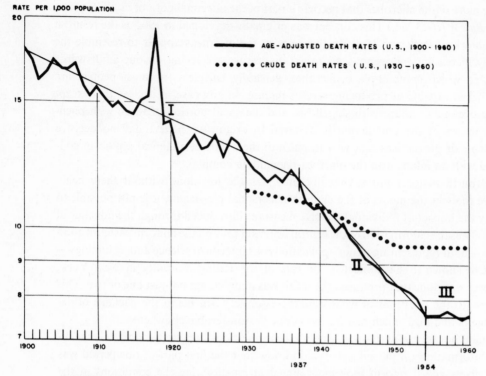

RATE PER 1,000 POPULATION

AGE-ADJUSTED DEATH RATES (U.S., 1900-1960)

• • • • • • CRUDE DEATH RATES (U.S., 1930—1960)

FIGURE 1-2. Crudely represents the influences of the nonclinical physician system and socioeconomic improvement. (Modified from National Center for Health Statistics: *Coronary Heart Disease in Adults.* Washington, D.C., ser. 3, no. 1, March 1964, p. 3.)

A major influence obviously entered at this point and for the next 17 years there was a sharp drop in this age-adjusted mortality. This tells us that some fairly large age group, presumably not the very old people, was living longer and that something had happened at the beginning of 1937 to intensify this effect to a considerable degree. The dotted line shows the crude mortality. And as one can see, the age-adjusted mortality started pulling away from it and dropped down much faster from 1937 on.

What happened, of course, was the introduction, late in 1936, of sulfonamide, the first of the great antimicrobial drugs. The writer believes that virtually all of this substantial fall in age-adjusted death rate from 1937 to 1954, and its maintenance at a stable rate thereafter, represents the influence of the broad application of the products of biomedical science by the individual physicians of the United States through the clinical physician delivery system.

THE ANTIMICROBIAL DRUGS: POWER FOR THE INDIVIDUAL PHYSICIAN

The case is as follows: the greater part of what could be accomplished in reducing infant deaths by alteration of living conditions outside and inside the home had already been done in the previous era; the quality and the quantity of the food supply were adequate in both eras; the new scientific developments which tumbled out in rich profusion from the mid-thirties can be directly related in a specific and decisive way to a whole roster of diseases; and generally speaking, there was a well-educated medical profession and a sufficiently educated public to take advantage of it.

The flattening of the age-adjusted mortality from 1954 on does not mean that progress stopped in 1954, but merely that we are now up against a hard-core disease pattern, the nature of which will be considered in a later section.

As one might guess, a look beneath this substantial fall in age-adjusted mortality from 1937 to 1954 reveals that there has been a substantial transformation of the disease pattern of early and middle life. For example, in 1937 tuberculosis was one of the five leading causes of death in all age groups from 5 to 44. What is more, for each fatal case there were even more people in these highly productive years of life who were completely incapacitated for two, three, or more years by the disease and its treatment.

In the period from 1946 to 1953, the death rate from tuberculosis fell by more than 70 per cent, and it continued to fall thereafter. At the end of the period it was no longer in the first five causes of death in any age group. Although it is still an important disease, its therapy no longer requires a year or two of incapacitation. In 1965, there were 214 deaths from tuberculosis under the age of 25 reported in the 50 states, whereas three or four decades previously tuberculosis caused more than 100,000 deaths in this age group.

We have an immensely improved capability to control the major acute pneumonias of adult life in contrast to the situation in infancy. Before 1937, between one in five and one in three young adults with the commonest form of bacterial pneumonia—pneumococcal pneumonia—would die. Now they almost invariably recover after only a short illness. The commonest form of meningitis, that due to meningococcus, is now readily managed if discovered in time as it should be. The commonest form of a virtually 100-per cent fatal disease, bacterial endocarditis, is now usually well handled; indeed its actual occurrence is presumably reduced by the use of drugs to prevent it. Two formerly major forms of crippling and fatal heart disease have been greatly affected. One, syphilitic heart disease, has virtually disappeared; and the other, rheumatic heart disease, is showing a marked decline.

A major reason for the decline in rheumatic heart disease is probably the general control of streptococcal infections in young children; that is, school-age children. Acute glomerulonephritis has likewise been affected in the same way. Along with tuberculosis, rheumatic heart disease was the major serious disease of youth at the beginning of this second era, and these two diseases together were really the ones that made up a great portion of the pattern of chronic illness before middle age. Ironically, at the same time that we have developed the ability to correct the late consequences of rheumatic fever by cardiac surgery, we are witnessing the almost complete disappearance of the acute form from our hospital beds. Syphilis of the brain, formerly a significant cause of stay in our mental hospitals, is now a great rarity.

The list of diseases, readily controlled or usually managed by therapy, includes the streptococcal diseases such as scarlet fever; the dreaded childbed fever, erysipelas; quinsy sore throat; many of the staphylococcal infections; typhoid fever; gonorrhea; brucellosis; adult dysentry; anthrax; syphilis and the other spirochetal diseases; all the forms of typhus fever and spotted fever; and a few of the important diseases due to fungi.

This capability to control, or in some cases prevent, these diseases in a decisive and purposeful way has had great effect on our disease pattern. If the writer were to make rounds on the same university hospital services where he was a student 35 years ago, he would find only a very few patients with the diseases he saw there as an undergraduate, and these marked changes all happened basically in that 17-year period that started in 1936–37.

Some of what has happened has not even been purposeful. There is the case of primary hematogenous staphylococcal osteomyelitis. Thirty-five years ago in the surgical outpatient department of a large general hospital—50 per cent of the outpatient visits were for the consequences of this infection of the bone. For this disease acquired early in life, leads to repeated crippling—and invalidism—thereafter. Now, it has virtually disappeared. No one knows exactly how it happened. Apparently it is a consequence of the rather widespread use of antimicrobial drugs for undiagnosed febrile illnesses in adolescents. Although this practice is not necessarily to be condoned, the example is cited simply to show that there may well be important social gains from the widespread use of biomedical science even when imperfectly applied.

But the over-all influence of the antimicrobial drugs on the disease pattern is far greater than this admittedly great impact on the diseases that can be directly affected. For in large measure it is these antimicrobial drugs that provided the key element in the technologic infrastructure on which is based virtually all the other great medical advances of the past 35 years. Thus every development, from viral vaccines such as the poliomyelitis vaccine and the measles vaccine to the use of corticosteroids, to chest surgery and open heart surgery, organ transplantation, and the modern work in genetics, all these would not have been possible had it not been possible for us to control infection easily both in patients and in artificial cultures as a consequence of the development of these drugs.

These other diseases will not be considered further because their qualitative effects on the disease pattern and the demographic pattern are as yet not great. But it was this capacity to control infection that led to all the rest. These developments have changed our disease pattern in the United States from one dominated by infection or its consequences, in which death or invalidism in childhood or early in adult life was not too uncommon, to one in which during the school years and in early middle life, the greatest risk is from accidents of some sort or another (see Chapter 12). Probably the most striking way to see the effects of this technology, applicable chiefly through the clinical physician system, is to review what happened to the United States population.

POPULATION INCREASE IN RELATION TO PATTERNS OF DISEASE

During the past 50 years and especially during the past 20, there has been little change in the United States crude death rate, yet a doubling of the United States population has occurred. This doubling has occurred not only with little change in crude death rate, but with a birth rate that would be classified as low; it never was higher than 26 and frequently was below 20. Immigration was sharply limited in 1921 at the beginning of the period. Thus, the principal way this doubling of the population could be attained was by minimizing the wastage of early death and by ensuring that each person born into this society had the maximal chance to survive through the child-bearing period and on into middle, or old, age. This involves the application of science and technology for the individual, and hence this population doubling represents the triumph of the clinical physician system to match the triumph of the non-clinical system in the preceding era.

The remarkable change in the disease pattern that has occurred in these two 35-year eras has thus been accomplished, broadly speaking, by the two quite different systems for the application of biomedical science and technology. As we have seen, most of what was accomplished in the earlier era, including the greater part of the extension of our life expectancy viewed from birth, represented a combination of broad socio-economic gains including imaginative use of the nonclinical physician system. It was Stage III medicine in a setting of broad economic development. In this second era, almost all the impressive accomplishment was the result of putting a decisive technology into the hands of the individual clinical physician; in terms of the model it was Stage IV medicine.

Although these two arms of today's dual system attained this technologic "decisiveness" in an historic sequence rather than in parallel, their respective influences are now operative simultaneously on each of us in our twin roles of being both an individual and a member of a group. With this dual system, the disease pattern or "level of health" in the industrialized countries has been modified to one that usually permits a long period of personal effectiveness and productivity. If one allows for the great diversity and size of the United States its "level of health" is at the top. But its over-all health level is definitely not at the top compared with what has been done in some of the small tightly knit nations of Europe; nor is it at the top in terms of what medical science now knows how to do. Our health challenge is thus of two sorts: one, to see to it that all of our people attain the same levels as are now enjoyed by our great majority; and two, to develop ways whereby certain key scientific developments can be utilized for the benefit of our majority and minorities alike. These are not easy tasks for they require thoughtful innovations—both administrative and technologic—in a complex, mixed private/public system with a strong negative tradition toward over-all planning. On balance this largely unplanned system, or collection of sub-systems, has served us well. Its "shortfalls" are considered in detail in certain of the chapters that follow.

When we turn from consideration of the contemporary disease pattern of the United States to the disease pattern of the economically underdeveloped areas, we are revisiting in large measure, the United States disease patterns of the nineteenth century. We are going from a world in which more than half the deaths are from cardiovascular disease—usually an affair of middle life or later—to a world in which more than half the deaths occur in people who are less than five years old. Obviously these are two quite different situations in terms of the biology of disease. Therefore, let us examine the degree of fitness of our two systems—the clinical physician system and the public or nonclinical physician system—to the substrate represented by the disease patterns in these economically underdeveloped or "overly traditional" societies.

As indicated diagrammatically in Figure 1-3, considered in broad terms, the disease pattern of the overly traditional societies has three components. One is the diseases of infants and young children—essentially the same diseases as those shown in Figure 1-1 for infants in New York City; the second is the adult diseases, including those treated surgically, that have been so well managed in our society from 1937 on. These two

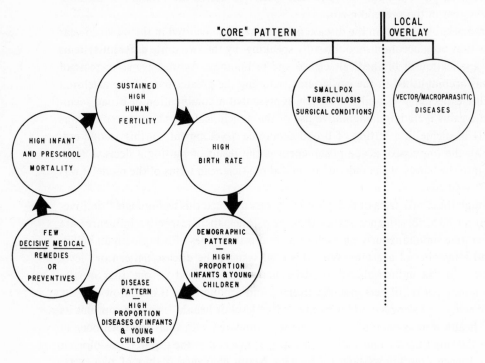

FIGURE 1-3. Demographic/disease pattern of an overly traditional society. (Modified from *Manpower for the World's Health.* Association of American Medical Colleges, Evanston, Ill., 1966, p. 139.)

components together represent the common "core" disease pattern present in all the impoverished areas of the world. The third component is the overlay of vector-borne and macroparasitic diseases that are present only when the environment has certain special characteristics.

When one looks at the core disease pattern, it becomes clear that it does not present an especially susceptible target to the technology of the clinical physician system. For the power of our biomedical technology depends on the nature of the substrate, namely the particular diseases that are present *in the particular people who are there to have them.* With annual birth rates as high as 40 to 50 per 1,000 population, half the population may be less than 15 years of age. In these circumstances, at least half of the target of the technology, i.e., the disease substrate, consists of the problems of infancy and the second and third years of life. When the community food supply is adequate, this half of the target is even more sharply limited to the first year. This general contour holds even if the vector-borne and macroparasitic diseases are being considered in addition to the core pattern. For example, at the Third National Public Health Congress in Lima in August 1968, it was reported (*The New York Times*, Aug. 20, 1968) that 50 of every 100 deaths in Peru are of children and that 30 per cent occur during the first year of life.

Within one half the population, therefore, almost all the diseases and deaths are clustered within a year or two of birth. In the other half there is a similar clustering within the seventh and eighth decades. Considering now only the core disease pattern, there is a general freedom from serious illness except for the results of trauma and the complications of pregnancy from the very early years to middle age. Moreover, the proportionately smaller number of adults in a rural overly traditional society usually have a diet low in fat, get plenty of exercise, smoke no cigarettes, rarely have hypertension, and are not exposed to the at least theoretical hazard of industrial pollution of the air.

As a consequence, many of the numerically important diseases of early middle age in an industrialized society are numerically insignificant in an overly traditional one. Once the spread of tubercle bacilli is interrupted, and surgical facilities, linked by a transport system, however rudimentary, are set up somewhere, those disease situations of the "adult" core pattern that could be decisively affected by our current technology are encountered with relative infrequency.

The total disease substrate represented by the core pattern thus consists of two quite distinct halves—the disease events of the very early years, principally the first year, and the diseases of middle age and thereafter.

With respect to the infant part of the core pattern, our relative lack of a decisive technology to put in the hands of the clinical physician faced with the particular conditions of the overly traditional societies has been previously discussed. In elementary terms, this is predominantly due to the relative inability of the clinical physician to alter what appear to be the two major factors that shape the pattern: the supply of food within the community, notably high quality protein; and the complex of structural and functional sanitary "housing" that are present in the domiciles. As both these factors, especially that of the protein, are considered in detail in Chapter 11, they will be considered here only in broad terms. With respect to the food supply, it is sufficient to point out that in the rural overly traditional societies, there are good reasons to believe that the height of the preschool, or actually the second-year mortality, is a reflection of the adequacy of the supply of food available within a community. For example, in the Manyfarms studies in a Navajo community,* the domicillary condition consisted of a complete absence of a set of structural and functional sanitary barriers, yet the food supply *in the community* was adequate. The infant mortality was high in these circumstances, but once past infancy, the mortality (except for trauma) was quite low into early middle age. By contrast, when protein-calorie malnutrition is present (see Chapter 11), the infant mortality may be four or five times that of a modernized society, but the second year or the preschool mortality may be higher by a factor of 20 or 30.

* Bruce Lecture, American College Physicians, Apr. 1, 1968, Boston, Mass.

CULTURE AND THE PATTERNS OF DISEASE

How do the domicillary sanitary "barriers" influence the situation? First it must be appreciated what kills these children under the age of five. Some are killed by diseases also present in adults, such as tuberculosis; others die from culturally linked diseases, such as tetanus of the newborn; and some are killed by vector-borne disease in those localities where such are present. Devastating as such diseases are, however, the observation all over the world has been the same, namely that the truly great killer throughout two thirds of the world is that same pneumonia-diarrhea disease complex that was described earlier in connection with early twentieth-century New York City. It may be recalled that the particular viruses and bacteria involved in this disease complex are not limited to the impoverished areas of the world. On the contrary they also are present in the affluent residential neighborhoods of an industrialized society. Indeed, they may be regarded as constituting some of life's inescapable microbial challenges. But in the overly traditional society the infant or two-year-old is wholly unprotected against these challenges and tends to receive them all at once. By contrast, in our society a set of structural and functional sanitary barriers have been erected whereby these individual challenges are stretched out over the whole childhood and adolescence of the individual. These barriers were developed in part unconsciously and in part by pediatricians and nurses; the barriers themselves are based soundly on biomedical science. They consist, in large measure, of the invention of a radically new kind of dwelling and of altering the events that go on within it. Among the structural changes are such inventions as windows that can be opened, central heating, hot and cold water, flush toilets, tables from which to eat, refrigeration, and paper towels. The functional change has been principally in the form of parents with at least enough education to enable them to manage the household machinery properly and to establish the hygienic practices within the home. This set of barriers, both structural and functional, is in continuous existence. Its effectiveness is readily visible; indeed, it is so effective that our military recruits in late adolescence are still experiencing new challenges by respiratory viruses. And, just before the introduction of the Salk vaccine, poliomyelitis had been transferred from a paralytic disease of young children to one affecting people in their twenties. In specific terms this set of structural and functional sanitary barriers is the difference between 54 and 5,000 cases of infant diarrhea per 100,000 infants each year. As the clinical physician in a modernized society is not pinned down by this load, both because of the household barriers and because he works in a society that is 10 per cent children rather than almost 50 per cent, the disease pattern he faces is quite different. It includes appreciable numbers of different diseases each of relatively low incidence. When these are drawn from across the entire age spectrum of what can be a larger population base (because of absence of the "load") there is formed a total group of diseases for which he has the technologic capability, medical or surgical, to take decisive action. Indeed this capability for decisive action for the benefit of an individual that is the hallmark of the clinical physician shows to best advantage among a people who are only intermittently at risk of developing serious disease, microbial or otherwise. This requires people who are properly nourished and who have survived beyond the physiological instability of early life. For those still physiologically unstable, notably the infants, the clinical physician system has little to offer in the way of specific drugs or vaccines *in the absence of these structural and functional sanitary barriers of a modern home.*

THE VICIOUS CYCLE—HIGH FERTILITY AND HIGH INFANT MORTALITY

In the writer's judgment the crux of the problem in the overly traditional societies lies in this fertility/disease relationship (Figure 1-4). Specifically, the sustained high fertility skews the disease pattern into one that is largely invulnerable, in a technologic

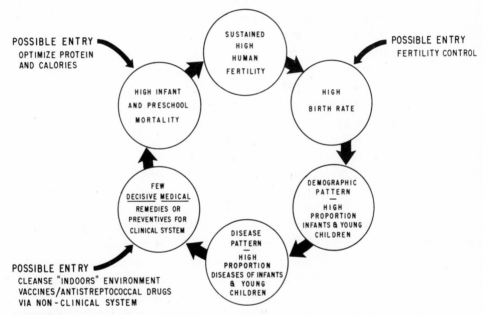

FIGURE 1–4. Fertility/disease circular relationship. (Modified from *Manpower for the World's Health.* Association of American Medical Colleges, Evanston, Ill., 1966, p. 151.)

sense, to the clinical physician system. The instrument of developing something called "the health team," including the use of paraprofessionals, does not usually alter this situation significantly, because what gets applied in this way is largely limited to what can be delivered through the clinical system. Because of this misfit between the disease substrate and the technology deliverable through the clinical system as well as the extreme unlikelihood of there being clinical physicians to man that system in the next one or two decades, a widespread impact on the disease pattern of sufficient magnitude to break into the fertility/disease circle does not seem very likely to happen. Yet until such a widespread modification of disease pattern occurs, the prospects for the limitation of individual family size on a mass basis are bleak.

The continued high infant and preschool mortality prevents the formation of one of the major preconditions necessary for the lowering of human fertility. It is in this way that it serves to reinforce the strong tendency toward high fertility. To reduce fertility requires a decision by an individual or by individual couples; for most birth-limiting techniques that individual decision must be made over and over again throughout several decades of adult life. In this, as in so many other activities in which a change in habit is desired, it is not enough to know how to accomplish a particular result, it is equally essential to know why the effort should be made in the first place. Once the know-why has been personally accepted, the know-how usually becomes of quite secondary importance.

In a society in which formal education is rare, a tightly totalitarian government might be able to effect a considerable reduction in births by a social policy in which births out of wedlock are frowned upon, or penalized, and marriage deferred until, let us say, the age of 25 for women and 30 for men.* But without such a widespread community pressure ultimately enforceable by government, it is necessary to depend upon individual decisions. In order to effect a widespread reduction in human fertility, therefore, it is first necessary to create a set of conditions in which the consequences of the high fertility come to *seem* disadvantageous to individual couples in almost infinite numbers. Yet in rural areas, where the majority of the people in the economically underdeveloped societies still live, high fertility can appear highly advantageous to the individual couple. Children commonly, even quite young children, are a useful part of the labor force in an agrarian economy. Without an organized system of social security for one's old age, about the only reliance for the parents and their only form of saving for the future is to have a few children survive to adulthood. And, it is essential that these children be male. To attain this goal in a situation in which there is a high infant and early childhood mortality, usually requires a relatively high level of live births per family. High fertility, therefore, is not something that is perceived as a drag or handicap; on the contrary, it definitely appears to the individual couple as something that is advantageous. To be sure, there is considerable evidence that many of the women would be happier with fewer pregnancies, but their views are not always taken into account. Moreover, males everywhere, including those in our own society, have fertility, sexual potency, and "manhood" all confused in their minds. Obviously, there are exceptions to this principle that high fertility appears advantageous to the individual couple in rural, overly traditional societies. For example, when land can be personally owned and transferred to children, family limitation may seem clearly advantageous. Even in this situation, however, because of the high early childhood mortality, it is necessary to have a fair number of live births in order to ensure that some of the males born alive survive to become adult heirs.

DEMOGRAPHIC CONSIDERATIONS

Without question, what can be termed "the population question" has suffered immensely from misleading simplifications. Nevertheless, the very broad generalization is essentially true, that as long as there continues to be high infant and early childhood mortality, it is very hard to make sustained high fertility seem disadvantageous.

* From the fragmentary information available, this is apparently the main thrust of the population-limiting program in mainland China.

Thus, the high early mortality blocks creation of the preconditions necessary for the reduction of fertility that is in itself necessary for the reduction of the early mortality.

It is to be emphasized that what is being discussed here is the situation among the largely uneducated rural populations of the economically underdeveloped world. In some of these countries with the beginnings of a middle class, or a trained labor force in large townships or cities, the situation is different, for the know-why is becoming generally prevalent and the preconditions have been established. But, increasing as such groups are in various parts of the world, they are still overwhelmed numerically by the largely uneducated rural residents. To these, the dangers of accelerating national population growth are very apt to seem an irrelevant abstraction, whereas for the successful preservation of their own family, a high fertility seems a good thing. This situation might be modified significantly by a major development in contraception technology, for example, a "pill" that need only be taken once per lunar month, or a chemical that could exert long enduring action following a single injection. Even here, however, the major impact at first would be on those segments of society, principally urban dwellers, to whom high fertility has already come to seem disadvantageous. For it does not profit a village woman to go in for contraception on the sly, so to speak, if she loses her husband in the process.

Where the preconditions have been established, programs based largely on contraceptive technology have met with a fairly good reception. Without the preconditions, however, programs largely based on contraceptive technology have had very little success.

This accelerating population growth in the economically underdeveloped regions—particularly in the rural areas where a majority of the population still live—is attributable to a reduction of death rates; this in turn, according to the "conventional wisdom," is a consequence of the application of modern medicine and public health. It goes directly opposite to the "conventional wisdom," therefore, to have the first steps in slowing population growth take the form of attempts to lower mortality still further. In actuality, except for malaria control, there is relatively little application of "modern medicine and public health" in these rural areas of the underdeveloped world considered as a whole; and what is being attempted faces formidable odds in a technologic sense. Moreover, when one considers the impressive population growth that occurred *before* we had any real understanding of how to alter the environment in a purposeful way to facilitate health, for example, the world's growth from 1650 to 1850, it seems likely that the "conventional wisdom" has grossly exaggerated the role of medicine and public health in the present accelerating growth in the rural areas.*

It seems much more likely that alterations of the environment made in the course of building the infrastructure—in effect, Stage I medicine—have been making the major contribution. It should be noted that this is quite a different situation from what has

---

* The total of African blacks forcibly transferred to what is now the United States is estimated as being no more than 500,000 (Curtin, 1968). Yet by the time of emancipation, roughly at the end of a 200-year period, the census of those of African descent was $4\frac{1}{2}$ million. This represented a seven-fold increase, with a doubling at least three times, in the approximately 200-year period. It must be remembered that malaria, yellow fever, cholera and smallpox were all part of the disease pattern of the United States throughout this period. Jennerian vaccination was available during the last 60 years; to what extent it was applied in the slave population is difficult to say.

happened in recent decades in the United States where it seems quite clear that the population doubling was largely attributable to biomedicine and was actually accomplished with no fall in crude death rate. Thus, the "conventional wisdom" that medicine and public health are largely responsible for the present accelerating rural population growth, and its implication that health programs are at cross-purposes with efforts toward socioeconomic development, is itself on quite a shaky foundation. These doubts coupled with recognition of the strong reinforcing tendency of high birth rates and high youthful mortality on each other (Figure 1-4), now make programs in health seem to offer the best hope of an entry point by which to break into the circular system. (Figure 1-4).

EARLY DISEASE AND HUMAN QUALITY

Whereas this need to create the preconditions for an effective program of family planning represents the major reason why a biomedical component is essential in a national program of socioeconomic development, there is a second reason, almost as compelling, that is likewise related to this high infant and early childhood morbidity and mortality. This has to do with the accumulating body of knowledge coming from research in biomedicine and in the behavioral sciences that a child entering school may have subtle brain damage resulting from a nutritional disturbance or certain kinds of illness in infancy. When the infant mortality is high, it is a safe assumption that the number similarly afflicted who did not die is considerably higher. To what extent the learning difficulties from this subtle brain damage can be overcome in the educational system and in what proportion of the "deprived" children they occur, is not yet established. But it is clear that we are beginning to get a solid scientific base for the concept that mental capacity and the capability to be educated can be permanently impaired by certain of the poverty-related conditions of late intrauterine life or early infancy. This concept is important, being the other major reason for a biomedical component in programs of socioeconomic development.

THE APPLICATION OF MEDICAL SCIENCE FOR THE INITIATION OF POPULATION CONTROL

For these two reasons (preconditions for family limitation, assurance of maximal educability), therefore, it is essential that the disease pattern of the overly traditional societies be sufficiently modified so that programs of socioeconomic development may proceed. As we have seen, the components of that disease pattern that most need modification, however, are not very susceptible to attack by the technology applicable through the clinical physician system. What are the prospects that the disease pattern can be appropriately altered by the application of science and technology through the other delivery system, the nonclinical system wherein the physician does not actually treat patients but organizes others to apply biomedical science and technology in a variety of ways? Based on what is available for application today, the prospects are only fair. Yet there are a number of things that can be done that are not now being done. Whether *in toto* their impact on the youthful morbidity and mortality would be sufficient to produce the changes necessary is anyone's guess, but it does not appear too likely. Nevertheless, they should be done pending the development of more effective measures. The respective approaches are presented here only in brief outline as this subject has been considered elsewhere in greater detail (McDermott, 1966). At least three approaches exist. The first and almost certainly the one of outstanding importance is to use our scientific knowledge to improve the total food supply for infants and young children, notably the supply of high quality protein.

A second approach through the nonclinical physician system is by the scientific manipulation of the extradomicillary, i.e., the "outdoors" environment. For certain diseases, notably malaria, this approach can be highly effective, but two qualifications have to be made. First, we have not yet developed satisfactory technology for the control of some of the most important of this vector-borne, macroparasitic group of diseases, e.g., hookworm or schistosomiasis. Second, because the core disease pattern is largely untouched by whatever successes are made in the local overlay disease pattern, the total gain in youthful lives saved is compromised to an extent not yet measured, by the phenomenon of "disease substitution." If 90 per cent of the smallpox deaths are in children and if the disease is causing one third of all deaths in children, as has actually occurred in certain societies, it does not follow that with the control of smallpox these children will necessarily survive. For, at least in the first year or two of life, they are almost continuously subjected to the other microbial challenges in the unprotected home. Disease substitution of this sort is not so much the case among the adults in whom a gain made from, say, malaria control, is apt to be maintained. But as previously discussed, it is the infant and early childhood deaths that are involved in sustaining the high fertility.

The third approach possible via the nonclinical physician system is a pluralistic program aimed principally at the core disease pattern that plays such a large role in the high youthful mortality. Basically the program consists of using carefully trained personnel other than physicians to apply what technology *is* available in the way of vaccines; to employ certain drugs on a mass rather than on an individualized basis principally to interrupt the "indoors" transmission of certain disease agents; and above all, to try to influence the events within the home both by education and by attempting to devise methods whereby the complex of nonspecific measures of known value in the pneumonia-diarrhea complex can be applied in proper time. Such a program would require considerable biomedical knowledge and imagination and an extremely well-organized effort. Whether it can be successfully done in the absence of change in the structure of the domicile and the educational level of its inhabitants is moot, for it has not yet been accomplished on any wide scale.

Of these three possible approaches via the nonclinical or public physician system (protein, extradomicillary environmental intervention, and alteration of the events within the home) only the first has at present received adequate attention in terms of biomedical science and technology. What is needed is a far greater program than it has been possible to mount to date on how science and technology could lead to the solution of disease problems, both those from the extradomicillary environment—vector-borne and macroparasitic diseases and those in the home—*within the economic constraints* of what it will be possible to allocate to programs in health. The question is not how can science and technology yield effective controls for particular diseases, but how it can be done by methods that can be financed when the total expenditure per capita for health will be of the order of one half to one United States dollar per year. This is the kind of question that is really new in biomedical research. Traditionally the development of cures or preventions has been carried on without much thought of cost and the research worker has left it to others to develop feasible methods of application. When a particular way of breaking a chain of disease causation was found, the tendency has been to go on to something else. What is needed now is something quite different, namely to search for other vulnerable links in the causation chain even though solutions technologically fitted to a modern society and its delivery systems already exist.

Let us assume that such a program based largely on new uses of biomedical science and technology met with enough success to reduce infant mortality to below 75 per 1,000 and preschool mortality to minimal levels. As this was occurring it would be accompanied by programs of contraceptive technology which eventually would attain acceptance, as family planning came to be perceived as something advantageous. A key question would be how long this process would require, because obviously until the preconditions were established the "conventional wisdom" that medicine and public health serve to encourage population growth would actually be the case. But once family planning did come to seem advantageous, the breadth of its use would be influenced by the availability and relative simplicity of the contraceptive technology. Inferences concerning the complex of factors that determine the birth rate of a whole nation are risky; yet it is noteworthy that the general availability of effective oral contraceptive and intrauterine devices in the United States has been associated with birth rates that are beginning to approach those of the Great Depression of the early nineteen thirties. Obviously in this case, the preconditions are there, and this is true even among the so-called "poverty groups." Experience with tax-supported family planning programs in the United States has been quite short, but from the preliminary indications it appears that family planning is being well accepted by the medically indigent as it already has been by the more affluent. In such an industrialized society the capability to space pregnancies and hence control family size not only has come to seem economically advantageous, but it is clearly a measure calculated to further the physical and mental health of children and parents alike. In short, it is a health measure of demonstrated effectiveness as it would be also in the economically underdeveloped world.

The question arises, however, as to whether acceptance of family planning per se—in which the parents make a free choice as to family size—is also a hopeful method of population stabilization. There is some reason to believe that it is not. This question has been considerably illuminated by the provocative essay of Kingsley Davis (Davis, K., 1967) in which the extraordinarily harsh social choices that will almost certainly have to be faced are sharply identified. He states—

The things that make family planning acceptable are the very things that make it ineffective for population control. By stressing the right of parents to have the number of children they want, it evades the basic question of population policy, which is how to give societies the number of children they need. By offering only the means for couples to control fertility, it neglects the means for societies to do so. . . . The unthinking identification of family planning with population control is an ostrich-like approach in that it permits people to hide from themselves the enormity and unconventionality of the task.

In so clearly distinguishing between family planning on a free-choice basis and population control. Professor Davis has performed a most useful service. For, as set forth above, whereas there is considerable reason to doubt that biomedicine per se has made much of a contribution to the presently accelerating population growth in the economically underdeveloped societies, there is every reason to believe that it has been the major factor in the most recent doubling of the United States population despite its relatively low birth rate. Thus the question of what are socially desirable population densities is something that sooner or later will have to be faced by us all.

On even the most superficial analysis, however, it is clear that we have no credible indices by which to determine what would constitute a socially desirable population density. In a nonagrarian economy it is clearly not to be measured in terms of land; even in an agrarian economy the proper population-to-land relationship would be widely variable depending on the degree of sophistication of the agricultural technology. From studies with small animal models it seems clear that there are "crowd diseases" and patterns of abnormal behavior that are independent of microbial pathogens or the food supply. Are certain of the components of the urban disease pattern of the industrialized societies today the "crowd diseases" of man or have we yet to face essentially new forms of disease? Would not the socially desirable population density be a value that would vary considerably in the same place at not too separated points in time? Above all, by what sort of political institutions could these values for population densities be set and compliance obtained?

Merely momentary consideration of such questions on population density along with the possible implication of such biologic phenomena as the effects of deprivation on brain growth, reveal the very considerable complexity of the biosocial problems that our science-based ability to intervene will force us to face in medicine and public health.

In a thoughtful and perceptive essay Morison, (1967) has discussed some of these issues under a title that in itself tells our story—"Where is Biology Taking Us?" Much of the scientific knowledge most relevant to these problems is set forth in the subsequent chapters of this book. It seems unlikely that we in medicine, having developed this scientific knowledge by which to act, will abstain from acting. But in order to act without causing harm of other sorts, we will have to develop whole additional bodies of knowledge. The broad challenge can be stated bluntly: Somehow we must learn how to "play God" and still maintain the essential elements of a free society.

REFERENCES

CORIELL, L. L.: Clinical syndromes in children caused by respiratory infection. *Med Clin N Amer*, **51**: 819–29, May 1967.

CURTIN, PHILIP D.: Epidemiology and the slave trade. *Political Science Quarterly*, **LXIII** (2) 190–216, June, 1968.

DAVIS, I.: Population policy: Will current programs succeed? *Science*, **158**: 730–39, 1967.

GORDON, J. E., *et al.*: Acute diarrheal disease in less developed countries. I (Gordon with Béhar, M., and Scrimshaw, N. S.) An epidemiological basis for control. *Bull WHO* **31**:1–7, 1964. II (Gordon with Guzmán, M. A., Ascoli, W., and Scrimshaw, N.S.)

Patterns of epidemiological behavior in rural Guatemalan villages. *Ibid.*, 9–20. III (Gordon with Béhar, M., and Scrimshaw, N. S.) Methods for prevention and control. *Ibid.*, 21–38.

GORDON, J. E., Chitkara, I. D., and Wyon, J. B. Weanling diarrhea. *Amer J Med Sci*, **245**: 345–77, March 1963.

McDERMOTT, W.: The role of biomedical research in international development. *J Med Educ*, **39**: 655–69, July 1964.

———: Medical institutions and modifications of disease patterns. *Am J Psychiat*, **122**: 1398–1406, June 1966.

———: Modern medicine and the demographic-disease pattern of overly traditional societies: A technologic misfit. Part 2. *J Med Educ*, **41**, September 1966.

MORISON, R. S.: Where is biology taking us? *Science*, **155**:429–33, 1967.

2

Genetic Determinants of Health and Disease

Alexander G. Bearn
and Edwin D. Kilbourne

Only recently has it been appreciated that "genetic disease" in man is more than an occasional bizarre curiosity of the clinic and that deleterious genes are universally distributed throughout the human population. The disciplines of both medicine and public health have been concerned traditionally with environmental agents of disease—particularly the infections. Control of the most devastating of these infections and the recent explosion in genetic knowledge have combined to shift attention to the intrinsic nature of man himself (i.e., his genetic endowment) in relation to his susceptibility to disease and his inheritance of it.

In a sense, public health is already the beneficiary of empirically based moral and religious proscriptions against marriage between closely related persons. These proscriptions relating to consanguinity have legal sanction and endorsement in the laws of the United States. (One third of the states forbid first cousin marriages.) The screening techniques of public health (see Chapter 8) have already been applied to the identification at birth of infants with phenylketonuria, and indeed testing for this trait is required by law, just as the administration of penicillin eye drops is legally required for the prevention of gonorrheal ophthalmia. It should be emphasized, however, that some of the variations detected by genetic screening programs are benign and the institution of dietary control before the presumptive diagnosis is confirmed is to be deprecated.

There is no doubt that the identification of genetically determined traits and diseases will progress rapidly in the next few years through the use of biochemical and cytological techniques and that preventive medicine and public health will become more and more involved in the implications of this expanding knowledge. Another dimension is added to epidemiology by recognition that individuals under study are unique, despite similarities in age, sex, ethnic background, and environment. The detection and identification of nondiseased (heterozygote) carriers of recessive traits is increasingly possible, and will influence eugenics and premarital counseling, as a form of preventive medicine. An understanding of the principles of genetics will, therefore, become crucial to a comprehensive understanding of public health, and appreciation of the concepts of population genetics will be directly relevant to planning of health services, demographic surveys (Chapter 1), and human evolution itself.

The Duality of Human Inheritance

As the only animal with an appreciation of the past and an awareness of the future, man has a cultural as well as a genetic inheritance. This cultural inheritance is important in the genesis and epidemiology of disease and in its containment. There is also an inherited "culture of poverty" that influences the pattern of disease and the problem of bringing health services to the people (see Chapter 1). The cultural inheritance can dictate whether the individual lives in a city or in the country and therefore whether he is at risk from air pollution or brucellosis; it can, through religious proscription, limit his choice of marital partners and so influence the genetic potential of his offspring. Thus, cultural and genetic inheritance are not completely separable. Neither can environmental influences on the expression of genetic endowment be assessed readily. But first, the genetic basis of heredity must be defined and understood.

The Genetic Basis of Human Heredity

Through the process of meiosis, or reduction division, the 46 *chromosomes* of the immature germ cells of man and woman are halved in number. Thus, each *gamete* (mature germ cell: i.e., sperm or egg) which will fuse in conception to form the new individual (*zygote*) is haploid and bears 23 chromosomes. The act of fertilization then restores to the zygote the full *diploid* complement of 46 chromosomes, which will subsequently characterize all its somatic cells. During the growth and development of the embryo, this full complement is maintained by mitosis—cellular division which, if normal, does not change the chromosome number of the daughter cells. The mechanics of meiosis, which is actually a two-stage divisional process, result in a reshuffling and a recombination of the genetic material. (Stern, 1960.)

The recombining of genes in meiosis explains why each child of a couple, excepting identical twins, has many genetic characters that other brothers and sisters do not have. Even if individuals lived for geologic periods and had a litter of children each year, the chance of forming two identical gametes would be so small as to make it practically certain that no two children would have the same genotype.

Any deviation in the fundamental process of meiosis and mitosis may lead to recognizable and characteristic abnormalities of the zygote produced, and the anomaly so produced may be heritable. It is now known that *nondisjunction* or failure of chromosome separation in the meiotic formation of the egg, may occur before or after conception leading to *trisomy* for one chromosome in the developing ovum; thus, the chromosome count is 47 rather than the normal diploid number of 46. This divisional aberration may result in mongolism (Down's syndrome), a relatively common mal-formation usually characterized by profound idiocy, which occurs in about 0.15 per cent of births in white populations. The greatly increased incidence of the disorder in the children of older mothers (but not fathers), especially after 35 years of age, is in accord with the theory that it is defective division in the formation of the female gamete which is responsible for the anomaly. Other accidents of chromosomal distri-bution leading to atypical numbers of the X and Y sex chromosomes may be associa-ted with abnormalities in sexual and skeletal development (e.g., Klinefelter's and Turner's syndrome). The recent observations that XYY males are frequently tall, aggressive, and predisposed to antisocial or even criminal behavior indicates the importance of chromosomal abnormalities in certain behavioral disorders. It has been estimated that chromosomal abnormalities are responsible for approximately 20 per cent of abortions in the first trimester of pregnancy. It should be emphasized, how-ever, that an abnormal chromosome count may be compatible with viability of the fetus, as in mongolism. Moreover, it appears likely that studies of large numbers of apparently normal people will reveal some persons with minimal structural chromoso-mal rearrangements, particularly small deletions with no stigmata of disease.

The 23 sets of chromosomes that an individual possesses (one set of 23 from each parent) differ significantly in morphology (Fig. 2-1) and may be distinguished from

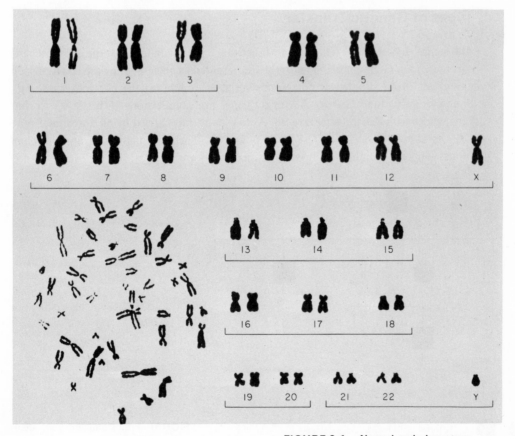

FIGURE 2-1.   Normal male karyotype.

one another by careful study. The *genes*, which are the basic units of heredity, are arranged in linear fashion on the chromosomes. It has been estimated that there are approximately 50,000–100,000 genes in the human chromosome set—one set from each parent. The corresponding genes from each parent located on corresponding chromosomes are termed *alleles*, or allelomorphs, and control the same hereditary characteristic or trait.

The chemical basis of heredity resides in DNA (deoxyribonucleic acid). The *gene* may be considered as the unit of inheritance responsible for the synthesis of a specific polypeptide (Bearn, in Beeson and McDermott, 1967). One strand of the double helix of DNA induces the intracellular synthesis of a messenger ribonucleic acid (*m RNA*) that transcribes the genetic message for protein synthesis. Transfer ribonucleic acids (*t RNA*) function by carrying amino acids to sites of protein construction on the ribosomes of the cell. *Structural genes* determine the sequence of amino acids in the polypeptides, while *control genes* quantitatively regulate their production. Mutations of structural genes obviously can lead to disease by modifying the structure of key proteins such as hemoglobin. Control genes can also have marked effects by critically diminishing the amounts of a protein that is synthesized. The impact of genetic mutations on evolution and natural selection will be discussed further.

Types of Genetic Transfer

Autosomal Inheritance.   *Autosomal* inheritance is mediated by the 44 (nonsex) chromosomes. Genes in man are doubly represented as alleles—one derived from each parent and each situated at corresponding sites or loci on the chromosomes, e.g., A and a. Individuals bearing AA or aa genes are homozygous with respect to that gene; those with Aa are *heterozygous*. A dominant trait carried by an autosomal gene *allele* is almost always manifest in its possessor. The transmission of an *autosomal* (nonsex-linked) dominant trait is diagramed in Figure 2-2.

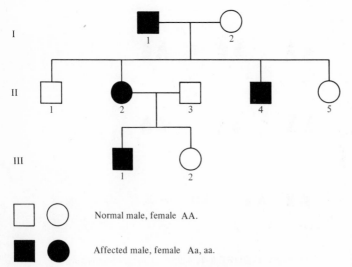

Normal male, female AA.

Affected male, female Aa, aa.

FIGURE 2-2. Dominant trait, idealized pedigree.

Recessive traits are apparent only in the homozygous individuals; it would not be expressed in the heterozygous individual, who therefore is an undiseased *carrier* of this trait—capable of transmitting the abnormal gene to his offspring (Figure 2-3). It is

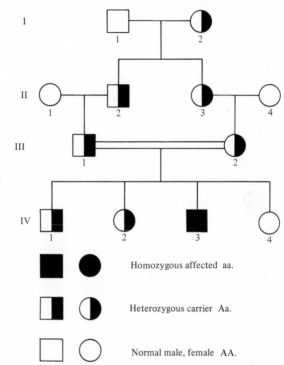

FIGURE 2-3. Recessive trait, idealized pedigree.

becoming clear, however, that recessiveness is a poor term, because it merely reflects the insensitivity of methods used to test for the abnormal gene—i.e., biochemical or cytologic testing can often demonstrate abnormality in the heterozygote who does not have clinically apparent disease. For example, the carrier of the abnormal gene for galactosemia can be shown by a "loading" test to have an abnormality in galactose metabolism. Therefore the detection of this trait is a matter of threshold. The genes involved might better be represented as having "single or double dose" effects, rather than as *recessive*. Detection of the heterozygote carrier is very important if the potential of the disease is to be known and if counseling is to be placed on a rational basis.

Sex-linked Inheritance (X-linked). Transmission of traits by genes located on the two sex chromosomes XX (female) and XY (male) are designated *sex-linked*. Only a few traits have been linked to the Y chromosomes, therefore the term *X-linked* is often used synonymously with sex-linked, and is more precise in most instances. X-linked traits may be *dominant* or *recessive*, as are autosomal traits. Dominant X-linked traits are rare, so that by implication most X-linked traits are recessive. The transmission of the sex chromosomes is illustrated simply in Figure 2-4. The Y chromosome is carried only by the male and transmitted only from father to son. X chromosomes are carried by both male and female and go to offspring of either sex.

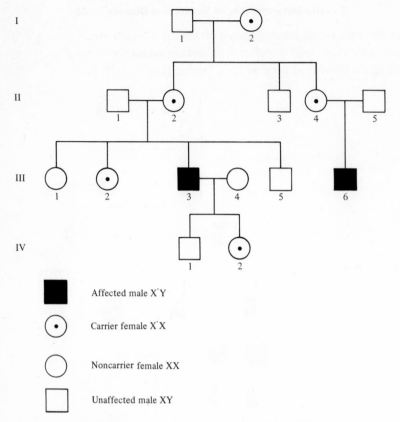

I

II

III

IV

■ Affected male X'Y

(•) Carrier female X'X

◯ Noncarrier female XX

▢ Unaffected male XY

FIGURE 2-4. X-linked recessive trait, idealized pedigree.

X-linked recessive traits are more frequently evident in the male because he is the recipient of only one X chromosome which is not "counterbalanced" by the normal allele of another X chromosome—as in the heterozygous female. Only the female who is homozygous in her inheritance of the recessive trait (having acquired abnormal recessive genes from both parents) may be affected. The affected male, who bears only one X chromosome, is said to be *hemizygous*.

Color blindness and hemophilia are classic examples of X-linked recessive traits. The extreme rarity of hemophilia in women is related to the statistical improbability of marriage between an affected individual and a carrier of this rare trait.

Expression of the Gene

It is possible for an individual to possess an abnormal gene which is clinically unexpressed. In genetic terms, the *genotype* (genetic constitution) may not be evident *phenotypically*. This is obviously true of the heterozygote in whom an abnormal recessive trait is balanced by a normal allele on the other chromosome. The total genetic endowment of the individual as well as environmental influences can also affect the functioning and expression of the abnormal gene. The term *penetrance* is a vague but widely used term applied to the degree to which the properties of a gene are evident or expressed. It is very important to note that the expression of the gene can be modified, this simple fact offers hope for prevention and therapy of diseases that

34

have heretofore seemed to be inexorable or "inborn." The example of phenylketonuria has already been cited as an instance of a biochemical metabolic defect that can be detected promptly and modified by diet.

Consanguinity and the Risk of Recessively Inherited Disease

The legal restrictions already mentioned forbidding marriage of individuals closely related by blood have a rational genetic basis. In autosomal recessive diseases the affected individual has inherited one abnormal gene from each parent. The probability of inheriting the same allele from each parent obviously is increased in proportion to the probability that the parents have genes in common, i.e., in proportion to how closely they are related. Thus, first cousins will have $1/8$ of their genes in common while their progeny will share $1/16$ of genes derived from a common ancestor. (Parent, child, and sib have $1/2$, grandparent and child $1/4$ of their genes in common). In evaluating the public health importance of a rare recessive condition, and in judging the adequacy of sampling and survey techniques, it is important to estimate the frequency of the gene in the general population as well as the frequency in small genetically isolated groups.

The frequency of occurrence of an abnormal gene in the general population (including, of course, carriage by the unaffected heterozygote) can be estimated. If the frequency of a recessive disease $(q^2) = 1/10,000$, then frequency of gene $(q) = 1/100$ and the frequency of the heterozygotes will be $2pq = 1/50$ (2 chromosomes, $1/100 + 1/100$), since if q is rare $p = 1$.

Thus heterozygous carriers of rare genes are widely distributed in the population. Indeed, it is estimated that each person has 3–7 genes in a single dose that, if they were present in a double dose, would be lethal. The implications of gene distribution are discussed below under *population genetics*, *mutation and selection*, and *congenital abnormalities*.

Population Genetics

Because public health is concerned with the fate of people in numbers, it is inevitably concerned with the distribution and flux of genes in large groups or populations. Elementary *population genetics* is a science based on the binomial theorem which permits the quantitation and estimation of gene frequencies and the testing for genetic equilibrium.

The basis of population genetics is the *Hardy-Weinberg* law, which assumes random mating in the human population. If the frequency of a given gene (allele) A is p, and p varies from 1 to 0, then the frequency of its alternate allele, a, is $1 - p = q$. The three possible genotypes in the population are homozygous individuals AA and aa, and heterozygous individuals Aa. In a randomly mating population, the frequency of these genotypes will be in the proportion p^2 (AA), $2pq$ (Aa) and q^2 (aa). For example, if the frequency of genotype AA is 36 per cent, Aa 48 per cent, and aa 16 per cent, the frequency of gene A and gene a can be readily calculated if the frequency of gene

A = p and the frequency of gene a = q, then p = frequency of AA individuals +1/2 frequency of Aa individuals = 0.36 + 1/2(0.48) = 0.6 and q = frequency of aa individuals +1/2 frequency of Aa individuals = 0.16 + 1/2(0.48) = 0.4, thus, $p + q = 1.0$.

If mating or the uniting of gametes occurs at random, then

$$P^2 = 0.36\text{AA}, \quad 2pq = 0.48\text{Aa}, \quad q^2 = 0.16\text{aa}, \quad p^2 + 2pq + q^2 = 1.00.$$

In the next generation

$$p = 0.36 + 1/2(0.48) = 0.6,$$

$$q = 0.16 + 1/2(0.48) = 0.4 \quad \text{and} \quad p + q = 1.0.$$

Thus, with continued random mating the frequency of the genes p and q *has not changed.*

Racial Stratification

Racial stratification reflects nonrandom mating and the existence of different subpopulations in which gene frequency varies. It is clearly essential that the existence of such subpopulations must be recognized when estimates for the gene in the general population are being calculated.

Genetic Drift

Genetic drift, the so-called "Sewall Wright effect" refers to a change in a population's genotype that results from the chance sampling errors in gene distribution that arise from the interbreeding of small populations or "breeding units." When a gene has

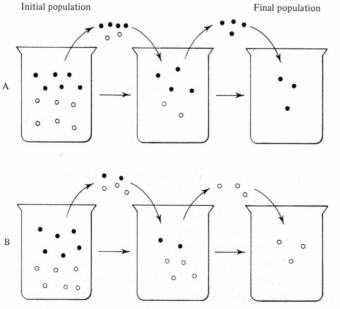

FIGURE 2-5.   Gene fixation.

reached a frequency of 1 it is said to be "fixed," when it reaches 0 it is "lost." This effect is readily understood if one randomly removes samples from a jar of white and black marbles (Figure 2-5). If a small number are picked (e.g., 12) then the probability of removing an equal number of each type is reduced. Thus, distortion of the original gene pool can lead to gene loss or *gene fixation*, and therefore a deviation of this population from the genetic norm of the general population. In a small population, an advantageous gene may never get established, and a deleterious gene may remain "fixed." Decrease in the frequency of the deleterious gene may be effected by simply increasing the size of the mating population.

Assortative Mating

The mating of parents is frequently not made at random, but according to their phenotypic resemblances. This mechanism predisposes to genetic stratification. For example, people of similar intelligence, religion, or socioeconomic group often mate preferentially. Assortative matings will not influence gene distribution unless the determining characteristics are genetically based.

Racial Admixture and Gene Flow

The merging of races through interbreeding can be measured by an ascertainment of gene frequency, using a marker gene that differs in prevalence in the two subpopulations. Such *racial admixture* has been quantitated in the case of the American Negro— the product of interbreeding by Caucasians and African Negroes. The frequency of the Rhesus gene R_o is much higher in the African population than in the American white population. If these differences are known quantities, the admixture of white and Negro genes in the hybrid population can be calculated (Table 2-1).

TABLE 2-1

Admixture of White and Negro Genes in the American Negro

American White Population	African Negro	American Negro
Frequency of R_0 gene $= 0.028$	0.63	0.446
Proportion of "African" gene in American Negro	$= \dfrac{0.446 - 0.028}{0.630 - 0.028} = 0.70$	
Therefore per cent white admixture $= 1 - 0.70 = 30$ per cent.		

It is of interest that approximately the same percentage admixture of "white" genes in the North American Negro is found using a variety of genetic markers (e.g., Sickle cell hemoglobin, haptoglobin type).

QUALITATIVE VARIATION IN GENOTYPE—THE "INBORN" METABOLIC ERRORS

Individual variation in physical traits has long been linked, at least, in part, to genetical influences. Individual biochemical variations have been less obvious, although they, too, may be associated with some physical variation. When single genes produce a variety of phenotypic effects, they are said to exert a *pleiotropic* effect. The pioneering work of Garrod at the turn of the century introduced the concept that genes control the synthesis of enzymes and that a metabolic block might be due to a deficiency in synthesis of a single enzyme. Metabolic or molecular disease thus can result from the ensuing disruption or block in a metabolic pathway.

Many inborn metabolic "errors" result in biochemical variations that are not associated with disease. It is probable that the variation in enzyme or protein structure demonstrable in the human population provides a potential for adaptation to changed environmental circumstances, in some instances the "abnormal" protein may represent a biochemical relic from adaptation to a previous environment. Hemoglobin S, a hemoglobin variant associated with sickle cell anemia may indeed represent such a biochemical relic. The substitution of a single amino acid (valine for glutamic acid) is the basis of the difference of this protein from normal hemoglobin. Although both the heterozygous and homozygous individual bearing the allele are "diseased," the circumstantial evidence is persuasive that the heterozygote has a survival advantage over the normal in areas where falciparum malaria is prevalent. Where malaria has been eradicated the sickle cell hemoglobin is slightly less efficient than normal hemoglobin even when present in the heterozygous state. A very large number of hemoglobin variants, over 150, have been identified in man, and these multiple types constitute a *polymorphism* (literally, many shapes or forms). These variations provide a series of choices for human adaptation. Proof that a variant protein form is truly part of a pattern of *polymorphism* that is *balanced* demands that this rarer allelic form be demonstrable in a frequency of more than 1 per cent—that is, at a rate greater than could be accounted for by recurrent mutation, and in which the influence of genetic drift can be discounted.

Other inherited biochemical polymorphisms of man include the common blood group antigens (ABO, MNS, Rh), leucocyte groups, and serum proteins. More than 50 enzymatic deficiencies associated with human disease have been identified.

PHARMACOGENETICS

The increasing use of drugs and chemicals constitutes a real change in the environment of man. This "pharmacologic environment" has revealed additional human biochemical variations, many of which cannot be detected in the absence of drugs. "Drug idiosyncrasy" or intolerance to a commonly used drug by a few individuals frequently proves to have a genetic basis, the biochemistry of which is definable in a number of instances. More subtle, are quantitative differences in drug-inactivating enzymes that may influence the incidence of drug toxicity in different racial groups (see discussion of isoniazid inactivation).

Inherited Differences in Response to Drugs

As a relatively nontoxic and widely used drug for the prevention and therapy of tuberculosis, isoniazid has been well studied with respect to its pharmacology. There is considerable individual variation in the rate of metabolism of isoniazid, and this variation is usually associated with differences in the rate of acetylation of the drug. Individuals can be divided into two nonoverlapping classes, i.e., "slow" and "rapid" inactivators. There is some evidence that the "slow" inactivators, because of their higher blood levels of drug, are more apt to suffer pyridoxine deficiency and therefore neurotoxic effects.

Metabolism of isoniazid is controlled by an autosomal dominant gene. Persons who are homozygous for this gene acetylate isoniazid more rapidly than the heterozygote; those who inactivate isoniazid slowly appear to be homozygous for a gene that does not synthesize the acetylating enzyme normally.

It is interesting that the slow inactivator trait is rarely observed in Eskimos and Japanese but is common to about 50 per cent of American Negroes and Caucasians. Clearly, the trait must have been selected by some environmental factor other than the relatively new drug, isoniazid.

Abnormal Reaction to Drugs in Inherited Diseases

In certain instances of abnormal reactions to drugs, the abnormal genotype is associated with clinical disease, as in the case of porphyria. In porphyria the administration of barbiturates can precipitate severe or fatal attacks of this disease by affecting the synthesis of a liver enzyme that controls the synthesis of porphyrins. Interbreeding of a small subpopulation in South Africa (40 original families) has increased the prevalence of porphyria in this country to 3/1,000 so that a blood test for detection of the trait is now required before the prescribing for barbiturates. This represents a new type of public health screening and preventive medicine directed at a special segment of the population (see Chapter 8). A devastating and unexplained outbreak of porphyria in Turkey in 1955 was eventually traced to the introduction of a fungicide—hexachlorobenzene. This fungicide was employed to improve the wheat yield in the eastern part of Turkey where bread represents the staple diet of the peasants. The severe toxic effects of hexachlorobenzene were not recognized as the agent responsible for the outbreak until 1959. As soon as the fungicide was prohibited, no further cases of porphyria occurred. This tragic episode, for more than 5,000 children still have symptoms of porphyria, is a vivid example of an environmental agent mimicking an inherited disease.

Drug-induced Disease in Susceptible Genotypes

An X-linked deficiency in erythrocytes of the enzyme glucose-6-phosphate dehydrogenase is like sickle-cell hemoglobin, a notable example of balanced polymorphism associated with increased resistance to falciparum malaria. Ironically, in a world in which the antimalarial drug primaquine is part of the environment—particularly in malarious areas—individuals with this trait are predisposed to hemolytic anemia when the drug is given. Thus, a trait with positive survival value becomes, through environmental change, a trait with negative survival value. This is particularly true of glucose-6-phosphate dehydrogenase deficiency in individuals that have migrated from malarious areas, for even common drugs, such as phenacetin, can also induce the hemolytic reaction.

QUANTITATIVE INHERITANCE

Inborn errors of metabolism are usually *attributable* to a single gene defect that is inherited in a simple autosomal or X-linked recessive fashion. In contrast, the role of genetic factors as etiological determinants in common diseases is often difficult to evaluate. Although there is a hereditary component in the etiology of all diseases, the relative importance of genetic and environmental factors is difficult to determine. In many common diseases the incidence of the trait in first-degree relatives is greater than can be expected by chance and suggests an inherited component. Familial clustering of this type, however, may be due to environmental or genetic factors. If, as is often the case, many genes exert a small effect, the condition is said to be multifactorially inherited. If the genes are additive, the cumulative influence may determine the presence or absence of a disease that is predominantly environmentally determined. Diabetes and essential hypertension are both common diseases that have been extensively investigated from a genetical viewpoint with little unanimity of opinion concerning their mode of inheritance. Although some physicians believe these conditions are inherited in an autosomal recessive fashion, it seems more reasonable to assume that their expression depends on a number of genetic and environmental influences, which are almost impossible to disentangle with existing methods of analysis. Falconer has constructed a graph that, given certain assumptions, enables an estimate of the "heritability" of a disease to be made provided the incidence of the disease in the general population and the incidence of affected relatives is known. Using this graph it can be calculated, for instance, that if a condition occurs with an incidence of 1 per cent in the general population and 8 per cent in first-degree relatives of the affected, then genetical influences account for 70 per cent of the etiological determinants. These estimates, however, do little more than express in rough quantitative terms the degree to which genetic factors may be important.

GENETIC DETERMINATION OF RESISTANCE TO INFECTIOUS DISEASE

Although it is only reasonable to suppose that the infectious diseases of man have played a major role in his evolution and adaptation, there is surprisingly little direct evidence for genetically related factors in resistance to human infection. This subject is discussed in full in Chapter 3.

CONGENITAL DEFECTS

Congenital defects or congenital abnormalities are not necessarily entirely dependent on genetic factors, but represent the sum of genetic, environmental, and cultural influences. Congenital malformations represent the consequences of developmental unpunctuality. They are abnormalities of structure present at birth and attributable to faulty development. Estimates of prevalence vary but abnormalities detectable at birth occur in approximately 15 of every 1,000 live births. If abnormalities detected in the first year of life are included the incidence is 4–5 per cent.

The relative importance of congenital malformations as a cause of infant mortality has increased enormously since the control of infectious diseases. In 1964 malformations accounted for 25 per cent of infant mortality compared to 3.3 per cent in 1900 (Table 2-2).

Those defects occurring with a frequency of more than 1:1,000 include anencephaly, cardiac disease, mongolism, trisomy 18, hare lip, and cleft palate. The corollary to this statement emphasizes the fact that many congenital abnormalities are quite uncommon.

There are interesting but unexplained geographically related differences in the prevalence of certain of these disorders. Thus, anencephaly occurs with a frequency of 30/10,000 births in northwestern Europe, but at only 10 per cent that frequency (3/10,000) in Sweden. Hare lip and cleft palate are three times as common in Japan as in the United States, and congenital dislocation of the hip (see below) is common in Japanese, Chinese, and certain American Indians.

TABLE 2-2

Increase in the Relative Importance of Congenital Malformations in Infant Mortality

		1900	1964
	Congenital malformations	5	5
Infant mortality rate per 1,000 live births	Total	150	20
	Per cent	3.3 per cent	25 per cent

ARE CONGENITAL ABNORMALITIES GENETIC?

The best evidence that some congenital defects may have a strong genetic basis derives from experiments with animals. However, at least one type of human hydrocephalus is due to a gene on the X chromosome. Certain cases of ectrodactyly (lobster claw deformity) are due to a single autosomal gene. Indirect evidence that genetic influences are important stems from the observation that the offspring of first-cousin marriages are more liable to exhibit congenital defects.

The Influence of the Environment

Dietary deficiencies and dietary excess (in the form of vitamin D) have been implicated in the genesis of congenital defects. Hormones, specifically follicle stimulating hormone (FSH), and cortisone can induce congenital defects. In experimental animals multiple births are commonly observed following FSH and cleft palate frequently occurs following large doses of cortisone. Chemicals, and such physical agents as radiation, hypoxia, and increased CO_2 tension may also cause abnormalities in intrauterine development.

Infection, notably infection with rubella and cytomegalo-viruses is an important cause of congenital defects, especially when it occurs in the first trimester of pregnancy.

In contrast to the nonspecific effects of nutritional, hormonal, and physical agents, the lesions arising from rubella are specific and reflect the time of involvement of differentiating germ layers, which are demonstrably infected with the virus. A spectrum of congenital defects is now apparent after rubella. Cataracts, deafness, and heart lesions are the well-known stigmata of rubella infection. Recent prospective studies, however, with modern virologic techniques in the large epidemic of 1963 indicate that less obvious disorders such as enlargement of the liver and spleen and slowing of mental development may also follow the intrauterine infection.

Congenital Hip Disease in the Navajo—An Example of the Interplay of Environmental and Genetic Factors in Congenital Disease

Congenital dislocation of the hip is uncommon in most populations; e.g., it occurs with a frequency of 1.3 per 1,000 live births in New York City. Because the disease is usually treated, the natural history of the untreated disease has been in doubt, although it has been suspected that spontaneous remission to normality may occur in some instances. A unique epidemiologic study of this disease was conducted in a population of 2,300 Navajo Indians at Many Farms, Arizona. This study, which was both prospective and retrospective in its orientation, represented a collaboration of physicians, epidemiologists, and anthropologists who considered all discernible factors in the etiology and evolution of the disease. The prevalence of the disease in this population proved to be exceedingly high, as had been suspected. Both adults and children had prevalence rates for dysplasia and dislocation of 3–4 per cent. However, the adult group (30–50 years of age) had a higher percentage of *dislocation* (the more severe manifestation of the disease) than the children, while dysplasias were nearly five times as common among children as among adults. Careful study of the pedigrees of this scattered but accessible inbred population produced evidence of hereditary transmission of the disease. Incidentally, the tracing of kinship was greatly facilitated by the Navajo's own intrinsic interest in his blood lines. Study of pedigrees did not provide clear indication for a simple recessive or dominant trait carried by a single gene. Rather, the conclusion was drawn that the defect was multifactorially determined (i.e., related to more than one gene) and expressed in varying degrees. Of great interest in the prospective study of the untreated disease in the children was the tendency to spontaneous improvement. In the absence of treatment, 10 of 14 children with hip dysplasia progressed to normal during a two and one-half year period. Thus a *decreased* prevalence of dysplasia occurred with increasing age. Therefore, the significantly *greater* prevalence of hip dislocation in the adults presented a paradox for interpretation. The investigators entertained two hypotheses: (1) that the over-all disease rate had been much higher 30 to 50 years ago in the study population (thus accounting for the higher rate in adults), and (2) that the basic prevalence in infants had not changed, but rather environmental influences had changed. A pertinent, perhaps critical, determining factor may have been the introduction of diapers. These tokens of civilization hold apart the legs of infants strapped on the traditional cradle board, and thus may have counteracted the opposite or adducting tendency of the cradle board itself. This latter hypothesis, although unproved, is highly plausible and was favored by the authors of the study.

This study of congenital hip disease makes several cogent points with respect to congenital disease in general, and indeed to all genetic diseases: (1) the true prevalence and natural history of a disease may be difficult to establish and will require the enlisting of several scientific disciplines in its investigation, (2) prevalence may be quite different as revealed by prospective or retrospective study, or study of different age groups, (3) environmental influences may contribute either to the emergence or the suppression of a genetically engendered disease, and (4) congenital "disease" may disappear spontaneously without specific treatment.

EVOLUTION AND SELECTION IN HUMAN DISEASE

Although space does not permit a detailed account of human evolutionary change as it pertains to public health, the principles underlying natural selection will be discussed briefly. It is clear that evolution requires the twin forces of mutation and selection. Mutation provides the essential phenotypic variation upon which selection operates. Most new mutations that arise confer a distinct disadvantage to the species and are rapidly eliminated; a smaller number that may be advantageous for a particular environmental circumstance will be retained and incorporated into the genome. Not all mutations are point alterations in the DNA itself; chromosomal duplications and rearrangements are not uncommon and provide, in a single step, a variety of phenotypic effects that offer the organism a spectrum of variation on which the forces of natural selection can operate. Evolution itself is a process that proceeds slowly, and calculations based on the number of mutant proteins suggest that, on the average, one gene substitution per locus occurs per ten million years.

The most significant evolutionary change in recent years of concern to students of public health is the radical alterations in the birth and death rates throughout much of the world. These demographic changes have occurred not only because of the delivery of modern medicine to a progressively larger segment of the world's population, but also owing to profound social and cultural changes, the details of which are seldom completely understood (see Chapter 1).

In genetic terms a gene can be regarded as advantageous only if the individuals carrying it differentially contribute to the next generation. Crow has introduced the useful concept of the *Index of Opportunity for Selection* to consider the genetic consequences of the changing patterns of birth and death rate. It is defined as the ratio of the variance in the number of offspring per parent to the square of the mean of children per parent. I (Index of Opportunity for Selection) $= V/M^2$. The total index I can be further subdivided into the Index due to mortality I_M, and that due to differential fertility I_F. Clearly I_M has decreased in proportion to the fall in death rate, but interestingly I_F, that fraction of the Index due to *prenatal* mortality, has changed hardly at all.

A recent study from Chile (Crow, 1966) will illustrate the variation in the Index of Opportunity for Selection in three different populations: (1) the inhabitants of a sea coast industrial town, (2) dwellers in an agricultural village, and (3) a nomadic shepherd tribe (Table 2-3). It will be apparent from examining Table 2-3 that the

TABLE 2-3

Variation in the Index of Opportunity for Selection in Three Different Chilean Populations (After Crow, 1966)

	Mean	Variance	Proportion Surviving to Adult Life	I_M	I_F	I
Industrial town	4.3	8.5	0.87	0.15	0.45	0.67
Agricultural village	5.9	7.5	0.75	0.33	0.22	0.62
Nomadic tribe	6.1	6.4	0.142	1.38	0.17	1.78

total I was largest for the nomadic tribe even though the variance of the mean number of progeny per parent was lowest in this group. Thus it is evident that the Index of Opportunity for Selection may remain high in the face of a low death rate and decrease in the birth rate. The variation in the family size is more critical in determining I than the mean family size.

The Effect of Modern Medicine on Natural Selection

It is evident that the introduction of medicine has resulted in a profound relaxation of selective pressures. Thus, the development of myopia, which would confer considerable disadvantage to a hunting-gathering society, and which has a strong heritable component, can be completely "cured" by the use of spectacles. It is likely that myopia, particularly in women, first began to become less disadvantageous when village life became established and the need for sewing, weaving, and other fine work could be delegated to women.

Color blindness, for which modern medicine has no treatment, is conventionally regarded as a disadvantageous trait. This X-linked trait occurs in some 6 per cent of normal American males, and its frequency decreases sharply in overly traditional societies. The lowest frequency that has been recorded exists among the Australian aborigines and the natives of Brazil and Fiji. Although it is reasonable to assume that this trait, like myopia, is most disadvantageous in a hunting-gathering community, the disadvantages of the color blind at the increasing number of street intersections marked by traffic lights is apparent. It is noteworthy that color-blind individuals were highly prized as observers during the last war when detection of camouflaged enemy activity was essential.

The high frequency of diabetes poses a particular problem for the population geneticist. How can such a serious and presumptively inherited disease achieve a frequency of 5 per cent in the general population? An intriguing explanation has been advanced by Neel. If there were an increased level of circulating insulin in prediabetics, food available on a "feast and famine" basis would be more effectively conserved. On the other hand, in a culture in which food is always available, the continued production of excess insulin may elicit the production of insulin antibodies and diabetes may then develop as a consequence. This attractive hypothesis, at least in its simplest form, is probably incorrect but is cited to emphasize the need to examine the problem in the light of the knowledge that for more than 99 per cent of the time that man has been on this planet he has followed a feast, famine, hunting-gathering existence.

The relative importance of genes and environment has reached its apogee in a consideration of intelligence. The simple concept that because there is frequently an inverse correlation between intelligence and family size, a progressive decrease in intelligence will be an inevitable consequence has proved false. Although it can be shown on the assumption that intelligence is controlled by a small number of genes and there is strong assortative mating, that this is genetically incorrect, the important role of cultural inheritance has still not been sufficiently emphasized. Indeed, recent investigations on the fertility differential between "successful" and "unsuccessful," graduates of Harvard, Princeton, and Yale suggest that since 1945 the tendency for those with the least intelligence to have the most children has been arrested.

EUGENICS AND EUPHENICS AND GENETIC COUNSELING

Before discussing the more general aspects of this problem, a number of consequences of a decrease in selection pressure due to the introduction of modern medicine will be considered. Let us assume that a recessive disease with a gene frequency of 1/1,000 is of such severity that affected homozygotes never reproduce. It can be shown that it would take approximately 40 generations or nearly 1,000 years for the frequency of the gene to double (Crow, 1966). Recognizing the great rapidity of medical progress, it is clearly needless to worry about the long-term genetic consequences of treating recessive traits.

If a gene were responsible for a dominant lethal trait, however, and the disease were completely cured, the generation following the institution of treatment would have twice the gene frequency of the preceding generation. Most autosomal dominant traits, however, are not lethal, so in practice the change in the second generation will be significantly less than 2.

The increased realization that it is not possible to agree on what genetic goals are desirable for any particular population, and the even greater concern that the definition of "desirable genes" could be the prerogative of a few politically influential individuals, has resulted in a refusal of thoughtful persons to embrace programs of so-called positive eugenics. However, there is general agreement that negative eugenics, an attempt to decrease the incidence of seriously disabling inherited disease by counseling based on genetical principles, could play an important and useful role in decreasing mankind's genetic load.

It should be emphasized that, even in those instances in which general agreement can be reached subsequent offspring face a significant genetic hazard, the *decision* must be made by the parents and not by the genetic counselor. Genetic counseling must always extend beyond the realms of the probable risk calculations for autosomal dominant, recessive, and X-linked diseases to include a sympathetic appraisal of the total situation.

It is paradoxical that so-called genetic counseling clinics are usually concerned with counseling individuals with predominantly nongenetic disorders. Patients attending a genetic counseling clinic usually present complex problems of gene-environmental interactions, such as hare lip, cleft palate, congenital dislocation of the hip, and non-specific mental retardation. For these conditions, a variety of empiric risk figures are available, but whether they can be directly applied to the patient under consideration is always less clear, for empiric risk figures vary widely in different parts of the world and in different ethnic groups. Perhaps, the most important aspect of a genetic counseling clinic is diagnostic; unless good diagnostic facilities are available such clinics can be devastatingly harmful. Genetic counseling without a thorough clinical examination of the affected individual and an extensive inquiry into the family history is inexcusable.

MAN'S GENETIC FUTURE

The possibility that man might be able to influence his heredity is a direct outgrowth of the spectacular advances of molecular genetics in the last decade. Studies with microorganisms have amply demonstrated that it is possible to insert new genetic determinants into a recipient genome (see Chapter 3). Genetic manipulation of the human genome, however, is not yet practical. Although the brave new world of Genetic Engineering is still a long way off, it would be unwise to assume that techniques for altering the genetic material already well developed for some organisms will not be applicable to diploid organisms such as man. For the present, it would seem that efforts should be directed to altering the expression of the mutant phenotype by modifying the intracellular environment. The elimination of phenylalanine from proved phenylketonurics, and of galactose from galactosemics, point the way to a future in which, without direct manipulation of the primary genetic material, it may be possible to alleviate the effects of seriously disadvantageous genes.

REFERENCES

BEESON, P. B., and McDERMOTT, W. (eds.): *Cecil-Loeb Textbook of Medicine*, 12th ed., 1202–16. W. B. Saunders Company, Philadelphia, 1967.

CROW, J. F.: The quality of people: Human evolutionary changes. *Bioscience*, **16**:863–67, 1966.

FALCONER, D. S.: *Introduction to Quantitative Genetics*. Ronald Press Company, New York, 1960.

Genetics and the epidemiology of chronic disease. Public Health Service Publication no. 1763, 1965.

STERN, C.: *Principles of Human Genetics*, 2nd ed. W. H. Freeman and Company, San Francisco, 1960.

THOMPSON, J. S., and THOMPSON, M. W.: *Genetics in Medicine*, W. B. Saunders Company, Philadelphia, 1966.

3

Genetic Interaction of Man and Microbes —Implications of a Changing Ecology

Edwin D. Kilbourne

All living things are subject to mutation and selection. Thus, not only man but the microorganisms in his environment undergo genetic change. In the case of the human parasites, the intimacy of their relationship with man provides abundant opportunity for selection pressure to operate in either of two directions: man may influence or select microbe and microbe may influence or "select" man. So long as ecologic change is slow, host and parasite can come to terms and endure—neither drastically changing nor eliminating the other. The mutational capacity of the unicellular organisms or viruses is quite different from that of man, but the short generation time and enormous reproductive yields of the former are balanced in part by the far greater number of genes carried by man as a complex multicellular host.

It is unlikely that until recently there have been any truly "new" infections. New *diseases* based on a changed relationship of host and parasite leading to an increased and, therefore, detectable incidence of disease (e.g., poliomyelitis) have appeared in this century. However, pictorial evidence of the occasional occurrence of poliomyelitis in the past indicates that this infection is ancient. The fact that mammalian species suffer from analogous infections strongly suggests that at least certain parasites (e.g., salmonella, pox viruses) have evolved from a common ancestor as variants adapted to different species. Man has smallpox, and the mouse ectromelia (mouse pox); dogs and man carry different (but related) adenoviruses. Thus, the viruses especially show a high degree of host specificity under natural conditions. Yet this specificity is not absolute in most instances but hinges on a delicate balance determined by the numbers or dose of the infectious agent, on environmental conditions that affect the act of

47

transmission, and upon the multiple factors that comprise the "resistance" or immunity of the challenged host. Indeed, immunity is rarely absolute and can be overridden in part by a large enough dose of the infectious agent. So, while man is ordinarily immune to equine influenza, he *can* be infected and diseased by large amounts of virus administered by artificial aerosol. So too, can human influenza virus infect the horse, but apparently only under artificially created conditions. In general, most of the infectious agents of man except for certain intensely obligate viruses, can be made to infect animal species below him in the phylogenetic scale. The viruses borne by arthropods move freely from species to species, and man is no exception to their incursions. However, the susceptibility of man to microbes seemingly confined under ordinary conditions to lower animals has been demonstrable from time to time by accident in the laboratory. Interspecies transfer of infection is now of increasing concern as a risk from new biologic products and vaccines of animal origin. Indeed, many of the viruses that now cause concern were not even recognized to exist prior to the development of tissue-culture techniques for the preparation of poliovirus vaccine. Living cells are needed for the propagation of virus—including vaccine strains. A convenient source of such cells is the kidney of the rhesus monkey. But, when such cells are transplanted to the test tube, viruses not demonstrable in the living intact monkey may be reactivated from a latent or dormant state in tissue culture and thus become a contaminant— sometimes unrecognized—of virus vaccines produced in such cells. Literally scores of *simian viruses* have now been isolated under these conditions. In the case of many of them, even their relation to disease in the monkey is unknown. At least some of these viruses have escaped inactivation during vaccine preparation and have actually infected man.

Thus, the unique capacity of man to change his environment and to bring about bold and striking changes in his ecology has led him into a changed relationship with the microbial species of his environment. Such ecologic changes and their potential are peculiarly important when compared to the inert nonmultiplying toxins of the environment. The air contaminant may injure and disease the human being, but the action is largely one-sided. Within the body the toxin may be neutralized and detoxified, but no true interaction with the possibility of a second step or selection of a new toxin occurs—at least within that individual. It is the *plasticity* of the human-microbial relationship—the mutual adaptability of man and virus—that will be considered here in some depth. For the limitations of the classical public health techniques of isolation, vaccination, and eradication procedures are now being recognized as new problems in infective diseases continually emerge in this era of sanitation and chemotherapy.

THE DECLINE OF THE EPIDEMICS

The great plagues of mankind have all but disappeared from industrialized society. Bubonic plague flares sporadically in the East in times of war and stress, as it did recently in Vietnam. Smallpox and cholera lie endemic throughout Asia—a constant threat to the West but held at bay by immunization and quarantine practice. Yellow fever, no mere exotic curiosity in New York and Philadelphia two centuries ago (see

Chapter 5), is a lingering problem in jungle areas of the New World but can no longer occur in great urban epidemics.

The more chronic pestilences of malaria and tuberculosis are very much with us—but the morbidity and mortality of malaria have been halved during the past decade through the efforts of the World Health Organization, and the National Tuberculosis Association talks seriously of the possibility of eradicating tuberculosis.

Less dramatic than the great plagues, which killed large numbers of young and old alike within short periods of time, were the epidemics of scarlet fever and diphtheria, which studded the graveyards of New England with tiny tombstones. These epidemics too have declined and all but disappeared in industrialized societies, as have typhoid fever and bacillary and amoebic dysentery. All but disappeared—but none has.

In the industrialized society the massive machinery of environmental sanitation effectively limits typhoid and most of the enteric infections. But New York City had 21 cases of typhoid fever in 1967. Diphtheria is a rarity in children—but is a growing problem in adults whose artificially induced immunity is impermanent and subject to decline. Scarlet fever is less common and is treatable when it does occur, yet it still occurs. Pandemic influenza remains a recurrent threat, despite intensive study of the virus and the availability of specific vaccines for 20 years. Thus, the "conquest of the

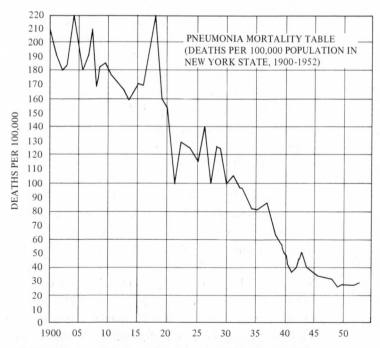

FIGURE 3-1. Curve compiled from *70th Annual Report of the New York State Department of Health* and *Monthly Vital Statistical Reviews* from the same source. New York State was selected as representative of the decline in pneumonia mortality over the last 50 years because of the relative accuracy of the statistics compiled by the New York State Department of Health. (Reproduced from "*Pneumonias, Management with Antibiotic Therapy*." Charles Pfizer and Co., 1953.)

infectious diseases" has a hollow ring, although the victories have been many. The reasons for the striking decline in human mortality from infectious diseases are considered in detail in Chapter 10. In summary, technological advances of urbanization present barriers to the acquisition of microbes from the environment—notably those carried by animals or arthropod vectors or derived from human wastes. The impact of artificial immunization has been less striking, with smallpox almost an exception as a "great plague" principally controlled by that technique. Chemotherapy and the antibiotics have had even a lesser impact on the life-threatening epidemic diseases despite their undeniable and dramatic effect on the bacterial infections, including pneumonia, meningitis, and tuberculosis (Figure 3-1).

The Unknown Factors

But if one considers the mortality rate of certain diseases *not* subject to control by traditional environmental sanitation or immunization, it becomes clear that unidentified factors have influenced the evolution of disease. The sudden introduction of a microorganism into a population that has had no recent experience with it often results in severe epidemic disease, despite the seeming avirulence of the same microorganisms (e.g., measles virus) in populations in which it is widely prevalent. There are numerous examples of such epidemics, notably involving the transmission of tuberculosis, measles, and smallpox from Europeans to American Indians and South Sea Islanders (Dubos, 1965). After the initial high mortality associated with such epidemics, the surviving population tends to come into balance with the parasite—to learn to live with it, and the severity of disease declines. Presumably, this coming to terms with the infection results largely from acquired specific immunity and shifts in the age distribution of cases of infection to a pattern more typical of societies endemically infected with the infectious agent. Thereafter the introduction of susceptibles is more gradual, principally by birth, so that a persisting but antigenically unchanging parasite never again confronts simultaneously in that society a large population of nonimmune subjects.

Less easy to explain is the decline in mortality in the present century from a number of infections common to industrialized European communities *in the absence of specific measures of control* such as sanitation, artificial immunization, or chemotherapy. Thus, tuberculosis—often epidemic in the nineteenth century—began a precipitous decline in England Wales in the 1850's, which continued into the first half of the twentieth century, well before effective antimicrobacterial drugs were developed (Wilson and Miles, 1946, cited by Magill, 1955) (Figure 3-2). Now, the pendulum has swung, so that tuberculosis is no longer a ubiquitous (but generally well-tolerated) infection. Rather, it is now so uncommon (Table 3-1), that a large reservoir of susceptibles exists even in urban communities almost comparable to that which used to characterize isolated populations. Yet other concomitants of our civilization—nutrition, housing, higher "standards of living"—serve to limit the prevalence and severity of tuberculosis.

It is interesting too, that when the influence of diphtheria antitoxin (introduced in 1895) on the case fatality rate of diphtheria is studied, one finds that a downward

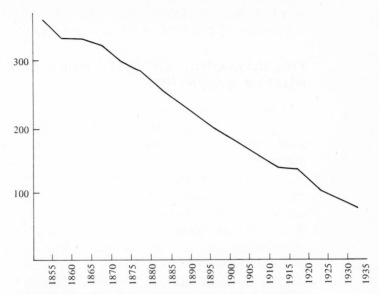

FIGURE 3-2. Mortality per 10^5 living in England and Wales 1851–1935. (Reproduced from T. P. Magill, *J Immun*, **74**:1, 1955. © 1955, The Williams and Wilkins Company, Baltimore, Md. 21202, U.S.A.)

TABLE 3-1

The Changing Incidence of Tuberculin Reactors Among Students Entering Cornell University Medical College, New York*

Year	Number Positive	Per Cent
1952	18	21
1953	14	17
1954	5	6
1955	3	4
1956	6	7
1957	6	7
1958	4	5
1959	8	10
1960	8	10
1961	5	6

*Unpublished data, courtesy Dr. J. R. McCarroll.

trend in mortality had begun ten years *before* the introduction of this specific therapy (Wilson and Miles, 1946, cited by Magill, 1955; Frost, cited by Maxey, 1941). The death rate from measles—another ancient disease—has declined almost parallel with that of diphtheria, beginning in the 1880's and dropping steadily up to the present time.

It is most unlikely that the lessened severity of these infections is related to a simultaneous reduction in the intrinsic virulence of three unrelated microparasites. It is equally unlikely that Western man has simultaneously developed genetically based resistance to these differing microorganisms. Rather we must suspect that no single factor has been responsible. The balance of this chapter will examine the interplay of host and parasite as affected by the environment of both (i.e., the ecology of infections) in order to show that the ecology of human infection is far from static and that new and unsuspected problems are arising as the great epidemics disappear.

THE INFLUENCE OF INFECTIOUS DISEASE ON HUMAN VARIATION

Certain infections of man are ubiquitous and universally distributed throughout human populations in all parts of the world. This kind of distribution is characteristic of most of the obligate human parasites—those bacteria and viruses that multiply only in man, that require man for their continued existence, and that are transmitted directly from man to man as "contagious" infections without the necessary intercession of intermediate hosts, arthropod vectors, or prolonged survival in the environment. These contagious, universal, and endemic infections are caused by microorganisms as diverse as the spirochete of syphilis, the typhoid bacillus, and the adenoviruses. Using these three examples, one can point out that in fact modern chemotherapy has altered the clinical nature of syphilis (if not its epidemiology (see Chapter 10), that environmental sanitation has drastically restricted (but not eliminated) the threat of typhoid, and that adenovirus infection—like infection with most human viruses—is probably unchanged in incidence and character. Thus, infections of this sort represent a continuing but variable potential influence on all human populations. The selective pressure on man of syphilis and adenovirus infection is probably minimal because these infections are rarely fatal and hence do not affect human reproductive potential. On the other hand, although it seems likely that typhoid, in common with other diarrheal diseases, has had an important impact on human survival and has exerted centuries of selection pressure, the effects of such selection are difficult to measure because of the universality of the disease.

Rather, association of infectious disease and human genetic variations must be sought in the case of endemic or epidemic infections that are restricted to certain geographical areas, that cause appreciable mortality before the reproductive age, and that occur with high prevalence or incidence, respectively. When these conditions are met, then the characteristics of the populations in such areas can be contrasted with those of unaffected populations and possible traits determining resistance to infection may be uncovered. In fact, it is the great plagues of man—malaria, smallpox, and bubonic plague—that satisfy these requirements and that have been best studied for their possible selective or winnowing effect on human populations.

Human Variation—How Determined and How Related to Infectious Disease

Human genetic variation is most obviously reflected by extremes of skin color and other physical characteristics that define race. But such characteristics have no reasonable link to resistance to disease. The so-called racial susceptibility to tuberculosis of dark-skinned peoples is probably nongenetic and is based rather on circumstances of crowding and poverty under which many such people are often forced to live.

The human blood group antigens (ABO) discovered by Landsteiner in 1900 are discrete, unambiguous, genetically determined markers that are readily identified by serological surveys and have been conjecturally linked with the past prevalence of infectious disease. To begin with, the distribution of the ABO blood groups is not uniform. Much of the nonuniformity is attributable to genetic drift (see Chapter 2) and the gene sampling variation that often occurs with small inbreeding populations. For example, the frequency of blood group A is 80 per cent in the Blackfeet, but only 2 per cent in Ute Indians of North America (Muschel, 1966).

Balanced Polymorphism. When in several large populations differences in gene frequency have been noted they have corresponded not with race but with geographical area and with the prevalence of certain infectious diseases. In areas where smallpox has been most prevalent (India, Arabia, and tropical Africa) the frequency of the gene for blood group A is low. A correlation has been made between this finding and the purported possession by variola (smallpox virus) of an antigen similar to the blood group A antigen. It is reasoned that individuals of A blood type would be unable to produce anti-A antibody in response to smallpox infection or might initially be more susceptible to infection because of their intrinsic lack of the antibody. Thus A-group individuals would be under selective pressure and at a survival disadvantage in small-pox areas. They would tend to be eliminated from the mating pool and thus the frequency of the A gene population would be reduced. Stated in another way (Figure 3-3), individuals of blood type B and O would be at a *relative advantage* in the presence of smallpox because of their anti-A antibodies, which might afford some humoral protection against a virus bearing the A antigen. Attractive as this theory is, it is weakened by the lack of good evidence that the virus in fact possesses an antigen cross-reacting with the blood group A antigen. Nevertheless, the incidence of smallpox scars is higher among individuals of A blood group in India and Pakistan, and the incidence of vaccination reactions is higher among such individuals in Germany (Pettenkoffer *et al.*, 1962). It has been argued that antibody plays no role in recovery from virus diseases and furthermore that experimentally induced anti-A serum does not neutralize vaccinia virus. The first point ignores the protective role of pre-existing antibody in preventing virus infection, and the second does not belie the possible effect of non-neutralizing antibody directed against a minor virus antigen (Jahiel and Kilbourne, 1966). Furthermore, vaccinia is not variola (smallpox virus). The pros and cons of this argument are reviewed here in order to demonstrate the difficulties involved in this kind of important but often inconclusive epidemiologic research. It should be mentioned that at least one careful study of smallpox does not substantiate the foregoing hypothesis (Downie *et al.*, 1965).

A similar case has been made for the reciprocal association of the former high prevalence of plague in Mongolia, Turkey, and North Africa and the reduced incidence in these ancient plague centers of blood group O (H gene). Again, there is equivocal evidence that the smooth virulent form of *Pasteurella pestis* contains the O or H antigen, and it is again presumed that individuals carrying this blood group antigen will be unable to respond to the exogenous introduction of the antigen in the form of the plague bacillus.

The evidence that common pathogens possess blood group antigenic reactivity has been summarized by Athreya and Coriell (1967) who also point out an interesting correlation between B gene frequency in population groups in various areas and the

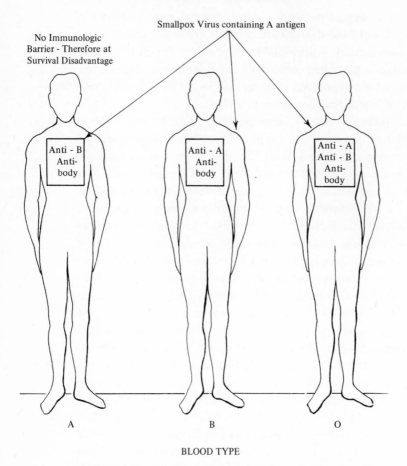

FIGURE 3-3. Possible selective survival advantage of individuals of blood groups B and O in milieu of smallpox challenge.

presence of endemic malaria. Indirect evidence (marked increase of anti-A titers after infection) suggests that the *Plasmodium falciparum* contains A-antigen and that individuals bearing the reciprocal B-gene are better equipped to deal with its incursions.

The Sickle Cell Gene and Resistance to Malaria

Better than any other disease, malaria illustrates the possible survival advantage of balanced polypmorphism (see Chapter 2). In certain southern European, Asian, and African populations, an abnormal hemoglobin is detectable in certain individuals by the tendency of their erythrocytes to assume a sickle shape *in vitro*. In those who are homozygous for this trait, sickling can occur at physiologic partial pressures of oxygen, whereas sickling in heterozygotes occurs only at considerably reduced oxygen tension. Chemical analysis proves that all hemoglobin in homozygotes is abnormal (hemoglobin S), but that in heterozygotes there is both abnormal and normal hemoglobin present. Homozygotes are afflicted with sickle cell anemia and its attendant complications, but heterozygotes are usually free of the disease.

It is remarkable that the geographic distribution of indigenous populations possessing the sickle cell gene corresponds closely with areas in which falciparum malaria is hyperendemic or holoendemic (transmitted throughout the year). In such areas infants and children are intensely infected, and many die before they can gradually develop specific immunity to the parasite. In children one to five years old, development of immunity is manifested by a decrease in parasitemia and a decrease in illness in the presence of any remaining parasites. The state of hyperimmunity that is attained by school age is maintained throughout life in those who continue to dwell in the endemic area.

In the newborn in whom parasitemia is very high and in individuals more than five years of age in whom specific immunity has developed, the parasite counts in sickle cell heterozygotes do not differ significantly from those of persons with normal hemoglobin. However, in the critical age range between one and four years, children heterozygous for the sickle cell gene have significantly less *Plasmodium falciparum* in their blood. Because fatality in falciparum infections is closely associated with high parasite counts, it has been inferred that the reduction in parasitemia associated with the sickle cell trait is protective and has definite survival advantage for the host. Sickle cell trait carriers are also known to incur the potentially fatal complication of cerebral involvement less frequently. Sickle cell hemoglobin (hemoglobin S) and normal hemoglobin differ only in the substitution of a valine for a glutamic acid residue in each half molecule (Allison, 1961). If, as indirect evidence suggests, this minor chemical modification is sufficiently inimical to the parasite to influence the survival of man, it is a dramatic illustration of the effects on a human population of a biochemically expressed genetic mutation.

In summary, it seems probable that under the influence of malaria favorable selection of children bearing the protective sickle cell trait has occurred; a heterozygous child has a greater chance than the nonsickler or the intrinsically diseased homozygote to reach reproductive age and thus perpetuate the trait. This expectation is actually borne out by surveys of the ratios of normal homozygotes and heterozygotes in infancy and at the reproductive age. In the presence of malaria, the increasing frequency of the sickle cell gene through increased survival of heterozygotes tends to be limited by the deleterious effects in homozygous individuals who are subject to actual sickle cell disease before the beginning of their reproductive lives.

When malaria no longer exerts its influence on populations carrying the sickle cell gene, it seems probable that the trait—no longer possessing survival value—will eventually disappear. One also wonders whether the heterozygote bearers of the sickling trait might actually be at a disadvantage in the new environments of the forthcoming air and space age in which exposure to reduced oxygen tension can be anticipated. It is ironic that the bearers of another biochemical trait thought to be protective against malaria (a deficiency in activity in the red cell of the enzyme glucose-6-phosphate dehydrogenase) are peculiarly vulnerable to toxicity effects from certain antimalarial drugs. Thus, in the modern environment with its new drugs, the cure might be worse than the disease—in those persons selected by previous environmental pressures.

Other Evidence of Blood Group Polymorphism and Susceptibility to Virus Infections

In studies of air force recruits in the United Kingdom, it was found that significantly more individuals of type O than type A blood group were infected with influenza A_2 virus, as determined by antibody response. Influenza, indeed, produces fatalities in the young and hence might be responsible for genetic selection in man. But the troublesome question arises: Does this prove that the O group subjects are more susceptible (more showing serologic evidence of infection) or that the A group are less able to form significant amounts of antibody against the virus? In any event, these differences from expected attack rates merit further study and do suggest that blood group antigens are at least associated with differing responses to infection.

It should be noted that at least one infectious agent, a parainfluenza virus, (Isacson and Koch, 1965) has been shown to have an antigen identical with blood group B substance. Furthermore, this antigen is truly a viral, not a host-derived antigen. The implications of this homology of microbial and human antigens are profound but again—in the present state of knowledge (or ignorance)—are hard to assess. This virus with its host-homologous antigen might be better tolerated by humans of group B blood type, or contrariwise might induce more severe disease by evoking less antibody response.

In conclusion, it seems only reasonable that the infectious diseases with lethal potential have exerted selective pressure on the human population. Considerable suggestive, but inconclusive, evidence has been adduced in support of this concept. When the efforts of public health alter the prevalence of such diseases as malaria and the hypothetical selective pressure of these diseases has been reduced, then the genetically selected individual will no longer have a peculiar survival advantage. Indeed, as mentioned earlier, he may be at a disadvantage in a new environment lacking plasmodia but containing drugs and chemicals.

THE EFFECT OF HUMAN PHENOTYPE ON MICROBIAL VARIATION

Just as man's microbes appear to exert selective and evolutionary pressure on his genes, so does he unwittingly influence the multiplication and genetic selection of his parasites. Those microorganisms which are obligate human parasites (i.e., which infect only man and require him for their growth and survival) are obviously most susceptible to changes in those aspects of the human phenotype that determine resistance to infection. Change in human phenotype in contrast to genotype occurs constantly and readily in response to infections as specific *acquired immunity*—reflected by the development of immunoglobulins (antibodies) in blood and secretions. With most infections, such specific antibody acts as a barrier to reinfection and proliferation in the individual host, or indeed, may limit transmission of infection to susceptibles by a herd immunity effect (see Chapter 7), even if only a portion of individuals in the community become immune. Nevertheless, even the obligate human parasites manage to survive

—either by persisting after the act of infection in immune hosts (as with herpes virus) or through a chain of transmission from susceptible to susceptible without necessarily producing any clinical signs of infection or any manifest community-wide epidemic. Such microorganisms, including the viruses of mumps, chickenpox, and measles, appear to survive and persist in human populations without the need for significant genetic change. Having evolved with man through the centuries, they do not exhibit wide swings in virulence. (The virulence of measles in isolated primitive communities is compounded of such host and environmental determinants as malnutrition, age-related effects, and secondary bacterial pneumonia.)

However, in the case of influenza, the virus seems to be peculiarly vulnerable to shifts in population immunity, so that within the last three decades of modern virology, two subtypes of influenza A virus have disappeared as causes of natural infection and new subtypes have replaced them in succession. The reciprocal correlation of the disappearance and appearance of these viruses and changes in the antibody patterns or "immune phenotypes" of the human population is striking.

The Apparent Influence of Human Immune Phenotype on the Influenza A Viruses of Man

The virus of influenza is unique among infectious agents in its capacity to infect within a short period of time virtually the entire population of the world to produce pandemics of disease. Pandemics are associated with marked mutations of the virus to an antigenically new type and with the disappearance of the older type against which population immunity has gradually increased. The introduction of the new strain is followed first by universal or pandemic infection and then by a series of recurrent, more localized epidemics that become progressively less extensive (Figure 3-4). Correlated with the decline in the severity of the epidemics is an increase in the population

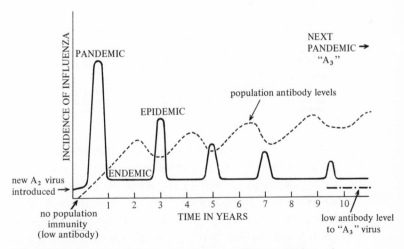

FIGURE 3-4. Schematic representation of the correlation of influenza incidence and mean population antibody levels after introduction of a new influenza A variant. (Reproduced from E. D. Kilbourne, *Sandoz Panorama*, **6** :7, 1968.)

in humoral antibody to the original variant virus and a gradual antigenic change in the virus recovered from these later epidemics. During the interpandemic periods, however, these mutations of the virus are relatively minor so that all strains are recognizable as variants of the same subtype (Table 3-2) and are neutralized (although less effectively) by antibody to the initial variant. It seems only reasonable, however, to conclude that this antigenic variation increases the ability of the virus to infect the partially immune, and hence to survive. A point is finally reached at which extreme change in the virus is required for it to surmount the increasingly effective immunity of the population, and at this point an antigenically "new" virus emerges to which the population is essentially not immune. Whether or not a pandemic then ensues will depend upon the transmissibility and virulence of the new strain.

TABLE 3-2
A Summary of the Influenza Viruses *

Subtypes human	Influenza A Prevalence	Influenza B	Influenza C
A_0	1933–46	Subtypes not well defined	No subtypes
A_1	1947–57		
A_2 ("Asian") 1957-present time ‡		Epidemics mainly in children and adolescents	Rare cause of epidemics (in children only)
Animal			
Fowl	Present time	Probably *not* a cause of pandemics	No animal prototypes
Swine †	Present time		
Horse	Present time		
All above are antigenically very different (noncross-immunizing) but are classified together because they do have (minor) and core antigens in common		No animal prototypes Completely distinct from A strains	

N.B. Since 1957 only influenza A_2 (Asian) virus has been isolated from cases of human disease.
* Reproduced from Kilbourne, E. D.: *Sandoz Panorama*, **6**:4, 1968.
† The virus of Swine influenza (discovered in 1931) is probably similar to the virus of the pandemic of 1918.
‡ The "Hong Kong" variant of 1968 represents another major mutation, but cross reacts with earlier A_2 strains through a shared antigen—the viral neuraminidase (Schulman and Kilbourne, 1969).

It is not known whether the radically different pandemic virus arises by a multistep mutation from animal reservoirs or by genetic recombination of human and animal viruses (Kilbourne, 1968). In any event, the pattern of simultaneous emergence of the new virus and disappearance of the old strongly suggests that the two events are related; the new virus has an obvious survival advantage over the old in the face of immunologic barriers that are restrictive principally to the latter. Thus, a nonheritable change in human phenotype (namely acquired immunity to influenza A) may dictate the pattern of microbial mutation and survival—in this instance to the disadvantage of man.

MICROBIAL VIRULENCE AND HOST SUSCEPTIBILITY AS RECIPROCALS

If disease is an expression of the interaction of host and parasite, then its severity will be a function of the virulence of the parasite and the suceptibility of the host. But from this simple and obvious reciprocal relationship it is often difficult to draw conclusions concerning the absolute or intrinsic pathogenicity of the parasite, because virulence is measured usually by evaluation of disease severity in nonuniform hosts of varying susceptibility inoculated in nature with undefined and unstandardized doses of the infectious agent.

It has been mentioned that the "virulence" of measles virus in certain populations —expressed as more severe morbidity and increased incidence of complications and deaths—is almost certainly dependent on environmental and host factors. The same virus in the same epidemic but involving well-nourished, well-housed children will present the customary patterns of disease. Even with influenza—probably the most changeable of human pathogens—viral virulence is remarkably constant, even in pandemics, and mortality is almost invariably linked to secondary bacterial pneumonia or to pre-existing cardiovascular disease. The strikingly different outcome of infection of two individuals in the same focal hospital epidemic is illustrated in the clinical charts of Figure 3-5.

The survival of the obligate human parasite is dependent upon the maintenance of an optimal level of virulence—virulence sufficient to damage host cells and to provoke expulsion and transmission of the agent, but insufficient in most instances to kill the host. Therefore, the burden of proof should be borne by those who propose altered microbial virulence as an explanation for changes in the severity of disease. Rather, the entire complex ecology of host and parasite must first be examined.

Myxomatosis—A Model of Host-Parasite Accommodation

The proper study of mankind is not necessarily man—Alexander Pope to the contrary —but may sometimes be the rabbit, or indeed the mouse (see Chapter 7). The study of myxomatosis in Australia is one of the great biologic experiments and illustrates quite clearly the bilateral adaptations that must occur in host and parasite when a virus of high virulence is introduced into a highly susceptible host population (Fenner and Ratcliffe, 1965).

Myxomatosis is a poxvirus infection apparently native to the South American rabbit (actually a hare, *Lepus sylvilagus*). In this host the infection results in a mild, rarely lethal disease that is probably transmitted by mosquitos. In contrast, when the virus is introduced inadvertently or in the laboratory into the so-called domestic or European rabbit (*Oryctolagus cuniculus*) a devastatingly rapid lethal disease ensues (Figure 3-6). For a time this observation was a laboratory curiosity and an occasional economic threat to breeders of domestic rabbits in the Americas. However, the potential of the virus as an agent of biologic warfare did not go unremarked for long.

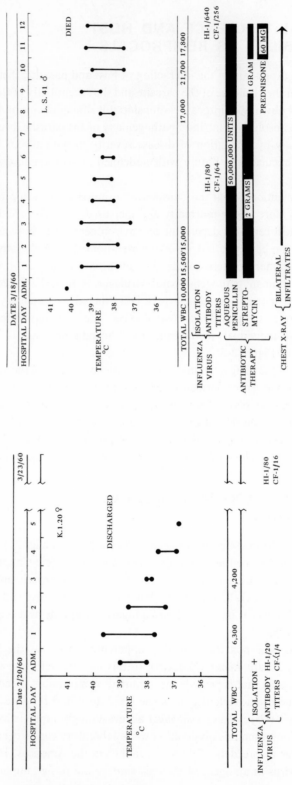

FIGURE 3-5. Clinical charts of two cases of influenza of contrasting severity caused by the same strain of influenza virus. (Reproduced from Kaye *et al. Amer Rev Resp Dis,* **85** :11, 1962.)

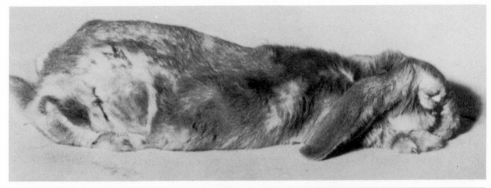

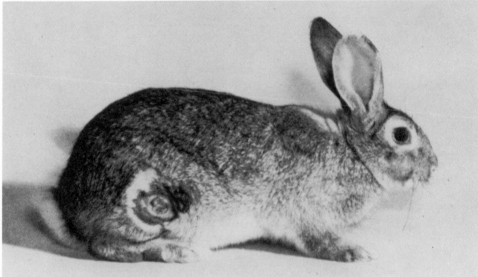

FIGURE 3-6. Rabbits infected with myxoma virus. These photographs demonstrate the influence of high and low environmental temperatures on the symptomotology of myxomatosis. The rabbit in the upper photograph had been held in a cold room after infection while the rabbit below, infected with the same amount of virus, had been held in a hot room. (Reproduced from I. D. Marshall, *J Hyg*, **57**:484, 1959.)

In Australia, the importation of the European rabbit for the benefit of sportsmen has had serious economic consequences for this wool capital of the world. Sheep-grazing ranges were destroyed by the rodents, and the defoliation not only reduced the food supply but led to soil erosion as well.

Myxoma virus was introduced on a pilot basis in the summer (December–January) of 1950–51 and produced an enormous epizootic in which the lethality rate was 99.5 per cent. Thus, *most, but not all* rabbits were destroyed. Thereafter, the infection recurred almost annually and in some areas was reintroduced by man. Yet, despite the continuing decimation of the rabbit population, the disease appeared to be progressively less lethal and the virus less effective in curtailing the population. Had the virus changed in antigenicity or in virulence? Antigenic variation among all existing strains was found to be slight. Selection by host antibody was deemed unlikely; most infection occurred in annual epidemics so that interim breeding had produced a large supply of young nonimmunes in which the virus replication cycle could be sustained without the necessity for antigenic deviation of the virus.

In fact, the virus had changed in *virulence.* An exhaustive analysis was made of virus strains collected between 1951 and 1959. These strains were tested for virulence, employing small doses of virus in *laboratory* rabbits (not subject to the impact of the previous epizootics). The strains were grouped in five categories ranging from very high to very low virulence. Figure 3-7 demonstrates that a progressive shift in the

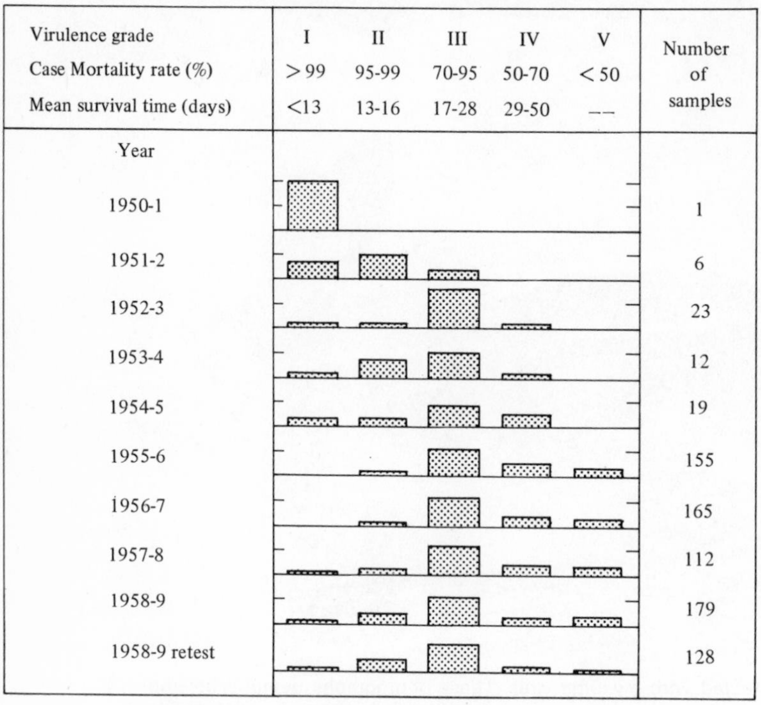
Virulence grade
I
II
III
IV
V
Case Mortality rate (%)
>99
95-99
70-95
50-70
< 50
Mean survival time (days)
<13
13-16
17-28
29-50
——
Number of samples
Year
1950-1
1
1951-2
6
1952-3
23
1953-4
12
1954-5
19
1955-6
155
1956-7
165
1957-8
112
1958-9
179
1958-9 retest
128

FIGURE 3-7. Histogram showing the virulence of Australian field strains recovered between 1951 and 1959. (Reproduced from F. Fenner, and F. N. Ratcliffe, *Myxomatosis.* Cambridge University Press, New York, 1965. Data from Marshall and Fenner, 1960.)

proportion of virulent and avirulent strains occurred during the decade after the initial introduction of the highly virulent strain of 1951. At the end of a decade, strains of moderate virulence predominated and highly virulent strains had virtually disappeared.

The factors that operated to select virus of intermediate virulence have also been studied. Because myxoma virus is transmitted mechanically by a mosquito vector it is reasonable that those virus strains that can persist in cutaneous lesions for the longest periods of time will be most likely to be picked up by the vector and transferred to another host. As illustrated in Table 3-3, it is strains of intermediate virulence that satisfy this requirement. The virulent strains achieve high concentrations in the lesions but kill the host promptly so that virus is available for transmission only briefly. The avirulent strains persist longer but only in low titer.

TABLE 3-3

Natural Selection of Myxoma Virus

Virulence*	Lethality	Host Survival Time	Virus Titer	Highest Probability of Vector Selection
I	+++++	+	+++++	
II	++++	++	+++++	
III	+++	+++	+++++	+
IV	++	++++	++	
V	+	+++++	+	

* I = most virulent.
  + = lowest lethality, lowest virus titer.
After data of Fenner and Ratcliffe (1965).

The foregoing experiments answered only the question concerning change in viral virulence. But had the rabbits as well as the myxoma virus been changed genetically by this encounter of a new virus with a suceptible host? To begin with, it could be reasoned that a highly virulent virus is a poor selector of genetically resistant rabbits. The lethality of this attack left few animals alive to propagate and many surviving bucks were sterile. Therefore, the next generation would be sired by normal (un-selected) bucks that had escaped infection. The susceptible progeny would then be wiped out by the next epizootic—if caused by a virulent strain. On the other hand, selection by a less virulent strain is plausible as such strains do not produce male sterility. Young rabbits—the progeny of the survivors, in epidemic areas, and hence "selected,"—were first tested for antibody to establish whether or not they had specific acquired immunity to myxomatosis. Those without antibody (hence, not previously infected) were challenged with either (1) the original highly virulent virus or (2) the virus currently circulating in nature. Results were compared with challenge of labora-tory (nonselected) rabbits. In brief, the results of a field challenge experiment indicated that the progeny of the survivors of the epizootic were more resistant to myxomatosis.

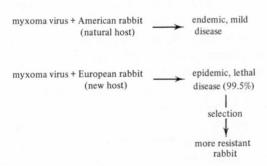

In summary, then, the introduction of an alien and extremely virulent virus into a genetically susceptible rabbit population *almost* eliminated both the rabbit population and the virus. However, within a remarkably short period of time, coincident natural selection occurred of less virulent virus and less susceptible host.

EVIDENCE FOR GENETICALLY DETERMINED RESISTANCE TO INFECTIOUS DISEASE

Genetically related resistance or susceptibility to infection in man is a subtlety. Among human populations, races or ethnic groups, the differing expression or effects of infections are not absolute and are usually explicable as being principally related to environmental rather than to genetic factors. As mentioned previously, such factors as crowding and malnutrition that attend the conditions of poverty result in a greater risk of tuberculosis and in fact a greater incidence of tuberculosis in the black American. But white Americans living in similar conditions are also demonstrably at jeopardy, so that the contribution, if any, of genotype to susceptibility to tuberculosis cannot be assessed merely from an examination of morbidity and mortality statistics.

Yet, although one cannot say, for example, that "Chinese don't get the common cold," or that "Caucasians are immune to syphilis," the preceding discussion of the blood protein polymorphisms has illustrated the great impact of *relative* resistance to an infectious disease (e.g., malaria). Also the earlier discussion of myxomatosis in the European rabbit has pointed to the role of the host's genes in preventing its eradication by a new and alien virus. Thus, the genetic determinants of resistance to infection are no less important because they may be difficult to discern.

It is, of course, not a simple question of either heredity or environment. Returning to the example of tuberculosis, in which environmental factors are clearly important, evidence from studies of identical (monozygotic) twins indicates that their susceptibility to tuberculosis (measured by the incidence of overt clinical disease) is much more similar than the susceptibility of nonidentical twins or siblings (Kallman and Reisner, 1943). Earlier studies have suggested concordance not only for the frequency of tuberculosis in identical twins but in the expression and localization of the disease if it occurred. These observations cannot be dismissed on the basis that identical twins are more likely to share the same environment, because sometimes they did not and yet were affected almost simultaneously while resident in different environments. Possibly relevant to these observations are studies of cutaneous hypersensitivity to tuberculin in identical and nonidentical twins; the difference in response was less in the identical twins. This latter point is interesting because it hints at a possible mechanism for the genetically determined defect. Studies of other types of delayed hypersensitivity with other microbial antigens would be important to assess the specificity of this reaction.

Other studies on identical twins (cited by Stern, 1960) suggest concordance for susceptibility to paralytic poliomyelitis but not for measles.

It may be concluded that genes determining resistance to infectious diseases are present and operative in man, and that the phenotype of resistance can be recognized in certain individuals under certain circumstances, i.e., in those rare human beings with close to identical genotype (identical twins) studied for similarity of fate with respect to a specific disease. But these limited studies provide little insight into the mechanism of genetic resistance, or into the relative importance of the genetic contribution to resistance to infection in any specific instance. In contrast, the approach of population genetics, cited earlier, has provided evidence for single gene defects (hemoglobin variation and falciprum malaria) that have probably had important selective and evolutionary effects.

Finally, there exist genetic deficiency diseases in which undue susceptibility to infection is either a direct or an indirect consequence of the deficiency. Hypogamma-globulinemia is a rare disorder carried by an X-linked gene in which deficiency in antibody-forming cells results in increased susceptibility to pyogenic bacterial infections. Interestingly, recovery from viral infections is normal in affected individuals —suggesting that antibody is not essential in determining the outcome of viral diseases.

Fatal granulomatous disease of childhood is another X-linked genetic disease in which resistance to bacterial infection is seriously impaired. In this case the deficiency is localized to the polymorphonuclear leukocyte, which is metabolically deficient and demonstrably defective in its ability to kill certain bacteria *in vitro* (Windhorst *et al.*, 1968). A less direct relationship of genetic deficiency to decreased resistance to infection is illustrated by cystic fibrosis of the pancreas (mucoviscidosis). In this heritable disease of unknown cause the basic genetic deficiency has not been defined. Patients with this disease have generalized bronchial obstruction and for this reason are unusually vulnerable to respiratory tract infections and particularly to infection with *Staphylococcus aureus*. In this instance, susceptibility to infection is obviously determined by nonspecific factors that determine the clearance of bacterial pathogens from the respiratory tract.

The Nature and Mechanisms of Genetically Determined Resistance to Infection

Understandably, studies of host resistance conducted in inbred laboratory animals under controlled conditions and with genetically characterized infectious agents have yielded more exact information than has been possible thus far in studies of human disease. Animal experiments are not only susceptibile to precise control but permit matings of animals of short generation time and crosses of progeny to produce F-1 and backcross generations (cf. Chapter 2). Analysis of the outcome of infection in a group of animals reveals whether susceptibility in a given disease is determined by single or multiple genes. A bimodal or trimodal distribution of susceptibility (Figure 3-8) is consistent with a single gene effect. A continuous distribution curve in plotting of susceptibility indicates a lack of segregation of susceptibility that is characteristic of the contribution of multiple genes (polygenic resistance).

If, once again, we consider the case of genetic resistance to tuberculosis—this time experimental tuberculosis of mice—it is clearly demonstrable that hereditary factors influence susceptibility. As illustrated in Figure 3-9, the crossing of resistant (Swiss) mice with susceptible (C-57-BL) mice with a short survival after infection, produced progeny demonstrating the wide distribution of susceptibility (as in the polygenic plot of Figure 3-8). Indeed, the mean resistance of the F-1 (progeny) generation was even *greater* than that of the more resistant Swiss parent. This effect may be ascribed to *heterosis*, or "hybrid vigor," and a favorable reshuffling and combination of multiple genes. However, an analysis of four successive backcrosses demonstrated a separation of backcross progeny into two groups, suggesting a segregation of genetic factors and

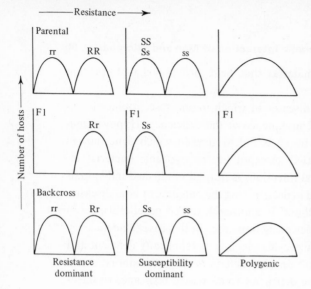

FIGURE 3-8. Diagrammatic representation of expected modes of inheritance against an infection on three hypotheses: *A* (left), that a single pair of alleles with resistance dominant makes an important contribution; *B* (middle), that a single pair of alleles with susceptibility dominant makes an important contribution; *C*, that many genes affect susceptibility. Upper curves show parental generations, with resistance plotted on the abscissa in arbitrary units (e.g., proportion of animals surviving a given virus dose, or dose of virus required to produce a particular response). Middle curves show progeny of matings of highly susceptible and highly resistant animals. Lower curves show back-crosses of F-I with suitable parental type. (Reproduced from A. C. Allison, *Arch ges Virusforsch*, **XVII**: 281, 1965.)

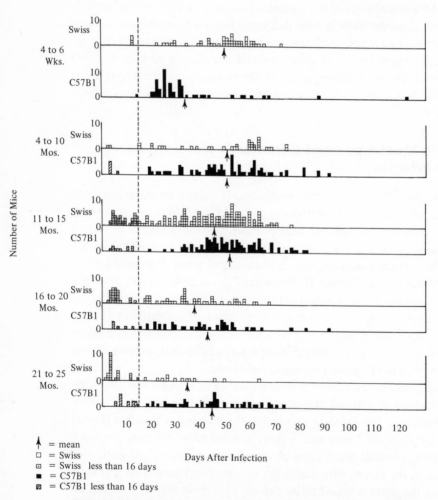

↑ = mean
□ = Swiss
▣ = Swiss less than 16 days
■ = C57B1
▨ = C57B1 less than 16 days

Days After Infection

FIGURE 3-9. Survival time of C-57-Bl and Swiss mice infected at different ages. Each mouse received intravenously 0.2 ml of a 1/50 culture dilution of *M. tuberculosis*. (Reproduced from C. J. Lynch, *et al. J Exp Med*, **121**: 1056, 1965.)

the dominance of a gene or many genes with linkage for resistance derived from the Swiss mice (Lynch *et al.*, 1965). These experiments did not define the mechanism of resistance nor the number of genes involved, but clearly demonstrated a genetic defect. In addition, the important points were made that susceptibility to tuberculosis in the two murine strains was (1) age conditioned and (2) dependent upon the number of organisms injected. Lastly, it was shown that the initial multiplication of the tubercle bacillus was similar in the susceptible and resistant animals. Thus, genetically determined susceptibility to tuberculosis even in the laboratory model is no simple thing.

The Specificity of Resistance and Susceptibility

In the experiments of Lynch and her associates cited above, there was evidence of a heterotic, or hybrid vigor, effect in the F-1 animals consistent with a general increase in resistance. For example, mothers of the F-1 generation had larger litters. This effect must always be reckoned with in genetic crossbreeding experiments. Yet the specificity of genetic resistance has been clearly shown in the case of several infections.

Virus Specific Susceptibility. That mice can be selectively bred for variation in susceptibility to viruses was demonstrated more than 30 years ago (Webster, 1937). This variation was also shown to be separate from bacterial resistance, was correlated with amounts of virus in the tissue, and was demonstrable *in vitro* in tissue culture. In later experiments by other investigators, it was shown that resistance to one group of viruses (namely, group B arboviruses) and resistance to mouse hepatitis virus (MHV) are separate and dissociable. Furthermore, two different mouse strains differ genetically in reciprocal fashion in their susceptibility to these two types of virus. (PRI mice are resistant to group B arboviruses and susceptible to MHV; C-3H mice are resistant to MHV and susceptible to the group B viruses.) Resistance, thus, has a measure of viral specificity, perhaps based on a single dominant gene in each case. Not surprisingly, the site of resistance to arbovirus and mouse hepatitis virus infections has been found by tissue culture experiments to be the cell. Susceptibility of mice in *in vivo* experiments correlates with the susceptibility *in vitro* of macrophages derived from them. This correlation applies as well to the susceptibility of mice (and cells) of the F-1 generation.

When comparison is made of genetic resistance to a leukemia virus in different strains of mice, the niceties of genetic resistance can be better appreciated. With a single strain of leukemia virus, three classes of resistance have been defined: Class I mice are highly susceptible as adults to the virus; Class II mice are relatively resistant as adults, but as infants are susceptible. Class III mice are highly resistant under all circumstances (Lilly, 1967).

A generalized nonspecific increase in resistance to all infections or even all viral infections has not yet been demonstrated. The implication for human disease is clear, namely, that separate and independent genes carry resistance that must be defined explicitly in terms of a given infection. Because these genes are not identified or presently identifiable we can only predict that efforts to identify or select populations that are generally "resistant to infections" will be meaningless.

Variation in Resistance of Human Cells in Vitro.   Not only the foregoing animal experiments but experiments with human viruses in human cells suggest that genetic resistance can be studied at the cellular level. Observations with poliovirus indicate that the essential step of attachment to cellular receptors occurs only with primate cells *in vitro*, thus mirroring the host susceptibility range of the virus. It is also well established that single gene defects affecting such enzymes as glucose-6-phosphate dehydrogenase are demonstrable in cell culture. Such biochemical lesions, of course, may underlie specific resistance to viruses.

The subtleties of the virus–host cell interrelationship—even in the *in vitro* environment are illustrated (literally in this case) by the differing destructive effects of several influenza virus strains in clones (subpopulations) derived from a single laboratory line of human conjunctival cells (Figure 3-10).

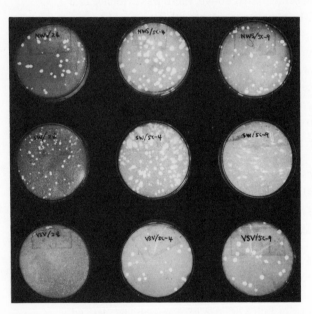

FIGURE 3-10.   Variation in plaque size of three virus strains (NWS, SW and VSV) inoculated onto monolayers of three human conjunctival cell clones (2B, 5C-4 and 5C-9). Note that susceptibility of the cells as measured by plaque size is dependent upon the virus inoculated. For example, NWS produces plaques of approximately the same size in clones 2B and 5C-9, but the plaques produced by VSV in these clones are markedly different. (From data of Sugiura and Kilbourne, 1964.)

HUMAN ECOLOGIC CHANGE AND THE EMERGENCE OF "NEW" INFECTIOUS DISEASES

As man has progressed to an increasingly urbanized existence, he has reduced his exposure to the microbes of both wild and domestic animals. The single exception is salmonellosis, a disease of increasing frequency that is actually fomented by the methods of modern food technology which include batch preparation and pooling of meat and poultry products (see Chapter 10). Therefore, the universe of potential microbial causes of human infection appears to be decreasing. It would seem that the liability of man to new infectious diseases would decrease as a consequence. But, in fact, new infectious diseases are appearing—not because of the *de novo* emergence of new parasites—but because of complex changes in human ecology that derive chiefly from man's manipulation of his physical and cultural environment.

An Unfavorable Effect of Change in the Physical Environment (Sanitation) with Postponement of Infection

Although environmental sanitation has been chiefly responsible for the control of such life-threatening enteric infections as typhoid fever, it has also lead, paradoxically, to an increase in poliomyelitis. In fact, poliomyelitis emerged as essentially a new disease in northern Europe and the United States at the end of the last century. Improved environmental sanitation reduced the probability of infection in infancy (when infection is best tolerated) and thus postponed infection to later childhood or adult life at which time infection is more often associated with overt paralytic disease. Stated another way, we can say that the change in human ecology associated with a more efficient pattern of waste disposal and personal cleanliness presented the infecting virus with a more vulnerable (namely older) human phenotype. No genetic change in either virus or man was responsible for the apparently increased severity of this infection.

The postponement of another enterovirus infection—Coxsackie B virus disease—may have serious consequences, not only for the adult but for the newborn infant. The neonatal period immediately following delivery is a period of maximum vulnerability to a number of infections. Transfer of antibodies from mother to child prior to delivery by the placenta and following delivery by the milk protects the infant for several months after birth. Viruses of the Coxsackie B group, which ordinarily cause mild febrile disease (pleurodynia) in childhood, may, if they infect the adult, cause more severe infection with carditis. If the pregnant woman is infected then her vulnerability is increased by her physiologic state as well as by her age. Furthermore, she may pass infection to her child either prior to delivery or afterward, and having no prior immunity, will be unable to transfer protective antibody. Under these circumstances the infant may develop fatal infection and myocarditis. Thus, myocarditis neonatorum may be another price of delayed infection in a society of adults not immunized by natural childhood infection (Table 3-4).

TABLE 3-4
Interrelation of Maternal and Neonatal Susceptibility to Group B Coxsackievirus Infection

	Maternal State	
	Immune	Nonimmune
Resistance to reinfection	+	0
Presence of humoral antibody	+	0
Transfer of maternal antibody to newborn	+	0
Resistance of newborn to infection	+	0
Susceptibility of mother to complications of infection	0	+*

* Apparently greater susceptibility to pericarditis in pregnancy (Plager *et al.*, 1962).

It is possible that the current increased incidence of hepatitis is in part a result of postponement of infection. Hepatitis in infants is less often associated with jaundice and it is milder than in adults. As with poliomyelitis, infection of the older subject is more overt and hence more easily detected.

Antimicrobial Drugs and the Changing Pattern of Bacterial Infections

Antibiotics and chemotherapeutic agents represent a man-made addition to the total environment of man and microbes. In restricted areas such as hospital wards, these drugs may actually become a significant part of the physical environment, but in most instances their effects are exerted indirectly through their use in chemoprophylaxis and chemotherapy. That is, the site of encounter of microorganism and drug is within the human host. The patient in whom an antimicrobial agent is circulating can be said to be altered (transiently) in phenotype. As a result of this alteration, the interaction of host and parasite can be affected in several ways. The most obvious result is prevention or cure of an infection caused by a drug-susceptible microorganism. This expected and happy result is not, however, without its consequences. A careful review of deaths on the medical service of a single large urban hospital during pre- and postantimicrobial periods demonstrated a reduction in the total number of fatal infections in the latter period. But microbial disease continued to contribute importantly to deaths in the medical unit.

Striking differences were noted between the two periods under study in the microbial parasites that produced fatal disease, the place where infection was acquired, and the presence of unassociated disease antedating infection.

In the pre-antimicrobial period the majority of fatal infections were produced by pneumococci, streptococci, tubercle bacilli, and staphylococci. These infections commonly arose in otherwise healthy persons in the outside community and were the direct cause of hospitalization. In contrast, fatal infections observed in 1957–58 were commonly caused by gram negative bacteria, staphylococci, viruses, and fungi. During this period, fatal infections commonly arose within the hospital in patients already compromised by other serious diseases (Rogers, 1959).

In a real sense, infection of the lung with microorganisms ordinarily present in the gastrointestinal tract is a new disease. Pneumococcal pneumonia "the old man's friend" has yielded to antimicrobial therapy, but the old, chronically diseased, and debilitated are now subjected instead to the less efficient slings and arrows of bacteria (the "gram negatives") that are not truly primary pulmonary pathogens. Thus, the modern hospital is hardly free of infectious disease problems—it is only that the problems are different.

Not only have bacteria that are intrinsically resistant to drugs filled the vacuum left by successful therapy of infections caused by drug-susceptible organisms, but the latter, through genetic mutation, have often managed to persist as a threat to human health. Virtually every genetic mechanism has been utilized by microbes in response to the inimical environment of the antibiotics. Microbial adaptation and mutation is not only a problem in therapy in the individual patient, but has serious implications for chemoprophylaxis of infection in the community. The past decade has seen the emergence of sulfonamide resistant meningococci and the return of epidemic meningitis as a threat to military installations.

There is no question but that we are better off for the discovery of antimicrobial drugs. But the predictions of the past for the "eradication" of infectious diseases and the inevitable triumph of chemotherapy were unrealistic and genetically naïve. It can be anticipated that present-day pathogens will continue their evolution and adaptation in the modern world of drugs and that organisms not presently recognized as pathogens may become so with changes in host and environment.

The Changing Cultural Environment and the Emergence of Serum Hepatitis

In a society in which piercing of the skin has become commonplace, serum hepatitis (see Chapter 10) appears to be a new disease. Although some evidence suggests that this infection may spread occasionally from person to person via the fecal–oral route, transmission depends principally on transcutaneous puncture with inadequately sterilized needles or instruments or by parenteral injection of human blood or its products. Again, a paradox of improved medical technology is the risk of hepatitis resulting from the development of special blood fractions for therapy and from the need for multiple transfusion introduced by the bolder techniques of modern surgery.

At the same time, the risk has been enhanced by the increase in drug addiction as a manifestation of social pathology. The addict himself (or even the occasional illicit user of drugs) is threatened by the use of shared unsterilized equipment, and serum hepatitis is clearly more common in such individuals. But recently it has been shown that the infected addict is a significant threat not only to other addicts but to the community at large. The impecunious addict—more liable than others to be carrying the virus of serum hepatitis in his blood—is often a commercial blood donor. Blood from a proprietary bank that was later found to have many addicts as donors produced hepatitis in recipients with six times the frequency observed in comparable recipients who received blood from hospital blood banks and from the American Red Cross (Cohen and Dougherty, 1968).

Thus, a cultural phenomenon (drug addiction) has had an important influence on the ecology of a microbial disease. The awesome potential of indiscriminate parenteral injection is discussed at the conclusion of this chapter.

Survival of the Unfit. Modern Surgery and the Emergence of Cytomegalic Inclusion Disease

The preservation of lives by modern surgery—particularly by the transplantation of vital organs—has required the use of highly toxic drugs for suppression of the immune response. A sequel of such immunosuppression has been the frequent activation of ubiquitously carried latent DNA virus, cytomegalovirus to produce serious and usually fatal pneumonia in patients who have had their primary disease "repaired" by organ replacement. This virus is also isolated from children with leukemia and from individuals of all ages with chronic disease affecting the reticuloendothelial system.

Like serum hepatitis, cytomegalovirus infection is socially influenced and is a risk of poverty as it occurs more frequently in institutionalized and indigent children (Li and Hanshaw, 1967). Also like serum hepatitis, the virus is a hazard of transfusion, particularly with fresh blood. The natural history of cytomegalovirus infection is only incompletely understood, but it seems to be yet another ubiquitous, chronically persistent microorganism that may evolve to pathogenicity as man's internal environment is manipulated.

WHAT HATH MAN WROUGHT? (NEW VACCINES, NEW VIRUSES, AND NEW PROBLEMS)

We have seen that virulence or pathogenicity as a characteristic of an infectious agent is a tenuous property that is subject to environmental influence and subtle host factors for its expression. Examples have been cited from studies of naturally occurring and experimental infection that verify the potential for virus-host interaction and reciprocal genetic selection. It is clear that viral parasitism has evolved to a state of relative stability in the context of an unchanged or slowly changing environment. Granted these premises, we may reasonably ask what will happen when (1) man changes his environment, (2) man changes his genetic endowment, or (3) man changes his viruses.

There is no question that the physical environment on earth has already suffered man-made change (see Chapter 4). In this new environment, in which concomitant cultural change has occurred, it is possible that new traits will have survival value and that susceptibility to infectious agents may be simultaneously influenced through pleiotropic genetic effects (see Chapter 2). In other words, the protein coded for by a gene important in adaptation to an atmosphere of increased SO_2 or radiation might also alter the resistance of the host (favorably or unfavorably) to an obligate human virus. The "bioengineering" or deliberate genetic repair envisioned for the future might well have similar side effects.

But the least speculative of the foregoing changes is the projection that man will be changing his viruses. This he has already done. In the United States, it appears that the vaccine strains of poliovirus are already supplanting the wildtype viruses. Even if these vaccine viruses do not become established endemically in nature they will still represent (directly from the bottle) a new part of man's ecology.

The New Viruses. I. LIVE (ATTENUATED) VACCINE VIRUSES. The great success of artificial immunization as a technique of preventive medicine has encouraged the belief that vaccines are the ultimate weapon against all infections. In this view, one has only to isolate all the human viruses, manufacture and administer the corresponding vaccines and illness will disappear. Of course, it is not that simple. Some 300-odd viruses produce disease in man and even the few vaccines now available have their limitations. In general, the inactivated (killed) virus vaccines have not produced enduring immunity. Furthermore, the abnormal parenteral route by which they are administered may induce (in the case of measles vaccine) a hypersensitive state that leads to severe reactions if the recipient is later exposed to the natural infection.

These problems with inactivated vaccines have shifted emphasis to the production of live virus vaccines. It is well to consider just what a live virus vaccine is. First, it is, in fact, a new virus changed in genotype and phenotype. The old term *attenuation* implies just this and not partial inactivation. Furthermore, because viruses require living cells for their multiplication, vaccine viruses must be grown in tissue or cell culture which are derived from alien (nonhuman) hosts, such as the chick embryo or the rhesus monkey.

II. THE LATENT VIRUSES IN VACCINE CULTURES.   The original fears about employing living vaccine viruses now seem simple and ingenuous when contrasted with the problems that have since arisen. In the case of polio vaccine, it was feared (1) that the relatively nonneurovirulent viruses might back-mutate to virulence, or (2) that extraneous viruses derived from the monkey kidney tissue culture might contaminate the vaccine. Elaborate screening and safety tests were designed by vaccine manufacturers and by the Division of Biologic Standards to guard against these possibilities. These tests were generally successful, but they could not detect the then undectable— a simian virus (SV40) that did not produce cytopathic effects in test cultures and which was so stable that it resisted inactivation even in *inactivated* Salk polio vaccine. SV40 was detected only retrospectively in stored lots of all three types of Sabin live polio vaccine and also in certain lots of inactivated polio and adenovirus vaccines also produced in rhesus monkey kidney tissue cultures and in seed stocks of respiratory viruses used

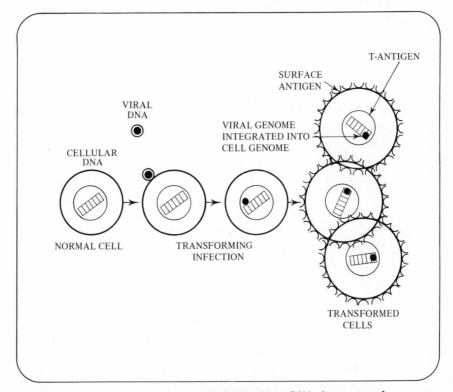

FIGURE 3-11. When a normal cell is transformed by a DNA virus, a part of the viral genome (or DNA) is integrated into the cell genome where it directs the production of new proteins called virus-specific cellular antigens. These include transplantation and surface antigens, located on the cell surface, and T (tumor) antigens in the nucleus. (Reproduced from *Progress Against Cancer.* A report by the National Advisory Cancer Council, 1967, p. 59.)

in volunteer experiments. It was then shown by antibody studies of sera from vaccinees and volunteers that infection of man with SV40 had actually occurred when the virus was inadvertently administered.

It has since been well established that SV40 is a DNA virus with oncogenic (tumor-producing) potential. It is a common contaminant of rhesus monkey kidney tissue culture. The natural role of the virus even in the monkeys which it latently infects is not clear; it does not seem to be a cause of cancer in its natural host, but it produces tumors in newborn hamsters and induces cellular transformation analogous to that seen in cancer in cultural cells of several species including man (Figure 3-11). In the course of polio immunization, the virus had been given inadvertently to millions of people. A follow-up was conducted of children who received Salk (inactivated) polio vaccine lots in 1955 in which SV40 contamination was retrospectively defined from stored samples. From cohort analysis of the years 1950–59 using cancer mortality data for children who were 6 to 8 (the vaccinee's age) in 1955, it was concluded that the vaccinees had no difference in mortality trends after 1955. Only unexplained increase in leukemia mortality was noted in both vaccinated and control groups. This interesting analysis, however, provides only a limited answer to the question of SV40 carcinogenicity in man, as the follow-up period of this study was brief, namely, four years, for a disease that may have a very long incubation period.

The Potential of Familiar Viruses in New Guises

In man's vaccine-oriented manipulation of his infectious environment, he must be concerned not only with unrecognized alien viruses of dire potential, but also with the risks of his new and abnormal relationship with familiar viruses of his own. A case in point is the adenoviruses, a family of viruses originally identified as causes of mild respiratory disease in children and acute epidemics in military recruits (see Chapter 10). Certain types of adenovirus, however, can induce the formation of tumors in newborn Syrian hamsters, and like SV40 can transform cells into malignancy in tissue culture. Among the oncogenic types is adenovirus type 7—an important cause of respiratory disease in the military. The practical question arises—should the use of adenovirus type 7 vaccine be prohibited? In short, what is the relevance of tumor production in the newborn hamster inoculated parenterally with large quantities of live virus to the risk of inoculation of an adult man with an inactivated virus? Caution still prevails at this writing—as well it should. It is not enough to contend that natural infection with adenovirus may be ultimately carcinogenic and that therefore the use of a preventive vaccine is justified. For on the other hand, the oncogenicity of adenovirus preparations that have been tested may be related to their unnatural tissue culture origin or to the abnormal transcutaneous route by which they are administered. Indeed, the carcinogenicity of at least some strains of adenovirus 7 is clearly related to an unprecedented biologic event—the genetic interaction and hybridization of this human virus with simian virus SV40 in tissue culture.

Viral Hybridization and Its Potential

A strain of adenovirus type 7 grown for vaccine production in rhesus monkey kidney cells induces tumor formation in baby hamsters—but the tumor contains the distinctive tumor antigen of SV40 virus—not the antigen of the characteristic tumor-forming adenovirus. This effect is not the result merely of the presence of contaminating SV40 virus particles in the adenovirus preparation. Rather it has been demonstrated in several laboratories that certain of the adenovirus particles contain some of the DNA and, hence, the genetic information of SV40 (Figure 3-12). Furthermore, these hybrid particles are defective in the sense that they can multiply only in the presence of non-hybrid adenovirus. Thus, the hybrid particles are difficult to isolate and study.

The implications of these rather esoteric observations are profound. In this instance, a virus propagated for the production of vaccine has undergone genetic recombination or hybridization with a virus latently infecting tissue culture cells used for vaccine production. Furthermore, the "piece" of viral DNA acquired from the latent SV40 virus is capable of coding for the tumor-associated antigen of that virus. This is a subtle kind of contamination, indeed. One must wonder what other more cryptic genetic messages can be transferred by vaccines. As indicated earlier in this chapter, the myxoviruses carry constituents derived from the host cells in which they replicate, but these constituents are polysaccharide or lipid. The carriage of alien nuclei acid— either cellular DNA of another mammalian species or nonvaccine viral nucleic acid— has the awesome potential of transplanted genes. The proposed use for vaccine production of human diploid cells with normal chromosome complement may answer the problem of inadvertent inoculation of alien nucleic acid. But the introduction of homologous human DNA may not be free of risk nor can one be sure that such cells are free of latent viruses.

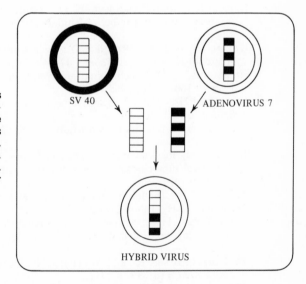

FIGURE 3-12. When SV40 and adenovirus 7 are present in the same culture, a tumor-producing hybrid virus may be formed. The new virus consists of a core of nucleic acids from both the SV40 and adenovirus 7, wrapped in the protein outer coat of the latter. (Reproduced from *Progress Against Cancer*. A report by the National Advisory Cancer Council, 1967, p. 53.)

Clearly, research in artificial immunization must continue, and new vaccines must be produced. But at least some of the risks in all their subtlety and complexity are now apparent so that caution and careful evaluation of each result is necessary. It is also necessary to determine for each infection whether other methods of control such as environmental sanitation or chemoprophylaxis are feasible as better alternatives to immunization.

If eventually man can select his microbes, substituting immunizing but domesticated species for the virulent strains in nature, he must be aware of their and his continuing capacity for genetic variation and interaction.

REFERENCES

ALLISON, A. C.: Genetic factors in resistance to malaria. *Ann. NY Acad Sci*, **91**:710–29, 1961.

————: Genetic factors in resistance against virus infections. *Arch Ges Virusforsch*, **XVII**:280–94, 1965.

ATHREYA, B. H., and CORIELL, L. L.: Relation of blood groups to infection. I. A survey and review of data suggesting possible relationship between malaria and blood groups. *Amer J Epidem*, **86**:292–304, 1967.

COHEN, S. N., and DOUGHERTY, W. J.: Transfusion hepatitis arising from addict blood donors. *JAMA*, **203**:427–29, 1968.

DOWNIE, A. W., MEIKLEJOHN, G., ST. VINCENT, L., RAO, A. R., SUNDARA BABU, B. V., and KEMPE, C. H.: Smallpox frequency and severity in relation to A, B and O blood groups. *Bull* WHO, **33**:623–25, 1965.

DUBOS, R.: The evolution of microbial diseases. In Dubos, R. J., and Hirsch, J. G. (eds.): *Bacterial and Mycotic Infections of Man*, 4th ed. J. B. Lippincott Company, Philadelphia, 1965.

FENNER, F., and RATCLIFFE, F. N.: Changes in the virulence of myxomavirus for oryctolagus cuniculus. In Fenner, F., and Ratcliffe, F. N. (eds.): *Myxomatosis*. Cambridge University Press, New York, 1965.

ISACSON, P., and KOCH, A. E.: Association of host antigens with a parainfluenza virus. *Virology*, **27**:129–38, 1965.

JAHIEL, R. I., and KILBOURNE, E. D.: Reduction in plaque size and reduction in plaque number as differing indices of influenza virus-antibody reactions. *J Bact*, **92**:1521–34, 1966.

KALLMANN, F. J., and REISNER, D.: Twin studies on the significance of genetic factors in tuberculosis. *Amer Rev Tuberc*, **47**:549–74, 1943.

KILBOURNE, E. D.: Recombination of influenza A viruses of human and equine origin. *Science*, **160**:74–76, 1968.

LI, F., and HANSHAW, J. B.: Cytomegalovirus infection among migrant children. *Amer J Epidem*, **86**:137–41, 1967.

LILLY, F.: Susceptibility to two strains of Friend leukemia virus in mice. *Science*, **155**:461–62, 1967.

LYNCH, C. J., PIERCE-CHASE, C. H., and DUBOS, R.: A genetic study of susceptibility to experimental tuberculosis in mice imported with mammalia tubercle bacilli. *J Exp Med*, **121**:1051–1070, 1965.

MAGILL, T. P.: The immunologist and the evil spirits. *J Immunol* **74**: 1–8, 1955.

MUSCHEL, L. H.: Blood groups, disease and selection. *Bact Rev*, **30**:427–41, 1966.

PETTENKOFER, H. J., STROSS, B., HELMBOLD, W., and VOGEL, F.: Alleged causes of the present-day world distribution of the human ABO blood groups. *Nature*, **193**:445–46, 1962.

PLAGER, H., BEEBE, R., and MILLER, J. K.: Coxsackie B–5 pericarditis in pregnancy. *Arch Intern Med*, **110**:735–38, 1962.

RIORDAN, J. T.: IX. Isolation of enteroviruses from sewage before and after vaccine administration. *Yale J Biol Med*, **34**:512–21, 1962.

ROGERS, D. E.: The changing pattern of life-threatening microbial disease. *New Eng J Med*, **261**:677–83, 1959.

STERN, C.: *Principles of Human Genetics*, 2nd ed. W. H. Freeman & Co., San Francisco and London, 1960.

WEBSTER, L. T.: Inheritance of resistance of mice to enteric bacterial and neurotropic virus infections. *J Exp Med*, **65**:261–86, 1937.

WILSON, G. S., and MILES, A. A.: Tuberculosis. In Topley and Wilson's *Principles of Bacteriology and Immunity*, 3rd ed. The Williams and Wilkins Company, Baltimore, 1946.

WINDHORST, D. B., PAGE, A. R., HOLMES, B., QUIE, P. G., and GOOD, R. A.: The pattern of genetic transmission of the leukocyte in fatal granulomatous disease of childhood. *J Clin Invest*, **47**:1026–34, 1968.

4

Influence of the Physical Environment on Health and Disease

James McCarroll

NATURALLY OCCURRING PHYSICAL INFLUENCES

As inhabitants of a solar planet, we are constantly subject to a variety of physical forces from both earthly and extraterrestrial sources. Some of these forces, such as magnetism, gravity, and cosmic radiation, are completely beyond our control and we have, therefore, tended to ignore their effect on human health. Only recently, as man has been able to escape from some of the terrestrial forces through space exploration, have we become aware of the very fundamental role they play in some of our basic physiologic processes. The physiologic effects of other forces, such as ultraviolet and infrared light, and extreme heat and cold, can be modified by erecting artificial barriers, such as clothing and housing, between ourselves and the environment, or by selecting areas of the globe for habitation where the extremes of these forces are avoided.

Electromagnetic Radiation

We are exposed to a continuous stream of physical radiation extending over much of the electromagnetic spectrum (Figure 4-1). Because most of this originates from outer space (cosmic and solar radiation), it is beyond our control, but the effects of certain portions of the spectrum can be modified by our activities. Our principal protection, however, against the more harmful rays is provided by our atmosphere, which effectively screens out those portions of the spectrum that would make life, as we know it, impossible on earth. Some portions of this spectrum are emissions of high energy and great penetrating powers, such as cosmic radiation. Against them, no practical

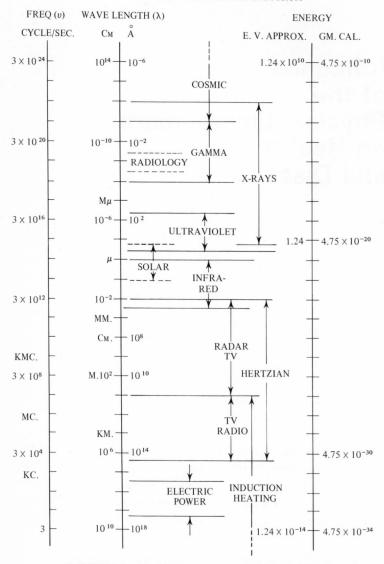

FIGURE 4-1. The electromagnetic spectrum. Energy from outer space, largely solar, reaches the earth as some form of electromagnetic radiation and is the fundamental source of power on earth. The energy delivered is directly proportional to the frequency (the higher the frequency, the shorter the wave length and the higher the energy transmitted). The wave length of a given emanation determines its specific characteristics. For all types of electromagnetic radiation, the wave length for a given frequency, multiplied by the frequency in cycles per second, is equal to the speed of light (3×10^{10} cm per sec). (Reproduced from Ferris, B. G., Jr.: *New Eng J Med*, **275** (20): 1100, 1966.)

type of shielding or protection is effective, but they are important to human health because of their ability to cause mutations in gonadal cells. Indeed, much of the spontaneously occurring genetic mutation in all forms of terrestrial life may be due to cosmic radiation. Although we cannot control our exposure to such naturally penetrating radiation, we can limit total human exposures by controlling artificial sources, such as x-rays and industrial radioisotopes, which add their effects directly to the background burden.

Ultraviolet Radiation

Other types of naturally occurring extraterrestrial radiation, such as ultraviolet and infrared waves, may be effectively controlled either by direct protective measures, or by natural physiologic adaptation. Tanning by solar ultraviolet rays is a spontaneous protective mechanism in most persons, limiting the harmful effects of sunlight. The same protective mechanism—deposition of melanin in the skin—has permitted dark-skinned races to spread successfully over the tropical areas of the earth, where the unprotected light-skinned man would be unable to thrive without the artificial protection of clothing and shelter. Ultraviolet radiation is blocked in large part by the atmosphere, so that the proportion reaching the earth is dependent largely on the angle at which the sun's rays strike the earth's surface, which determines the amount of atmosphere through which the rays must pass (Figure 4-2). For this reason, sunlight reaching the earth between 10:00 A.M. and 2:00 P.M. will contain a far higher portion of ultraviolet rays than early morning or late afternoon sunlight. Similarly, sunlight in summer, when the sun is more nearly overhead, will provide much more ultraviolet radiation than the lower-angled sun of the winter months. Contrary to popular impression, these rays are not appreciably reflected by water or sand, so that tanning on an ocean beach is dependent almost entirely on direct exposure. Snow, however, does reflect ultraviolet rays to an appreciable degree, so that skiers may typically develop sunburn on the tip of the chin and undersurface of the nose—areas not frequently exposed to direct sunlight.

Except in childhood, when some exposure to the sun's ultraviolet rays may promote good bone development by stimulating vitamin D formation, there is no known physical benefit derived by deliberate exposure to solar radiation (Buettner, 1951). Although a deep suntan is often considered cosmetically desirable, the health benefits popularly supposed to accompany it are nonexistent. Ultraviolet radiation can be definitely damaging to eyes and skin, accelerates aging changes of the skin and, occasionally, induces malignant neoplasms (Cogan, 1950). Skin cancers have been recognized for years to occur with greatly increased frequency in persons whose occupations expose them to intense sunlight. Recently, malignant melanoma has also been linked with exposure to sunlight, and in this case the tumors are as likely to appear on areas covered by clothing as on parts of the body exposed to direct sunlight. This would suggest that the effects of some types of physical radiation may be mediated through pathways other than direct exposure.

MINIMUM ERYTHEMA TIME
0° N. LATITUDE

(Direct sunlight and skylight on a horizontal surface)

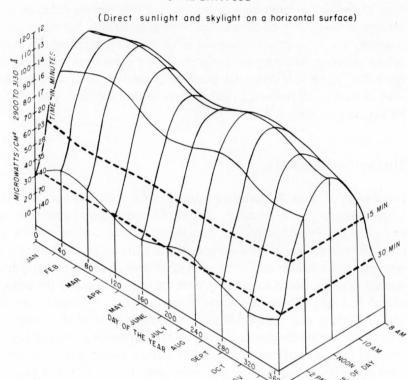

(a)

MINIMUM ERYTHEMA TIME
40° N. LATITUDE

(Direct sunlight and skylight on a horizontal surface)

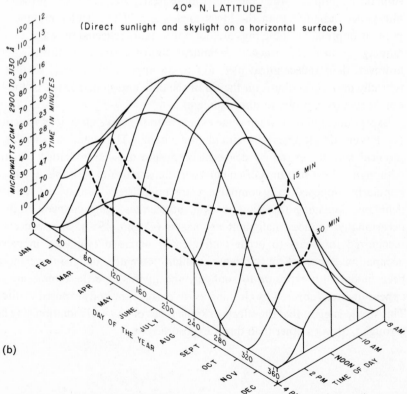

(b)

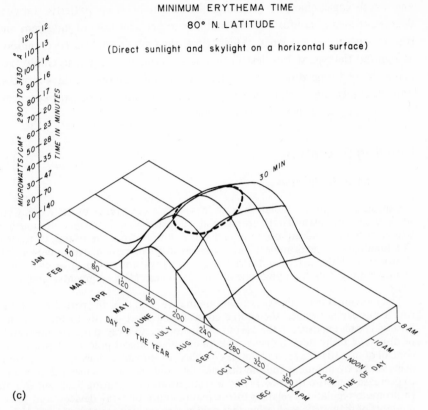

(c)

FIGURE 4-2. Ultraviolet Radiation. Ultraviolet solar radiation reaches the earth's surface in sufficient concentration to produce sunburn only when the sun is overhead. Earlier than 10 A.M., or later than 2 P.M., the rays traverse a sufficiently long course through the atmosphere to filter out much of the UV radiation. Moving north or south toward the earth's poles also increases the angle at which the sun's rays strike the earth's atmosphere, and similarly results in decreased UV radiation with increasing latitude. (a) UV radiation at the equator. (b) UV radiation at 40° latitude. (c) UV radiation at 80° latitude. (Reproduced from F. Daniels in S. Licht [ed.] : *Therapeutic Electricity and Ultraviolet Radiation*, 2nd ed. Elizabeth Licht, Publisher, New Haven, Conn., 1967.)

Light

Many basic physiologic functions are regulated by "biologic clocks," which depend primarily on day length for synchronization. Such bodily functions as temperature, pulse rate, certain types of hormone production, and a variety of other basic physiologic functions are controlled, at least in part, by sunlight as we unconsciously perceive it. If a volunteer is experimentally sealed in a chamber where he cannot perceive normal cycles of day and night, some of these bodily functions may gradually drift out of phase with others. Although some physiologic functions will continue on a normal 24-hour cycle, others gradually drift toward longer periods, and end up out of phase with other associated functions. The effects of abrupt disruption of these normal circadian (i.e., *circa dies* or daily) rhythms are seen with increasing frequency in today's jet airplane travelers who may cross many time zones within a few hours. Travelers experiencing this abrupt transition frequently notice a variety of physiologic and psychologic changes, including disruption of sleep patterns, fatigue, varying degrees of mental confusion, and inability to perform tests of judgment and concentration with usual efficiency. This "time zone syndrome" is so common and well recognized that many business firms and governments requiring employees to travel across several time zones will require them to journey several days in advance of an important meeting, so that their physiologic functions may become synchronized with the diurnal cycle of their new environment.

Ionizing Radiation

Kenneth G. Johnson

Exposure to ionizing radiation is an inescapable occurrence of daily life. Certain foodstuffs, such as cereals and nuts, are naturally radioactive, and man is continuously exposed to cosmic radiation and atmospheric and soil pollution from the testing of nuclear devices. For hundreds of years miners have been exposed to radioactive minerals (pitchblende, feldspar), and the list of industrial uses of x-rays and radioactive chemicals, in both manufacturing (photographic chemicals, ceramics, glass, pigments) and testing grows yearly.

The individual person's exposure is cumulative, and over the period of his lifetime, barring a nuclear holocaust, the source contributing most heavily to the total accumulated dose will be his exposure to the use of radioisotopes and x-ray in the diagnosis and treatment of disease, a technology indispensable in effective clinical practice. Thus, the problem of control of hazards due to radiation is complex: to eliminate unnecessary exposures as those experienced by luminous radium-dial painters and shoe-fitters using fluoroscopic devices, to decrease exposure to workers and investigations by requiring licensing and monitoring, to promote regulations relating to the manufacture of x-ray devices, and to seek refined methods of diagnostic evaluation that deliver a tolerable dose to both patient and operator without diminishing the information content of the procedure.

Known human biologic effects constitute the basis for the estimate for maximum permissible dose of external radiation. This estimate has undergone drastic reduction downward to the *average* level of 0.5 rad per year for the general public, and 5 rad per year, not to exceed 12 rad in any year, from age 18 on, for radiation workers (National Council, 1968). (The units of measure *rein* and *rad* are identical for the common types of radiation. *Roentgen* and *rad* vary within 10 per cent of each other and are in this discussion used interchangeably).

The biologic effects of ionizing radiation in the human being can be separated by chronicity. A whole body exposure to a dose greater than 100r (roentgens) is sufficient to produce the *acute radiation syndrome*. Nausea, vomiting, and weakness are experienced within a few hours. The patient may recover from this initial episode, but within the next two weeks malaise, fever, petechiae and painful ulcers of the skin, buccal and intestinal mucosa will develop. Epilation may occur within the third week at which time a profound leukopenia and thrombocytopenia are noted. Barring superinfection by microbial agents in the patient's environment, recovery from the acute illness may be complete.

Continuous, localized exposure to radiation may produce erythema of the skin, followed by atrophy and telangiectasia, and finally ulceration. Squamous cell epitheliomata may develop in the radiation scar and in the management of several cases amputation has had to be employed. This sequela is most often seen in radiologists and in other persons who have had multiple exposure to x-radiation, unfortunately, often for the treatment of benign conditions.

The biologic effects of radiation are related to dose and tissue sensitivity. The earliest observation of the association of human disease and ionizing radiation was made among the uranium miners of Scheneberg and Joachmistal in Saxony. Their pattern of mortality was considered unusual even in the sixteenth century and as late as 1900 these Miners developed lung cancer at a rate of 1 per cent per year (Hesse and Harting, 1962). In several other human populations, the survivors of the atomic bombings of Hiroshima and Nagasaki (Bizzozero *et al.*, 1966), British adults with rheumatoid spondylitis treated with radiotherapy (Court-Brown and Doll, 1957), American radiologists (March, 1961), infants whose thymus glands were irradiated (Murray *et al.*, 1959), leukemia has been the earliest effect noted. Peak incidence was noted in Japanese survivors eight to nine years after exposure (Bizzozero *et al.*, 1966), predominantly in persons who were less than 30 years of age in 1945, the year of the bombings. In addition to leukemia, the frequency of cancer of other sites (thyroid [Wood *et al.*, 1967] lung, [Wanebo *et al.*, in press], breast [Wanebo *et al.*, 1968]) has been found increased in A-bomb survivors within 1500 meters of the hypocenters. Japanese mothers at this distance and within the first 16 weeks of pregnancy were likely to have issue who were mentally retarded and/or who had a head size of minus 2 standard deviations from the mean of children who were not exposed *in utero* (Wood *et al.*, 1967).

Diagnostic roentgenography during intrauterine life and in early childhood has been shown in several studies to be associated with the subsequent development of cancer (Macmahon, 1962; Stewart *et al.*, 1958). One study suggests that even exposure prior to conception infers increased risk of cancer to progeny (Graham *et al.*, 1966). It is estimated that 10 roentgens delivered to the fetus is capable of producing all the cancers of childhood (Radiation Protection, 1966).

The gonadal or fetal dose delivered during a diagnostic procedure will vary with the type of radiographic technique and apparatus used. A fair estimate of the total gonadal dose to a woman during a single hospitalization that includes a chest film (0.3r), oral cholecysto-gram (0.1r), intravenous pyelogram (1.0r), upper GI series with fluoroscopy (2.0r), and a barium enema (6.0r) is approximately 9 roentgens. Because a clinical study of this extent is not unusual, careful inquiry should be made prior to radiographic studies for every woman of child-bearing age in order to avoid potentially disastrous teratogenic and carcinogenic effects in the fetus. The experience of a United States national sample of 4,096 women, representative of all women having liveborn infants during 1963 (Brown and Nelson, 1968) indicates that approximately 23 per cent had one or more x-ray examinations during pregnancy. One fifth of these examinations were performed *during the first trimester*, and of these first-trimester examinations, 2.5 per cent were pelvimetry, fetography, and placentography x-ray examinations. Most of these examinations were performed in places other than a physician's office (hospitals, clinics, mobile units, Public Health Departments, and so on). These observations are extremely important in pointing up an urgent need to protect the fetus during the critical period of organogenesis.

Leukemia and related disorders, cancer of the thyroid, lung, breast, lenticular opacities, and the intrauterine effects cited, are all obvious, easily recognized late effects of radiation. Court-Brown and his associates (Court-Brown *et al.*, 1965) and Bloom and his associates (Bloom *et al.*, 1966) have detected chromosomal abnormalities in persons as long as 20 years after exposure to ionizing radiation. These observations lend great support to the concept of total lifetime exposure of an individual.

The use of ionizing radiation has saved and prolonged countless numbers of lives. Nuclear energy has been harnessed to provide electrical power without polluting the air or depleting natural resources, and the new industrial uses of x-ray and radioisotopes undoubtedly have had substantial beneficial effects on the economy. Legal restraints on the manufacturers of x-ray equipment to produce better products, licensing of users of isotopes, and the discriminating use of diagnostic radiography, especially during pregnancy and early childhood, will go far in reducing the potential hazard of ionizing radiation.

Weather and Disease*

Dating from earliest human legends, weather has always been popularly considered as a major determinant of health and disease. Actual evidence for a direct causal relationship between changes in meteorologic conditions and specific human diseases is

* See also Chapter 7.

scanty and contradictory. Many diseases follow well-defined seasonal patterns, such as the peaks of respiratory illnesses in winter and spring, and the similar increases in gastrointestinal ailments in summer. Nevertheless, these seasonal occurrences may well be the result of factors other than the weather alone. Thus, increased crowding, with prolonged indoor contact in dry, steam-heated schools and offices, may be a more important factor in spread of respiratory infections than a lower outdoor temperature. Common colds in isolated arctic communities occur only when outsiders (carrying viruses) enter the area.

Some weather factors may favor the survival and transmission of certain infectious disease agents (see Chapter 7). The weather, itself, however, rarely causes the disease. It acts, instead, as one of a cluster of environmental factors uniting to favor initiation or spread of an illness. Thus, cold and damp weather and the notorious London fogs, for example, aggravate the effects of air pollutants and infectious disease agents simultaneously present, and result in more and severer respiratory disease during such episodes than might otherwise occur.

Although weather usually plays a secondary role in human disease, in special circumstances it may be the dominant factor. Periods of excessive heat, especially when coupled with high humidity, are one of the most stressful situations to which man is called to adapt. A severe heat wave in a major city will precipitate more immediate deaths than will a severe cold spell or any infectious disease agent commonly occurring in industrialized countries. These deaths, however, will be almost entirely among the elderly, or those with various chronic diseases. A direct effect on the health of well people has been frequently ascribed to special types of winds, peculiar to a few geographic areas—the foehn and the mistral of Europe, and the chinook of the American northwest. Unfortunately, these reports are highly subjective impressions of local residents, and no objective scientific evidence has confirmed actual physiologic changes in citizens of these areas during such episodes. Except for extremes in temperature, humidity, and wind speed, the principal direct effect of weather on health is probably psychologic. Certainly, a sunny day with moderate temperature and humidity is more pleasant than an extremely hot, cold, humid, or windy one. Indirect effects of weather on health, however, are common in that meteorologic factors are part of the constellation of environmental parameters affecting the prevalence and severity of many diseases.

Heat and Cold. With moderate variations in temperature, man's physiologic mechanisms of sweating, shivering, and increase or decrease of surface blood flow and metabolic rate can effectively maintain his homeostasis. As greater extremes of temperature are reached, he must add external buffers, such as clothing and shelter, between himself and his environment. The heat stress to which a man is subject at various temperatures may be quantitated by adding metabolic heat produced (M) to the heat lost by radiation (R), and convection (C), which will determine the amount of evaporation (E) by sweating needed to balance the equation.

$$M \pm R \pm C = E.$$

The maximum evaporative capacity will, in turn, be determined by dry-bulb temperature and relative humidity of the atmosphere, which determine the vapor pressure difference between the skin and air, and by the air speed. When each of these factors has been determined, it is possible to plot maximum evaporative capacity of a person against evaporation required to maintain a normal temperature and derive a heat stress index (Leithead, C. S., and Lind, A. R., 1964).

Clothing. Clothing may greatly accelerate or retard each of these factors, and the types evolved by different people in different geographic areas reflect their special needs. Arctic clothing is loose-fitting, light-weight, and moisture-proof, to form an insulating layer between the environment and the trapped, still air surrounding the body. The light weight of the animal skins used helps conserve the metabolic energy needed for motion.

In tropic areas, the type of clothing needed depends on humidity as much as temperature. In humid areas, scanty clothing of high porosity, to favor convection and radiation, is essential, and evaporation is assisted by materials that act as a wick to absorb sweat from the body and evaporate it to the environment. In desert areas, more covering is needed to protect the body from direct sunlight, but light color, loose fit porosity, and light weight are important. Evaporative cooling may be less important if insufficient water is available to replace that lost by sweating.

Housing. Housing—in effect a further extension of clothing—can also be manipulated to increase or decrease the efficiency of the same heat-regulating physiologic mechanisms. The thick-walled igloo, with minimum surface presented to the environment, and with little internal air motion, favors maximum heating from a single oil flame. When occupied by several people, the internal environment is virtually "tropical," so that Eskimos were described by early explorers as remaining virtually naked in comfort inside their igloos.

Similar insulating qualities are necessary in desert climates, so that the thick-walled adobe pueblo, or Navajo hogan, produces cavelike internal temperatures greatly modifying the wide diurnal fluctuation between extreme heat and cold. The thick walls, with few openings, also protect against wind and help maintain a higher humidity in the home. In the humid tropical jungle, overhead protection from direct sun and rain is of major importance. Walls are porous, with many openings, or absent altogether.

Naturally Occurring "Pollutants"

In only a few localized areas of the world are naturally occurring chemicals or elements present in sufficient concentration to affect human health adversely. In fact, the reverse is true; deleterious effects on health occur far more frequently from the absence of one or more important trace minerals than from excessive amounts present. In some areas, ground water contains sufficient amounts of sulfur, or other minerals, to be unpleasant to the taste or smell, and these are usually avoided. There are few other naturally occurring "pollutants" present in sufficient concentration to affect health. One exception is fluoride, which may be present in some water supplies at levels of three or more parts per million (ppm). At this concentration a slight brown mottling of the teeth may be noted, after prolonged exposure during the teeth-forming years. Accompanying this mild reaction, however, is a definitely increased resistance of the teeth to cavity formation. It has been found that this increased resistance to cavity formation can be preserved with water levels of only 1 ppm of fluoride, and that the mottling phenomenon does not occur at this low dosage. Small amounts of fluoride in water are therefore no longer regarded as a contamination of the resource. On the contrary, the absence of fluoride is now considered a defect to be remedied, and an increasing number of communities are adding small amounts of fluoride to deficient waters to increase the dental health of their children (Schlesinger, 1957).

Another important element missing in many environments is iodine. Deficient iodine in the diet leads to goiter and insufficient thyroid gland production. This problem is sufficiently common to cause salt producers to add, routinely, small amounts of iodine to table salt to assure an adequate iodine intake to everyone.

OUR ARTIFICIAL ENVIRONMENT

Most of the substances in our environment giving cause for medical concern are the results of man's activities. Deliberately or inadvertently, we add to the air we breathe, to the water we drink, and to the land on which we grow our food, a host of substances of suspected or proved biologic activity. Inevitably, these are introduced into our bodies, and to what extent they may be altering our health or functioning is one of today's most pressing questions. Because man is the only creature capable of altering his environment fundamentally, we have no precedent or animal model to guide us. The problem, furthermore, is quite recent in man's history, resulting directly from the twin phenomena of urbanization and industrialization that appear to be the destiny of virtually all nations. During most of his tenure on earth, man, like all other forms of life, has lived in balance with his environment. His activities and waste products did not alter the environment beyond its capacity to regenerate itself. In the past few decades, however, man has overloaded many areas of the world with the effluent of his industrial and social activities, so that natural forces can no longer cope with the volume of his discharges. The problem is further complicated by the artificial nature of much of this effluent. Every year we synthesize some 10,000 new chemical compounds, many of which find uses in various industrial processes or social activities. Inevitably, they are introduced into the environment and into us, where their effect may be unpredictable.

At the end of World War II, synthetic hydrocarbon detergents were introduced and rapidly replaced fatty acid soaps for many purposes. As tons of these compounds emptied into our rivers and streams, it became obvious that they lacked one of soap's inherent characteristics—the susceptibility to destruction by bacterial action. As the concentration of these compounds in streams receiving sewage grew, persistent foaming and frothing became a familiar sight at many scenic waterfalls. Once the problem was recognized, the detergent industry was able to remedy the situation by developing new detergents susceptible to destruction by naturally occurring bacteria.

Although this example of the introduction of a new chemical with unforeseen consequences was happily solved, the problems produced by other new compounds have not always ended in such a satisfactory solution. Thalidomide, a newly introduced tranquilizing agent, was found after some months of use to be associated with congenital deformities in children of mothers who had taken the drug early in pregnancy. Although such tragic effects are rare, they illustrate dramatically the potency of some of these newer chemical agents. The episode also illustrates how subtle and devious may be the pathways through which some of these compounds may affect our health. In this case, the effect was not evident until months after the drug was taken—and then showed up in a different person from the one using the medication.

This episode, and an increasing number of others, point out the urgent need to develop new methods of testing for such delayed and indirect reactions. Toxicity tests carried out on all new chemical agents that may be taken into the body are aimed primarily at determining acute toxic effects. Complicating this testing is the well-known variation between animal species in their reactions to different drugs. Nevertheless, the existence of acute toxic effects is relatively easy to determine when compared with possible long-term chronic or additive effects.

If a new drug or chemical has the potential of stimulating cancer formation when used over a long period, the effect may not be visible for many years. Thus, cigarette smoking was a common habit for a full generation before its role in lung cancer became apparent. A similar delay may be necessary before mutagenic or other serious effects of some compounds can be recognized.

The concentration by various organisms of some chemicals introduced into the environment in small amounts also poses a potential hazard. DDT, a highly effective pesticide, was widely used for 20 years in agriculture before being replaced by less persistent compounds. Although used on crops in relatively dilute amounts, rain washed the pesticide into streams and rivers where it was taken into the bodies of many forms of life. Many of these organisms—shellfish, crustaceans, and free-swimming fish—concentrated the chemical in their bodies so that the total body burden became many times higher than would be anticipated from the dilute solutions in which they were living. These higher concentrations proved lethal for several species, including higher forms of life using these lower forms as food. Progressing up the ecologic food chain, each form of life is found to contain appreciable amounts of DDT, resulting in part from this concentration process. Virtually all adult Americans now have 0.1 gram of this chlorinated hydrocarbon deposited in their fatty tissues as a direct result of this concentration process (Dale and Quinby, 1963). The compound is apparently inert and has not yet been shown to have any deleterious effects on man at this concentration. Nevertheless, its concentration and storage in our bodies, and its remarkable persistence there, point to the dangers of introducing new chemicals into our environment without fully studying their impact on our environment and on us.

DDT has been largely replaced by pesticides that are more readily destroyed, so that the effects of chronic accumulation of these compounds are of less importance than the possibility of acute toxic effects. Some of the organic phosphate insecticides, which are now widely used, in addition to the chlorinated hydrocarbon products, are dangerous to man at relatively low concentrations, and must be used with extreme care. Their danger, however, is primarily to the farmer applying the product, because relatively little residue will remain in the crops by the time they reach our table as food. A new hazard has been introduced, however, with some of the newer pesticide agents, because some of them are easily absorbed through the skin, as well as through the intestinal and respiratory tracts. Obviously, extreme care must be used in handling these potent products and their use should be restricted to those trained in using them.

Many other compounds are added to processed food and each of us continually ingests a continuous stream of synthetic chemicals which bleach, color, preserve, stabilize, flavor, clarify, homogenize, emulsify, and thicken our food. Each of these compounds is tested for acute toxicity, but the long-term chronic effect of repeated small doses of most of them remains to be determined.

Changing Concepts of Pollution.   Traditionally, we have assumed a pollutant to be a noxious substance added to the environment, which is either not normally present, or which occurs naturally in amounts too small to be objectionable. More recently, we have found it necessary to broaden our definition, as environmental changes have been found to be associated with several agents formerly considered innocuous. Carbon dioxide (CO_2), for example, is a normal—and essential—component of our atmosphere. Introduced into air by respiration of men and animals, and by combustion of organic material, it is absorbed by plant life in the process of photosynthesis and replaced by oxygen. A balance between plant and animal life has apparently maintained an atmospheric CO_2 level of about 300 ppm for most of recent geologic time. The concern has recently been expressed that the large and steadily increasing CO_2 emissions from man's industrial heating and power generating activities is increasing the total amount of atmospheric CO_2. Some have predicted this increase may reach 25 per cent by the end of this century, and this might significantly alter the heat balance of the earth, through the so-called "greenhouse effect." Carbon dioxide permits ready passage of the warming infrared rays of the sun through our atmosphere, but tends to block the waves reflected from the earth's surface, which dissipate part of the energy received. The net effect may be to increase the mean temperature of the globe the few degrees necessary to melt the Antarctic and Greenland icecaps which, in turn, could raise ocean levels sufficiently to inundate most coastal cities.

Whether such an effect could occur is disputed by some climatologists, who point out the colder arctic seas might be able to absorb any excess of CO_2 produced. Nevertheless, the question raised is a valid one: What is a pollutant? It is becoming apparent that some agents considered harmless, or even beneficial, can, in excess, alter our environment in unexpected ways.

Thermal Pollution.   Heat, which we produce at great expense by various means, can produce highly undesirable side effects when introduced into rivers and streams. Cooling of steam generators by such waters has raised the temperature of many American rivers sufficiently to alter greatly the types of life they can support. Game and food fish have been eliminated from many rivers and threatened in many more by such thermal pollution. The introduction of nuclear reactor power plants has expanded the need for water cooling, further aggravating the problem. In an attempt to prevent such thermal pollution, cooling towers evaporating thousands of gallons of water hourly have been designed. Although reducing the stream pollution problem, such towers may produce other types of pollution problems, with the enormous amounts of water vapor they release into the atmosphere. In a small valley, or in an area of low wind speed, heavy fogs could be produced, and in winter severe icing of surrounding roads and structures. Automobile accidents resulting from reduced visibility or icing might, in turn, be considered the result of another type of environmental pollution. Thus, each change in our technology alters our environment, and thus the potential for disease.

Noise. A final example of a "new" pollutant is noise. Many industrial processes expose workers to noise at levels sufficient to cause hearing loss. Often, this takes the form of a temporary threshold shift (TTS) from which the ear recovers, usually within an hour or two of the end of the exposure. Such a phenomenon, known as auditory fatigue, is a common experience after a noisy airplane flight and rarely occurs with sound pressure levels below 78 decibels (dB). Duration of sustained exposure to loud noise is a significant factor in hearing loss. A noise of 4,000 Hertz (cycles per second) that is not heard in alternate minutes would cause only half the TTS that the same noise would have produced if continuous. As exposure to excessive sound levels continues, permanent hearing loss may occur, usually occurring first in the 3,000 to 6,000 Hertz band (Figure 4-3). As the hearing loss progresses, loss at these higher

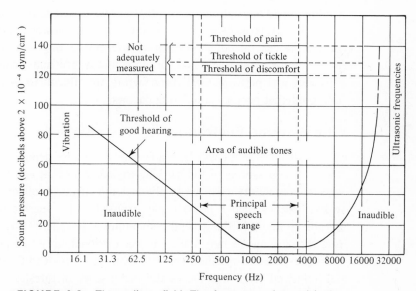

FIGURE 4-3. The auditory field. The frequency of sound is the number of times a complete cycle, which consists first of an elevation and then of a depression below atmospheric pressure, occurs in one second and is measured in cycles per second (c/s) recently renamed hertz (Hz). Normal hearing range extends from approximately 50–15,000 Hz. (Reproduced from World Health Organization: *CIS Information.* Sheet 17: "Noise in Industry." The Organization, Geneva.)

frequencies increases, and the loss is increasingly shifted to lower frequencies, including those of normal speech. Such hearing loss due to industrial exposure has become a major cause for claims under workmen's compensation acts, and most industries now attempt to protect exposed workers by requiring some combination of earplugs and ear muffs.

The American Conference of Governmental Industrial Hygienists, the organization that establishes appropriate industrial exposure limits for reactive chemicals and other industrial hazards, has recently proposed standards for noise exposure. These proposals are for a worker exposed 4–8 hours a day—92 dB; for a worker exposed 2–4 hours a day—97 dB; for a worker exposed 1–2 hours—102 dB; and for a worker exposed to noise less than one hour—107 dB. These standards have not yet been adopted officially but they represent the first nationwide attempt to set standards in this area.

In addition to occupational exposures to known sources of intense noise, concern is growing about the rising background sound levels in all of our cities and their possible effect on health and functioning. Most persons manifest progressively decreasing hearing acuity with advancing age. For men, this deterioration is first noticeable at about age 32, and for women at age 37. This hearing loss occurs even without high level exposure or ear disease, so that conservatively between 8 and 10 million persons in the United States are estimated to need hearing aids. How much of this hearing loss may be due to our noisy environment cannot be determined. It is of interest, however, that studies on isolated populations in environments free from modern urban noise show far less decrease in hearing with age. It is possible that the continuous background noise of urban areas, as well as the unpleasantly loud sounds of jet aircraft, large diesel trucks, and power lawn mowers, may contribute to hearing loss in the general population. In addition to hearing loss, exposure to continuous noise at moderate levels may produce annoyance and irritability interfering with efficiency and performance. These factors are difficult to evaluate and undoubtedly affect different persons in differing degrees.

The Working Environment

Although no attempt will be made here to discuss details of industrial toxicology, there are two aspects of the working environment that are important in considering general community exposure to physical and chemical influences. The first is that the worker spends only 8 hours a day exposed to his specific industrial hazards, and spends 16 hours in the general community atmosphere, where exposure to physical and chemical agents may add to his occupational stress. To protect the health of the worker exposed to specific chemical agents, the American Conference of Governmental Industrial Hygienists has established a series of threshold limit values (TVL) for nearly 1,000 commonly used chemical agents (ACGIH, 1967). This private organization, with members representing all the various professions concerned with industrial safety, regularly publishes a guide for recommended and intended values for all common industrial agents. These values refer to the airborne concentration of substances, and represent conditions under which it is believed nearly all workers may be repeatedly exposed day after day without adverse effect.

Recommended TVL's may vary from as little as 0.02 ppm for a highly toxic agent, such as toluene diisocyanate, to 5,000 ppm for relatively innocuous carbon dioxide. The list is reviewed annually and the TVL altered, if new information so indicates. These standards, however, are based solely on the eight-hour industrial exposure, and in some circumstances additional community exposures may be important. In the case of carbon monoxide, the TVL has been recently reduced to 50 ppm from 100 ppm. If, however, a worker is a heavy cigarette smoker, and perhaps drives an automobile with a leaky muffler, he may arrive at work with an effective carbon monoxide exposure (and hence a carboxyhemoglobin level) which adds significantly to his industrial exposure. It is, therefore, impossible to separate completely the working environment from the general community environment, and a man's exposure must be considered as a continuum extending throughout all 24 hours of the day.

A second feature of the working environment, which must sometimes be considered in assessing general community health problems, is the possibility of discharges from various industrial processes involving nearby residents who have no other contact with the industry. In early studies of beryllium and mercury, these two elements were recognized as highly toxic substances that could cause severe disease problems in exposed workers. It was also noted, however, that diseases associated with these metals could be detected among some residents of neighborhoods in which these industries were located (Eisenbud, 1949; Chesner, 1950).

A more recent example of the contribution of an industrial environmental hazard to disease in the general community is suggested by studies on asbestos. Workers with this mineral have been shown to be unusually susceptible to the development of a mesothelioma—a rare tumor of pleural and peritoneal surfaces. This tumor is so rare in the general population, and has such markedly increased frequency among those occupationally exposed to asbestos, that it has been considered almost certain evidence of exposure to the mineral. Reviews of a series of cases of mesothelioma have shown that, on occasion, no history of an occupational exposure to asbestos is present. Careful residential histories have shown that many of these people lived in the same house as an asbestos worker and may, therefore, have come in contact with the mineral brought in on the body or clothing of an occupationally exposed worker. A significant number of patients with mesothelioma, however, had no such direct household contact, but were found to have lived within one-half mile of an asbestos factory (Newhouse and Thompson, 1965). This involvement of ordinary urban residents in what is considered to be a strictly occupational problem indicates the close interrelationship of all features of our environment that must be considered in attempting to control environmental problems.

Exotic Environments

Without the aid of protective devices, man can exist and function only in the relatively narrow temperature and pressure variations of the more moderate portions of the earth's surface. With appropriately designed clothing and shelter, he has been able to inhabit most of the globe, excepting only the highest elevations and areas of unremitting cold. In the past two decades, he has started exploration of two completely new, widely disparate, and clearly hostile, environments—outer space and the depths of the sea. The maintenance of life in both these areas poses problems of synthetic gaseous environment, thermal protection, abnormal degrees of weightlessness, and numerous psychological problems. The most difficult feature in each environment, which must be controlled to permit life to continue, is pressure. This may range from the vacuum of outer space to as much as 30 atmospheres in underwater exploration. By manipulation of the gas content of pressurized environments, it has been found possible for man to live and work in a hyperbaric environment for periods of two or more weeks in an atmosphere many times denser than surface air. The atmosphere most commonly used for such prolonged high-pressure exposures is approximately 80 per cent helium, 16 per cent nitrogen, and 4 per cent oxygen. Four per cent oxygen at this pressure would be equivalent to 26 per cent oxygen at normal barometric pressures. The nitrogen component must be greatly reduced from the normal 79 per cent level, because of the rapid development of nitrogen narcosis at these high pressures. Helium, as an inert gas relatively insoluble in body tissues, provides a suitable component for the remainder of the atmosphere. This use of helium, however, introduces another complication. Because helium is a lighter gas than nitrogen, the molecules move more rapidly and impact with the human skin about 2.6 times as frequently. This carries off body heat more rapidly and requires chamber temperatures to be maintained between 85 °F and 91 °F, rather than the 72 °F which would be considered comfortable with normally balanced air (Bond, 1966). Thus, each change which we introduce into an artificial environment may have secondary effects, which must be controlled either by physiologic adaptation of the exposed individuals, or by further environmental manipulation.

Although specially conditioned and trained men, provided with elaborate artificial environments, have successfully withstood short periods both deep in the sea and in outer space, the problems of maintaining normal physiologic functioning in these artificial environments will apparently limit their use to highly specialized projects. The immediate effects and complications of these exotic environments can be fairly well controlled by constructing a synthetic microenvironment around the deep sea diver or astronaut. With such elaborate environmental manipulation, it is possible for these specially trained men to function with reasonable efficiency under these conditions for short periods. Short-term physiologic effects do not appear to be cause for serious concern. It is possible to minimize or eliminate such problems of a hyperbaric environment as oxygen poisoning, nitrogen narcosis, and "the bends," by use of artificial atmospheres and judicious decompression. Long-range effects on health in men regularly exposed to these stresses remain to be determined. Bone necrosis has been reported in men working under increased pressure in tunnel construction. Whether other physiologic abnormalities may occur as a result of long-term exposure to high pressures remains to be determined.

Weightlessness and some of the other physiologic problems of outer space exploration have proved to be more incapacitating than had been predicted. Under these artificial circumstances, the energy required to perform simple tasks is far greater than that needed on the earth's surface—a problem that may seriously limit the efficiency of space explorers. Unprotected by the earth's atmosphere, men in outer space may also be exposed to radiation in amounts and at frequencies never encountered on the earth's surface. The long-term effects of this exposure also remain to be determined, but the possibility of long-term existence in outer space for human life appears remote.

The General Urban Environment

Within the past two generations, America has become an overwhelmingly urban society, and the trend is rapidly accelerating. Within another generation, the vast majority of citizens of all developed countries of the world will be city dwellers. The problem is further accelerated by the rapid increase in total population of the world, and by the increasing industrialization of all countries. The steadily increasing demand for goods and services of all these people concentrated in urban conurbations will require a tremendous increase in industrial activity in the same areas. It has been estimated, for example, that our power requirements to serve this population will cause us to burn as much fuel oil during the next 10 years as we have burned in all of the past 150 years, since oil was first introduced as a source of energy. Most of this consumption, furthermore, will take place in the center of these population concentrations, so that the effluent of these processes will be part of the normal environment to which all urban residents are continuously exposed. These factors, plus the increasing use of synthetic chemical compounds previously discussed, result, in effect, in a new and artificial environment into which most of our citizens will be born and live out their lives. The effects on health of this continuous exposure to the pollutants and by-products of city living remain to be determined. Again, the problem of acute toxic reactions to these new chemical agents is relatively easily managed. The problem remains: What is the effect on health of continuous exposure to small amounts of these compounds over a lifetime?

Air Pollution

The problem of the possible effects on health of this artificial environment, and the difficulties inherent in determining these effects, are best illustrated by considering the problem of air pollution. Disposal of our solid waste products, although an increasingly severe problem in logistics, has relatively little importance in terms of human disease. Similarly, the problem of water, as a vehicle of disease in urbanized societies, has been largely solved by the application of appropriate environmental engineering techniques. Our problem with water in the future will be concerned largely with finding adequate supplies for our expanding population, and with maintaining potability as the water available is more frequently recycled.

Air pollution is a major problem of all urban areas with serious implications for human health. Air is an obligatory feature of the environment in which we live. Unlike water, supplies of air cannot be imported from uncontaminated areas, nor can we store air on good days to be released during times of high pollution. No type of purification or decontamination is practicable for our ambulatory urban residents. To keep alive, we must breathe the atmosphere around us at all times.

This urban atmosphere, loaded with all the effluent- and by-products of our cities, is furthermore presented to our bodies by the method that most favors its absorption into our bodies. The 15,000 liters of air we breathe each day is presented to 400 square meters of highly absorptive endothelium in the lung. Unlike the intestinal tract, where a large element of selection occurs in what is and what is not absorbed, the lung permits passage, in some degree, of almost all compounds presented to it. With no feature of our environment are we in closer contact than with the ambient air we breathe.

Although it is obvious we are continually absorbing into our bodies compounds of known biologic activity, specific effects on health of this exposure have been difficult to demonstrate. Part of this difficulty derives from our inability to duplicate in the laboratory the actual atmosphere, as it exists in our cities. We can study the effect of one or two pollutants on animals or human volunteers, and we almost invariably find that, at normal ambient air levels, healthy animals or men show no significant physiologic alteration. In the polluted urban environment, however, we are not exposed to one or two pollutants singly, but to a combination of many substances simultaneously present, that may produce synergistic or additive effects. It has been suggested that particulate matter and condensation nuclei—the minute particles produced by all forms of combustion processes—may act as carriers of gases or other substances to the lung, which would otherwise be filtered out by the body's protective mechanisms. Some disagreement exists as to whether this mechanism does, in fact, occur under normal weather conditions, but it is obvious that reactions to urban air pollution do occur that cannot be accounted for by any single known component of the atmosphere.

Until recently, much of our knowledge of the effects of air pollution on human health has come from the rare, but dramatic, "acute air pollution" episodes. These widely publicized occurrences, such as that in Donora, Pennsylvania, in 1948 (Schrenk et al., 1949), and in London in 1952 (Logan, 1953), caused the simultaneous illness and death of many persons. Virtually all persons dying during these episodes were already known to have serious cardiac or pulmonary disease. The effect of air pollution, in this case, was to aggravate an illness already present. The problem of acceleration of pre-existing disease by air pollution is of increasing importance, as the numbers of persons in our population with these disabilities increase. It is, perhaps, paradoxical that our successes in medical therapy of acute diseases have had the effect of creating, quite literally, a population with more and more chronic disease, which in turn may make them more susceptible to air pollution. Obviously, the needs of the millions of persons with these chronic disease conditions, as documented by our National Health Survey, must be considered in setting air quality criteria and standards (National Health Survey, 1960).

Another important consideration in studying these acute air pollution episodes is that the words *air pollution* do not appear on the death certificate of a single person dying during these disasters. Virtually all of them died of various chronic cardiac and pulmonary conditions that they were known to have, and nothing but their simultaneous deaths during the episode indicated that air pollution was in any way connected with their fate. Obviously, we need not look for a specific disease initiated by air pollution in order to judge its impact on our health. Hidden within many of the diagnostic categories to which we assign death certificates, there may be many deaths in which air pollution has been a factor.

In addition to the effect of air pollution in accelerating pre-existing disease, there is now developing information that air pollution may increase susceptibility to other disease agents. Many of the pollutants regularly present in urban air, such as sulfur dioxide, ozone, oxides of nitrogen, and various hydrocarbons, can be shown to affect adversely the various protective mechanisms of the respiratory tract, such as ciliary movement, mucous production, and pulmonary clearance of particulate matter. Obviously, any interference with these protective mechanisms leaves the respiratory tract less able to cope with infectious disease agents. Epidemiologic studies of exposed populations have shown significant associations between the incidence of respiratory illness and air pollution (Dohan, 1961; Mountain et al., 1968). Although these respiratory illnesses, such as the common cold, are not life-threatening experiences, they nevertheless represent the principal illness burden most of us bear, in terms of time lost from work or school, and days of decreased efficiency due to illness symptoms. The economic burden of such illness is, obviously, tremendous, and a portion of this may be charged directly or indirectly to air pollution.

In addition to the roles of air pollution in accelerating pre-existing disease, and in increasing susceptibility to acute respiratory illness, another—and perhaps more important—consideration is the possible role of air pollution in the initiation of chronic degenerative disease. These illnesses now include virtually all of our commonest causes of death, as well as our principal causes of prolonged disability. All of these diseases are problems of multiple causation, with a variety of factors acting together to produce a specific illness. In some of them, environmental factors, including chemical agents absorbed from the environment, undoubtedly play a role. One of the most rapidly increasing of these diseases—emphysema, perhaps better called chronic obstructive pulmonary disease—is our most rapidly rising cause of death, having increased more than ten-fold during the past 15 years. This disease is also the second most important cause (after arteriosclerotic heart disease) for disability payments under our federal Social Security system. How much of this increase may be related to environmental pollution is difficult to determine, but it has certainly occurred primarily in major urban areas, paralleling increasing industrialization, automobile usage, and all the other factors of our increasingly urbanized society.

The evidence for relating emphysema and other chronic obstructive lung diseases, such as chronic bronchitis, to air pollution is largely indirect and derives principally from epidemiologic studies. These studies in many different parts of the world point to a consistent trend greatly strengthening the suspicion that air pollution may be a factor in this emerging major health problem. The prevalence of chronic bronchitis has been clearly demonstrated to be associated with (1) population size of the community, (2) the amounts of fuel consumed, (3) levels of annual sulfur dioxide measurement in the ambient air, (4) levels of both settled and air-borne dust (5) decreased air visibility (Stocks, 1959; Fairbairn, 1958; Reid, 1958). All these factors are obviously related to the degree of air pollution to which the populations with increased chronic pulmonary disease are exposed.

A major complication in evaluating the significance of air pollution in such epidemiologic studies is the well-known effect of cigarette smoking in the genesis of chronic pulmonary disease. Tobacco has, of course, been demonstrated repeatedly to be a major factor in chronic bronchitis, pulmonary emphysema, cancer of the lung, and many other pulmonary diseases. It must be remembered, however, that all these diseases, like the other chronic degenerative diseases, are conditions with multiple causes, and the incrimination of one factor as a causative agent by no means eliminates others from a significant role.

The role of air pollution, as a predisposing or conditioning factor in the development of disease, has been demonstrated in studies of cancer of the lung among immigrants from England to South Africa and New Zealand (Dean, 1959; Eastcott, 1956). These persons spent the first portion of their lives in England, largely in heavily industrialized areas. They then moved out of this highly polluted environment to the relatively uncontaminated South Africa and New Zealand environments. Following this group over decades, it was noted that they developed cancer of the lung at a much higher rate than either native-born white South Africans, descended from British stock, or immigrants from other countries in the same age group. An important factor in these studies is that the effect of cigarette smoking was controlled. White South African males, for example, have long been among the heaviest cigarette smokers in the world. Comparing groups of native-born white South Africans with immigrants, by numbers of cigarettes smoked, showed a marked excess of deaths from cancer of the lung among those preconditioned by growing up in a heavily polluted environment, over their South African neighbors who smoked equal numbers of cigarettes, but had escaped this early imprinting. The role of air pollutants in potentiating the effects of other disease agents appears to be remarkably persistent.

The possibility of such "imprinting," or conditioning, during early life playing a role in subsequent illness experience is one of the most intriguing and potentially important suggestions of this, and many other, recent studies. Evidence has been accumulating suggesting that nutritional and, perhaps, environmental experiences of a person during his early formative years may determine, in some part, his subsequent illness experience throughout his life. Because most of our children in the future will be born into and grow up in the constant environment of air pollution, it is possible that we are creating new and entirely unanticipated health problems.

The fact that growing up in a polluted urban environment may cause permanent physiologic alteration in our children is a sobering possibility. At least three separate studies now underway in three very different parts of the world are producing evidence that this may be happening (Watanabe *et al.*, 1964; Toyama and Timono, 1961) These studies in England, Los Angeles, and Japan, are each comparing a group of children living in a heavily polluted area with another group of children of the same age and height living in relatively unpolluted areas of the same towns studied. Consistently, children living in the more highly polluted areas show decreased pulmonary function when compared to the children living in areas with less pollution. These studies effectively eliminate the influence of cigarette smoking, because they all involve children of ages before the smoking habit has become established.

Evidence that heavy metals in the air, even in extremely dilute amounts, may have some relationship to human health, has also been giving cause for concern. These elements are introduced into the atmosphere through smelting and a variety of industrial processes, as well as through activities in which we have a direct part, such as the tetraethyl lead added to the gasoline we use. A heated controversy has been going on over the past few years on the role of lead emitted from automobile tailpipes in relation to the accumulation of this element in the body (Advisory Committee, 1959). Lead, of course, has been recognized for several hundred years as a toxic element producing a variety of disease syndromes when concentrations in various organs reach critical amounts. Until recently, however, most lead entering the body came in through the gastrointestinal tract, which is actually a very poor absorber of the metal. The lung, however, does not have the same capacity for selective absorption permitted by our intestinal mucosa. Lead particles reaching the lung are, therefore, more readily absorbed, and may contribute to the total body burden far more than those present in food or water. Unfortunately, most of the lead that emerges from automobile tailpipes as a complex inorganic ion is of just the particle size to most efficiently reach the alveoli of the lung and be absorbed. Whether this does, in fact, contribute to increased body levels of lead is a controversial subject, but one which deserves serious consideration. Some recent studies suggesting that such heavy metals may, in some cases, act as mutagenic agents, producing congenital abnormalities, make this a subject of serious concern to all of us.

Another possible relationship of such elements in extreme dilution in ambient urban air to serious health effects has been suggested by recent studies on cadmium. This element is present in the air of all of our cities in highly variable, but extremely dilute, amounts. A recent study by the Public Health Service (Carroll, 1966) compared the levels of cadmium in the air of many American cities with a variety of health indices. Surprisingly, there was a direct correlation between ambient air cadmium levels and death rates from heart disease. Whether this is a cause and effect relationship, and the mechanisms through which such a relationship might occur, are not clear. The finding, however, is a real one and obviously deserves further investigation. It might be expected that the ambient-air cadmium levels were merely reflections of general atmospheric pollution, and that the association with heart disease might actually have been related to a variety of other compounds. This was apparently not the case. Cadmium levels in the cities studied appeared to vary independently of all other pollutants, except only for zinc—obviously a closely related element. Most disturbing were the absolute levels of cadmium monitored in these cities. In all cases, the metal was present only in extremely small amounts—ones which conventional toxicologic study would usually suggest could have no physiologic effect. Nevertheless, a statistically significant correlation was found, suggesting that even minute amounts of some pollutants may have significant effects on health.

Obviously, air pollution does not represent a single defined entity, but varies from place to place depending on local industry, population concentration, automobile usage, and local topography and meteorology. In general, however, there are two principal types of air pollution with their own special characteristics. One is the oxidizing atmosphere of photochemical smog, typical of Los Angeles. This pollution is produced primarily by unburned hydrocarbons and oxides of nitrogen emitted from automobile tailpipes. These undergo a complex series of reactions in the atmosphere, catalyzed by ultraviolet light from the sun, producing a variety of irritating oxidant compounds. Although this smog produces eye and mucous membrane irritation in many exposed people, it has not been demonstrated to be associated with excess mortality, or serious morbidity. There are indications, however, that it may play a role in physical fitness, as measured by athletic performance, as well as in reduced pulmonary function of exposed school children. Local meteorologic and geographic conditions play a large part in determining whether an area will have a significant photooxidizing atmospheric pollution problem, as will, of course, patterns of automobile usage and population concentration.

The second major type of pollution is that associated with the burning of fossil fuels—coal and fuel oil—which tend to produce a reducing atmosphere featuring particulate matter and oxides of sulfur as major components. Added to this, of course, are the effluents of whatever industrial processes may be present in the area, as well as the combustion of rubbish. It is this type of particulate-laden atmosphere with high concentrations of oxides of sulfur that has been associated with most of the acute air pollution episodes in which excess morbidity and mortality have been described. Obviously, much work remains to be done to determine the enormously complex and subtle relationships between disease in humans and air pollution. Nevertheless, the burden of evidence now leads to the conclusion that there are, in fact, associated— and even causal—relationships. The universality of the problem and its importance to our health, and that of future generations, does not permit us the luxury of temporizing until we have satisfied all the requirements for disease causality. We have sufficient evidence now that we must act rapidly and forcefully to protect our vital air resources.

A Critical Urban Mass?

The effects of the polluted physical environment on health of urban residents are often difficult to separate from the many other genetic, infectious, nutritional, and other factors involved in human disease. Even more difficult to evaluate, but probably of equal importance to effective functioning, are the less tangible factors of crowding and population pressures. Observations on wild animals show this problem to be solved by territoriality, whereby each animal or pack stakes out its own hunting area sufficient to meet its needs, and drives away all others of the same species. In captivity, animal colonies allowed to multiply without restriction in confined areas, demonstrate for each species a critical limit to the number of animals that can function effectively in a given space. As this limit is exceeded, the social organization of the colony disintegrates, and destructive and antisocial behavior predominate.

Whether man, too, has critical space requirements and reactions to crowding and population pressures will become a question of major importance as cities coalesce, and major urban conurbations sprawl over hundreds of square miles. Already, it is evident that all major American cities are faced with social crises of major proportions, as traditional social patterns fail to meet the rising expectations of poorer citizens. Much of this disruption of the social structure arises from the legitimate demands of minority groups to share more fully in the goods, services, and high living standards of most Americans. A significant part, however, may also derive from the psychologic and physiologic pressures and frustrations of crowding and inadequate living space. The direct correlations between frequency and severity of civil disorders and crime, and city size, suggest there may well be a critical mass for cities, beyond which population pressures multiply problems to almost insoluble proportions. The anticipated doubling of our population by the end of this century will require, at a minimum, the doubling of all our present housing, schools, factories, and institutions—in effect, the superimposition of a second America where we now exist. In planning for this expansion, we might well consider construction of new and wholly separate cities, rather than expansion of our already overcrowded megalopolises.

POLLUTANTS AS RESOURCES

The rapid rise in the world's population, and the hopes of all peoples to improve their standards of living, present serious problems in terms of resources available to meet these demands. Serious question has been raised and widely discussed as to the ability of the earth to produce sufficient food to support the populations projected for two and three generations from now. Similar shortages, which have not been as widely publicized, can be anticipated in a variety of the natural resources of this planet. Potable water is already a scarce commodity in many portions of the world, and available supplies are being used more rapidly than they can be replaced by precipitation. As the limited supplies available are recycled with increasing frequency, pollutants steadily build up to the point where the water is no longer usable for many purposes.

The atmosphere of the globe is also a finite resource, that must be protected. Already the quality of our lives in many urban areas has been adversely affected by using our air resources as a dumping ground for our wastes. If the process continues unabated, the adverse effects may be increasingly quantitative, as well as qualitative.

Supplies of many of the minerals and fossil fuels of the earth are being consumed at rates that promise rapid exhaustion of some of our most valuable resources. Up to the present time, advances in technology have managed to outdistance the increased consumption of most of these elements, but the tremendous increases in population may outdistance our ability to uncover new sources of materials.

Under these circumstances, we can no longer afford the luxury of the profligate use of our natural resources. The debris that we vent into our air, discharge into our streams, and strew across our landscape contains many useful compounds and materials that can be rechanneled into the resource cycle. We have given relatively little thought in the past to recovery of these items for productive use, because the cost of such recovery has usually exceeded the cost of new supplies. With finite resources, and a growing demand, however, we can no longer afford the luxury of disposing of these resources after a single use, but must devise ways to recycle them. Pollutants are merely resources in the wrong place. Each of them is of value, when properly used, and the only reason for calling a substance a pollutant is that it is in a place where we do not wish it to be in the resource cycle. The problem will obviously call for a totally new approach to resource management, but the change must be made if the quality and quantity of our environment and our lives are to be preserved.

REFERENCES

BIZZOZERO, O. J., JOHNSON, K. G., and CIOCCO, A.: Radiation-related leukemia in Hiroshima and Nagasaki 1946–1964: I. Distribution, incidence and appearance time. *New Eng J Med*, **274**:1095–1101, 1966.

BLOOM, A. D., NERIISHI, S., KAMADA, N., ISEKI, T., and KEEHN, R. J.: Cytogenetic studies in exposed survivors of Hiroshima and Nagasaki, *J Lancet*, **2**:672–74, 1966.

BOND, G.: Effects of new and artificial environment on human physiology. *Arch Environ Health*, **12**:85–90, 1966.

BROWN, M. L., and NELSON, A. B.: Medical x-ray visits and examinations during pregnancy. National Center for Health Statistics, Ser. 22, no. 5, 1968, 41 pp.

BUETTNER, K.: Physical aspects of human bioclimatology. *Compendium of Meteorology*, American Meteorological Society, Boston, 1951, 1315 pp.

CARROLL, R. E.: The relationship of cadmium in the air to cardiovascular disease death rates. *JAMA*, **198**:267–69, 1966.

CHESNER, C.: Chronic pulmonary granulomatosis in residents of a community near a beryllium plant. *Ann Intern Med*, **32**:1028–48, 1950.

COGAN, D.: Lesions of the eye from radiant energy. *JAMA*, **142**:145–51, 1950.

COURT-BROWN, W. M., and DOLL, R.: *Leukemia and Aplastic Anemia in Patients Irradiated for Ankylosing Spondylitis*. Medical Research Council Special Report no. 295, London, Her Majesty's Stationery Office, 1957.

———, BUCKTON, K. E., and MACLEAN, A. A.: Quantitative studies of chromosome aberrations in man following acute and chronic exposure to x-rays and gamma rays. *J Lancet*, **1**:1239–41, 1965.

DALE, W. E., and QUINBY, G. E.: Chlorinated insecticides in the body fat of people in the United States. *Science*, **142**:593–95, 1963.

DEAN, G.: Lung cancer among white South Africans. Report on a further study. *Brit Med J*, **5267**:1599–1605, 1961.

DOHAN, F. C.: Air pollutants and incidence of respiratory disease. *Arch Environ Health*, **3**:387–95, 1961.

EASTCOTT, D. F.: The epidemiology of lung cancer in New Zealand. *J Lancet*, **270**:37–39, 1956.

EISENBUD, M., *et al.*: Environmental studies in plants and laboratories using beryllium: The acute disease. *J Indust Hyg Toxicol*, **30**:281–85, 1948.

———, *et al.*: Non-occupational berylliosis, *J Indust Hyg Toxicol*, **31**:282–94, 1949.

FAIRBAIRN, A. S., and REID, D. D.: Air pollution and other local factors in respiratory disease. *Brit J Prev Soc Med*, **12**:94–103, 1958.

GRAHAM, S., LEVIN, M. L., LILIENFELD, A. B., SCHUMAN, L. M., GIBSON, R., DOWD, J. E., and HEMPELMAN, L.: Preconception, intrauterine and postnatal irradiation as related to leukemia. *Nat Cancer Inst Monogr*, **19**:347–71, 1966.

HARDY, H. L.: Beryllium poisoning: Lessons in control of a man-made disease. *New Eng J Med*, **273**:1188–99, 1965.

———, and TABERSHAW, I. R.: Delayed chemical pneumonitis occurring in workers exposed to beryllium compounds. *J Indust Hyg Toxicol*, **28**:197–211, 1946.

HESSE and HARTING (1879), cited by ROSTOSKI, N., and SANPE, N.: Die bergkrankheit der erzverglente in schneeberg in sachsen ("Schneeberg lungenkrebs"). *Z Krebsforsch*, **23**:360–84, 1962.

LEITHEAD, C. S., and LIND, A. R.: *Heat Stress and Heat Disorders*. Cassell, London, 1964, 304 pp.

LOGAN, W. D.: Mortality in the London fog incident, 1952. *Lancet*, **264**:336–38, 1953.

MACMAHON, B.: Prenatal x-ray exposure and childhood cancer. *J Nat Cancer Inst*, **28**: 1173–91, 1962.

MARCH, H. C.: Leukemia in radiologists, ten years later: With review of pertinent evidence for radiation leukemia. *Amer J Med Sci*, **242**:137–49, 1961.

MOUNTAIN, I., *et al.*: Air pollution and illness in a normal urban population. *Arch Environ Health* (in press).

MURRAY, R., HECKEL, P., and HEMPELMANN, L. H.: Leukemia in children exposed to ionizing radiation. *New Eng J Med*, **261**:585–89, 1959.

National Council on Radiation Protection and Measurements Report no. 33. Medical x-ray and gamma ray protection for energies up to 10 MeV. Washington, D.C., 1968, 66 pp.

National Health Survey: *Chronic Respiratory Conditions Reported in Interviewers, United States, July, 1957–June, 1958*. Public Health Service Publication no. 584–B12, 1960.

NEWHOUSE, M. L., and THOMPSON, H.: Mesothelioma of pleura and peritoneum following exposure to asbestos in the London area. *Brit J Industr Med*, **22**:261–69, 1965.

Radiation protection. International Commission on Radiation Protection Publication no. 8. Pergamon Press, Oxford, England, 1966.

REID, D. D.: Environmental factors in respiratory disease. *Lancet*, **1**:1289–94, 1958.

SCHLESINGER, E.: The medical aspects of water fluoridation. *Pediatrics*, **19**:156–61, 1957.

SCHRENK, H., *et al.*: *Air pollution in Donora: Epidemiology of the Unusual Smog Episode of October, 1948*. Public Health Service Bulletin no. 306, 1949.

STEWART, A., WEBB, J., and HEWITT, D.: Survey of childhood malignancies. *Brit Med J*, **1**:1495–1508, 1958.

STOCKS, P.: Cancer and bronchitis mortality in relation to atmospheric deposit and smoke. *Brit Med J*, **1**:74–79, 1959.

Threshold Limit Values for 1967. American Conference of Governmental Industrial Hygienists, Cincinnati, 1967.

TOYAMA, T., and TIMONO, Y.: Pulmonary ventillatory capacity of school children in a heavily air polluted area. *Jap J Public Health*, **8**:659, 1961.

U.S. Public Health Service, Advisory Committee on Tetraethyl Lead to the Surgeon General of the Public Health Service: *Public Health Aspects of Increasing Tetraethyl Lead Content in Motor Fuel*, Public Health Service Publication No. 712, 1959, 49 pp.

WANEBO, C. K., JOHNSON, K. G., SATO, K., and THORSLUND, T. W.: Breast cancer after exposure to the atomic bombings of Hiroshima and Nagasaki. *New Eng J Med*, 1968.

WANEBO, C. K., JOHNSON, K. G., SATO, K., and THORSLUND, T. W.: Lung cancer following atomic radiation. *Amer Rev Resp Dis*. **98**:778–87, 1968.

WATANABE, H., *et al.*: Effects of air pollution on health: I. On peak flow rates and vital capacity of primary school children. *Reports of the Osaka City Institute of Hygiene*, **26**:32, 1964.

WOOD, J. W., *et al.*: Thyroid carcinoma in atomic bomb survivors, Hiroshima and Nagasaki. Technical report to the Atomic Bomb Casualty Commission, Hiroshima and Nagasaki, Japan, 1967.

———, JOHNSON, K. G., and OMORI, Y.: *In utero* exposure to the Hiroshima atomic bomb: An evaluation of head size and mental retardation: Twenty years later. *Pediatrics*, **39**:385–92, 1967.

FURTHER READING

Air Pollution
HEIMAN, H.: Status of air pollution health research. *Arch Environ Health*, **14**:488–503, 1967.
STERN, A. (ed.): *Air Pollution*, Volumes I and II. Academic Press, New York, 1962.

Clothing
KELLY, J. B.: Heat, cold and clothing. *Sci Amer*, **194**:109–16, 1956.

Electromagnetic Radiation
FERRIS, B.: Environmental hazards: Electromagnetic radiation. *New Eng J Med*, **275**:1100, 1966.

Heat and Cold
LEE, D. H. K.: *Heat and Cold Effects and Their Control*. Public Health Service Monograph no. 72, 1964.

Housing

HERRINGTON, L. P.: *Biophysical Adaptations of Man Under Climatic Stress.* Meteorological Monograph no. 8, American Meteorological Society, Boston, 1954.

LANDSBERG, H.: *Bioclimatology of Housing.* Meteorological Monograph no. 8, American Meteorological Society, Boston, 1954.

Industrial Environment

POWELL, C., and HOSEY, A. (eds.): *The Industrial Environment–Its Evaluation and Control.* U.S. Government Printing Office, Washington, D.C., 1965.

Light

PATTY, F.: *Industrial Hygiene and Toxicology*, 2nd ed. Interscience Publishers Incorporated, New York, 1958.

Noise

BELL, A. (ed.): *Noise–An Occupational Hazard and Public Nuisance.* Public Health Paper no. 30, WHO, Geneva, 1966.

DOUGHERTY, J., and WELSH, D.: Environmental hazards, community noise and hearing loss. *New Eng J Med,* **275**:759–65, 1966.

Pesticides and Insecticides

AYERS, J., *et al.* (eds.): *Chemical and Biological Hazards in Food.* Iowa State University Press, Ames, Iowa, 1962.

GLEASON, M., *et al.*: *Clinical Toxicology of Commercial Products.* Williams and Wilkins, Baltimore, 1957.

Toxicity Testing

Guidelines for Pre-Clinical Toxicity Testing of Investigational Drugs for Human Use. Office of New Drugs, Bureau of Medicine, Food and Drug Administration, Washington, D.C., 1967.

Weather and Disease

LOWRY, W.: *Weather and Life.* Oregon State University Book Stores Incorporated. Corvallis, Oregon, 1968.

PART TWO

Public Health —Problems and Practice

SECTION I

Retrospect

5

Public Health in the United States —the Beginnings

Wilson G. Smillie

The Colonial Period and the Great Epidemics

The Colonial Period lasted about two hundred years, from 1607 to the end of the eighteenth century. The oustanding health crises that had to be faced were recurring epidemics that often reached disaster proportions. Chaos prevailed. Usually certain natural community leadership emerged and a highly autocratic organization was set up to meet the most pressing needs. Eventually the holocaust was stayed, or simply burned itself out. Nevertheless, some lessons were always learned from disasters. These lessons germinated slowly and did not always develop in direct ratio to existing community needs. For example, child health protection and promotion, greatly needed, did not develop effectively as a community function until the end of the nineteenth century.

Savage conditions, bitter struggles for life itself, left little time for consideration of community protection against disease. Physicians came with the first settlers, of course, but did not stay. When John Smith was wounded by a gunpowder explosion there was no surgeon in the Colony and he had to go home to England for treatment.

Dr. Samuel Fuller, the first American doctor who stayed, came on the *Mayflower* in 1620. In 1633, an epidemic of infectious fever occurred in Salem. Dr. Fuller went across the Bay to help the new settlement, developed the disease himself, and died. It probably was smallpox.

The most dreaded epidemic disease in the Colonies was smallpox. The Indians suffered even more than the whites. Even simple childhood diseases such as measles caused havoc among the Indians. The great epidemic among the Indians in 1618 was not smallpox, but measles.

Influenza, diphtheria, scarlet fever, and lobar pneumonia, as well as cerebrospinal meningitis added their toll in winter months, while typhoid fever and dysentry were scourges during the summer.

Several REASONS

Proving that Inoculating or Transplanting the *Small Pox*, is a Lawful Practice, and that it has been Blessed by GOD for the Saving of many a Life.

By *Increase Mather*, D. D.

Exod. XX. 12. *Thou shalt not kill.*
Gal. I. 10. *Do I seek to please Men? if I please Men, I should not be a Servant of* CHRIST.

It has been Questioned, Whether *Inoculating* the *Small Pox* be a Lawful Practice. I incline to the Affirmative, for these Reasons.

I. Becaufe I have read, that in *Smyrna, Conftantinople,* and other Places, Thousands of Lives have been saved by Inoculation, and not one of Thousands has miscarried by it. This is related by Wise & Learned Men who would not have imposed on the World a false Narrative. Which also has been published by the *Royal Society* ; therefore a great Regard is due to it.

II. WE hear that several *Physicians* have Recommended the Practice hereof to His *Majesty,* as a Means to preserve the Lives of his Subjects, and that His Wise and Excellent *Majesty King* GEORGE, as also his *Royal Highness* the *Prince* have approved hereof, and that it is now coming into practice in the Nation. In one of the Publick Prints are these Words, " *Inoculating the Small Pox is a safe and* " *universally Useful Experiment.* Several Worthy Persons lately arrived from *England* inform us, that it is a succefsful Practice there : If Wise & Learned Men in *England,* declare their Approbation of this *Practice,* for us to declare our Difapprobation will not be for our Honour.

III. GOD has graciously owned the *Practice of Inoculation,* among us in *Boston,* where some Scores, yea above an hundred have been *Inoculated,* & not one miscarried; but they BlefsGOD, for His difcovering this Experiment to them. It has been objected, that one that was Inoculated, died, viz. Mrs. D——ll : but she had the *Small Pox,* in the common way before, & her Friends and nearest Relations declare that she received no hurt by Inoculation, but was by a fright put into Fits that caused her Death. It is then a wonderful Providence of GOD, that all that were *Inoculated* should have their Lives preserved ; so that the Safety and Usefulness of this Experiment is confirmed to us by Ocular Demonstration : I confefs I am afraid, that the Discouraging of this Practice, may caufe many a Life to be lost, which for my own part, I should be loth to have any hand in, *because of the Sixth Commandment.*

IV. IT cannot be denied but that some Wise and Judicious Persons among us, approve of Inoculation, both *Magistrates* and *Ministers* ; Among Ministers I am One, who have been a poor Preacher of the Gospel in *Boston* above Threescore Years, and am the most Aged, Weak and unworthy Minister now

in *New-England.* My Sentiments, and my Son's also, about this *Matter* are well known. Also we hear that the Reverend and Learned Mr. *Solomon Stoddard* of *Northampton* concurs with us ; so doth the Reverend Mr. *Wise* of *Ipswich,* and many other younger Divines, not only in *Boston,* but in the Country, joyn with their Fathers. Furthermore, I have made some Enquiry, Whether there are many Persons of a Prophane Life and Conversation, that do Approve and Defend *Inoculation,* and I have been answered, that they know but of very few such. This is to me a weighty Confideratior. But on the other hand, tho' there are some Worthy Persons, that are not clear about it ; nevertheless, it cannot be denied, but that the known Children of the Wicked one, are generally fierce Enemies to Inoculation. It is a grave faying of Old *Seneca, Pessimi Argumentum Turba est.* For my part I should be afhamed to joyn with fuch Persons ; *O my Soul come not thou into their Secret, unto their Assembly be not thou United.* I am far from reflecting upon all that are against *Inoculation.* I know there are very worthy Persons (with whom I defire to Live and Die) that are not clear in their Judgments for it, and they are greatly to be commended and honoured in that they will not act against a doubting Conscience ; yet it may be some of them might change their minds, if they would advise with those who are best able to afford them Scripture Light in this as well as in other Cafes of Conscience.

Novemb. 20. 1721.

That the Cause may have Two Witnesses, here are subjoyned the Sentiments of another, well known in our Churches, of which I declare my hearty Approbation.

Sentiments on the Small Pox Inoculated.

A most Succefsful, and Allowable Method of preventing Death, *and many other grievous Miseries, by the* Small Pox, *is not only Lawful but a Duty, to be used by those who apprehend their Lives immediately endanger'd by the terrible Distemper.*

But the Method of managing and governing the Small Pox *in the way of* Inoculation, *is a most succefsful and allowable Method of preventing Death, and many other grievous Miseries by this dreadful Distemper. Therefore, 'tis not only Lawful, but also a* Duty *to make use of it. None but very foolish, and very wicked People will deny the* Proposition *in this* Argument ; The Assumption *is all that is disputed. But now, That this is a most* Successful Method *we have all the Evidence that Humane Reason can ask for.*

Men of Honour, and Learning, and Incontestible Veracity, not one or two, but a considerable Number of them, agree in the Relation they give us, of it's being used with constant Success *in the* Levant. *It has been used upon vast Multitudes, even many Thousands, and for some Scores of Years : And when regularly used, it yet appears not, that ever one* Person *miscarried of it, or had the* Small Pox *after it. We have sufficient Proofs that it is a growing Practice in those Countries. If it had been unsuccessful, or been attended with bad Consequences, it must needs have been put out of Countenance, and have ceased long ago. Such Testimonies on the other side, as our People have been frighted withal, are not worth a Straw. No Man of sense that considers them can lay weight upon them : Ask us not, why we say so !*

And we have an Army *of* Africans *among our selves, who have themselves been under it, and given us all the Assurance, which a Rational Mind can desire, that it has long been used with the like Success in* Africa. *Yea, Behold, ye yourselves have seen it. The Operation has been performed on an Hundred & more, in the Town of* Boston : *And not one of them has miscarried : They have every one of them hitherto done well. They all give Thanks to our Merciful Redeemer for leading them into it. They would every one of them rather undergo it again, and many times over, than suffer the* Small Pox *as People ordinarily suffer it in the common way of* Infection. *The Story of one Dying after it, is trump'd up with so much folly and falshood, that it is unworthy to have any Answer given to it. In fine ; Experience has declared, that there never was a more unfailing Remedy employed among the* Children of Men.

That this is an Allowable Method, is plain ; Because there can be no Objection brought against it, but what will also lie against the use of almost all the preventing Physick, *that is used in the World. The* Objector *must maintain, That it is unlawful for a* Man, *who would preserve his Life and Health, to make himself Sick in a way that constantly tends to Preservation. But a very Familiar Case will so illustrate the Matter, as to put it beyond all Dispute. Suppose, There is a Bloody Flux prevailing in the Town where I live, which proves Mortal to a great part of them that have it ; many more than Four Hundred perish by it in a Month. A Physician is Master of a* Purge ; *which whosoever takes it, is in an ordinary way, delivered from the danger of that Mortal Distemper. An Artificial Purge seasonably taken saves him from Death by the Natural Purge, which he is exposed unto. Will any scruple the taking of this Artificial Purge? Surely, None but such as want a Purge of* Hellebore ! *Here the* Man *makes Himself Sick, while He is well : and thinks that he is not the whole who has no need of a Physician, while he has the Humours in him which render him obnoxious to a Deadly Sickness. He won't think it*

his Duty to stay till God send the Sickness in another way upon him ; when it will be too late for him to seek relief ; But he will give Thanks to GOD *for teaching him, how to make himself Sick, in a way that will save his Life. He most properly takes* GOD's *Time to fall Sick : He does it seasonably, and in the Time when* GOD *has commanded him to do it.*

Many Good People, who are sensible how weak their own Judgments are, will for a Case of Conscience be much assisted by the Judgments of the most able Divines in the Country. Now every Body knows how they concur in their approbation of this Practice.

The Design and the Spirit, (evidently of no good Original) with which the fierce opposition to this Practice is carried on will also go a great way towards determining of Good People in Favour of it. The Conclusion will be Victorious ; That when People have their Lives endangered by the Small Pox *hovering about them, they not only may use the Method of Inoculation, to save their Lives, but they even ought to do it, if they can. They keep not in good Terms with the Sixth Commandment, if they do it not.*

INFERENCES.

I. HEnce *the Physicians may do well to beware, of going too far, and of taking wrong steps, for the frighting of People from this Practice, lest they Unawares have more to answer for than Men of their Profession should be willing to.*

II. *Hence, the Parents, and Masters, and Husbands and Wives, whose Relatives have beg'd as for their Lives, that they might have leave to save their Lives, by this Method, should not by their obstinate Violence hinder them from it, least on the Loss of their Lives they have sad matter of Reflection left unto them.*

III. *Hence, a People will do well, not to be too hasty in Resolves, that should forbid their Neighbours, to do what God has made their Duty for the Preservation of their Lives in this Method ; lest they do in Effect forbid Obedience to the Sixth Commandment. Especially, when the Bugbear of the Pestilential Consequences, is a Falshood, that has not the least shadow of Reason for it, and has the Experience of all the Countries under Heaven, where they use the Inoculation, to confute it. Nor has it ever been known of Later Ages, that the Plague ever began any where but in the* East-Indies, *from whence it has always been brought unto the Western World. And when the King, and Prince, and most Eminent Physicians in* London *and* Dublin, *and elsewhere, have declared their Approbation of it ; it seems not much for our Honour, to declare that we disapprove it.*

IV. *Hence to Rave, and Rail with such bitter Execrations, as are too commonly used, against the Ministers, and other serious* Christians, *who favour this Practice, is a very crying Iniquity ; and to call it a Work of the Devil, and a going to the Devil, is a shocking Blasphemy ; and much more likely to bring the Plague among us, than the Practice, which they so ignorantly and maliciously do charge with such Imaginary Consequences.*

FINIS.

BOSTON: Printed by S. Kneeland for J. Edwards at his Shop in King-Street. 1721.

Diagnosis of these epidemic diseases was inexact. Scarlet fever and diphtheria were both called "angina maligna." Malaria was confused with yellow fever. Typhus was not differentiated from typhoid fever until the early part of the nineteenth century.

Medical science was encompassed in a few texts—all written in Latin and Greek. The educated men of the day were clergymen and many of them practiced medicine. The knowledge and medical resources of the day were inadequate to deal with most crises, so that spiritual and practical leadership was often their primary contribution to the community.

The major public health activities that developed during the Colonial period were related to control of contagion. Usually these were philanthropic rather than official. They involved isolation of the sick and quarantine of contacts. Ship quarantine, particularly of ships from the West Indies, which brought yellow fever, was frequently carried out. Sometimes whole communities were placed under quarantine.

Smallpox.   Smallpox was the epidemic disease that was dreaded most by the Colonists. It struck time and again with devastating force. Cotton Mather describes a New England epidemic in 1689. "In a twelve month over a thousand of our neighbors were carried to their long home." Boston at that time had a population of only 7,000. Cotton Mather tells of a slave who stated that he would never have smallpox because he had been inoculated with the disease. During the smallpox epidemic of 1721, Mather inoculated his own son, Sammy, "with excellent outcome." In the same year, Dr. Zabdiel Boylston inoculated his only son. Boylston was mobbed by the populace but persisted in promoting the technique and in 1726 published a report of his work. Boston then had a population of 15,684 persons:

5,998 had had the disease.
1,843 fled the city to escape the epidemic.
5,545 developed smallpox in the natural way.
2,124 were inoculated.
  174 escaped infection.

The death rate in the uninoculated was over 10 per cent, whereas only 1.5 per cent of inoculated persons succumbed to the disease.

In 1796, an obscure practicing physician in England, Dr. Edward Jenner, introduced cowpox vaccine. Jenner conducted a well-planned experiment on ten persons who had had cowpox. He then inoculated them with smallpox and proved that they were immune to the disease. How different from our present caution in vaccine evaluation studies! (See Chapter 3.) Dr. Benjamin Waterhouse wrote to Jenner and received dried vaccine impregnated on silk thread. He vaccinated his son with this material and thus the child became America's first vaccinated person. Two years later Doctors John Warren, Josiah Bartlett, and Benjamin Waterhouse conducted a study of eleven boys at Noddles Island. All were vaccinated against smallpox and subsequently proved immune to the disease. The town of Milton, Massachusetts, was the first to organize an official vaccination clinic. The town arranged to vaccinate, for 25 cents each, all who would come to the schoolhouse. Within a few days 337 persons were vaccinated— more than one fourth of the total population. Thomas Jefferson, who later became

President, aided Waterhouse in promoting vaccination. He wrote a letter to Jenner in which he said: "Future nations will know, by history only, that loathsome smallpox had existed, and by you has been exterminated." A century and a half have passed, and although Jefferson's prophecy will eventually be realized, it is still far from fulfillment.

Nevertheless, a great page in history had been turned. There is no greater single triumph of man in his struggle to control his environment than the discovery and utilization of smallpox vaccination.

Yellow Fever.   Yellow fever struck the West Indies time and again with devastating force, beginning in 1647, but the Colonies escaped. In 1699, yellow fever struck Charleston. One hundred and fifty persons died within a few days. The same year, a ship from Barbados brought yellow fever to Philadelphia, which at that time had a population of 4,000. Over one third of the population developed the disease, and 220 died within a short time.

The disease struck New York in 1702 and 570 died. Norfolk and New Haven, as well as New York, were frequently invaded. The infection occurred only in the summer in the northern ports of America because *Aëdes aegypti* could not survive cold winters, but in southern ports, such as Charleston and New Orleans, the disease became endemic.

In Philadelphia in 1793, this "tropical" disease caused the greatest single disaster ever to befall an American city. Philadelphia, then the capital of the nation, had a population of 36,871. During the summer of 1793, some 13,000 people fled the city. Virtually all of the nonimmunes of the remaining population contracted the disease; an estimated 6,000 were ill simultaneously in October alone. Deaths totaled 4,044 giving a fatality rate for the epidemic of 15–20 per cent. French refugees, newly arrived from the West Indies, were immune to yellow fever and were indispensable in nursing the sick.

A "medical committee" drew up a list of sanitary rules:

1. Avoiding contact with a case.
2. Placarding all infected houses.
3. Cleanliness and "airiness" of the sickroom.
4. Hospital provision for the poor.
5. Keeping streets and wharves clean.
6. General hygienic measures, such as quick private burials; avoidance of fatigue of mind and body; avoidance of intemperance; accommodation of clothing to the weather.

All these well-intentioned measures may have prevented secondary epidemics of enteric diseases, but they surely had no influence on the impact of yellow fever, except to lessen somewhat the suffering of the sick. Mathew Carey, in discussing the cause of termination of the epidemic, finally concluded that it was an act of God. Temperature, he said, could not bring about an abatement of the disease, as there had been no cold and little rain. We find the answer to his questions at this late date from his own temperature records on the frosty nights of October 17 and 18. We now understand clearly what happened. We know that the daytime temperature was not so important as the night temperature. It was on the night of October 18 that the frost either killed or drove the *Aëdes aegypti* mosquitoes into hibernation, thus ending the epidemic.

Not until the Spanish American War in 1898, when General W. C. Gorgas discovered in Cuba that yellow fever was transmitted by a mosquito, was the disease brought under complete control in North America.

Other Contagious Diseases. The prevalence of many other communicable diseases that prevailed in the Colonies might be described. These would include tuberculosis, pneumonia, diphtheria, scarlet fever, influenza, venereal disease, and other infectious disease problems described elsewhere in this text (see Chapter 10).

Formally established community machinery for prevention of disease and for health promotion was slow to develop in the Colonies. Disease was believed to spread through decomposition of animal and vegetable matter. Epidemic diseases were called *zymotic* diseases (from Greek *zymos*—fermentation). These diseases were believed to be due to a fermentation of the tissues and to be always produced by an external stimulus. This miasma might be cosmic in origin and airborne, or it might be produced by man himself, by the products of his household, or by any type of decaying vegetable or animal matter. Therefore, municipal cleanliness was secured by community ordinances. Certain trades—such as tanning—were considered health hazards and were abated. Isolation and quarantine regulations were, of course, very early health measures.

Ship quarantine laws were initiated in 1700, and a ship quarantine hospital was authorized in 1736.

The Beginnings of Public Health Administration

In 1797, the first act that authorized Local Boards of Health was passed. In Boston in 1799, by special legislative act, a Board of Health was formed with Paul Revere as its chairman. The chief activities of the Board related to abatement of nuisances. Slight attention was paid to control of the individual as a means of protecting him from infection, or when he became infected, in preventing him from spreading disease. Attempts were made to control smallpox by isolation, quarantine, and immunization. Port quarantine in yellow fever was imposed many times. As mentioned earlier, Dr. Zabdiel Boylston had introduced smallpox immunization by variolation, but it was abandoned, because many patients became very sick and some died. Dr. Benjamin Waterhouse had obtained cowpox vaccine from Jenner in 1800; he vaccinated his son with good results and the procedure spread rapidly.

Scarlet fever was second as a cause of death from zymotic disease, and tuberculosis caused 3,000 deaths in Massachusetts in one year, a rate of over 300 per 100,000 population.

Little growth in public health administration occurred from 1800 to 1850. By 1845, New York had a population of 300,000. A city health inspector system was in vogue. Public health measures related chiefly to overcrowding in tenements, uncleanliness of the streets, regulation of public baths, slaughterhouses, pigstys, tanneries, and anything else that caused bad smells.

In 1850, Lemuel Shattuck, a bookseller in Cambridge, Massachusetts, wrote an extraordinary book, *Report of Sanitary Commission of Massachusetts*. This report recommended the establishment of a State Board of Health in each state with powers to appoint a well-qualified, full-time, well-paid secretary. Shattuck recommended also the establishment of nurses' training schools, the teaching of sanitary science to medical students, the incorporation of preventive medicine in clinical practices, the establishment of competent local boards of health in each community, and the inclusion of vital statistics as a function of the health department.

Shattuck was far ahead of his times and many years were to elapse before all these sound recommendations were put into practice. As a direct result of his recommendation, however, the first State Board of Health was organized in Massachusetts in 1869. Twenty-one cities, as well as a few smaller towns, had more or less active boards of health.

The American Public Health Association.   A group of farsighted public health men formed the American Public Health Association in 1872, and Dr. Stephen Smith was selected as president. To quote Mazyck P. Ravenel, a pioneer in tuberculosis control, "no more opportune time could have been chosen for the organization of . . . the Association. The art of medicine was becoming the science of medicine; modern preventive medicine was being born."

The first meeting of the Association discussed subjects that, after a hundred years, are still pertinent:

1. *Public health education*, which was considered of primary importance in public health affairs.
2. *Vital statistics*, racial and national, rural and urban factors relating to mortality.
3. *The germ theory of disease*, Pasteur's studies were just beginning to penetrate medical science.
4. *The epidemiology of typhoid fever*, with special relation to water supplies.
5. *Control of zymotic (infectious) disease*, particularly smallpox, yellow fever, and cholera.
6. Quarantine and disinfection.
7. *Water purification, street cleaning, and scavenging* (environmental sanitation).
8. *Organization* of local, state, and national boards of health.

A Dr. C. C. Cox presented a paper on "The Necessity for a National Sanitary Bureau." At that time (the last third of the nineteenth century) the national government had no health services and only two state boards of health were in existence.

Modern public health practice may truly be said to have been born at the first meeting of the American Public Health Association. Local boards of health began to require reporting of communicable disease about 1870. Environmental sanitation became a secondary activity of health departments.

Further Development of Public Health Practice—The Application of Science

Providence, Rhode Island, established the first diagnostic laboratory in 1888. Tuberculosis began to be recognized as a communicable disease and not a family trait (see Chapter 10) and was made reportable to health departments in 1895. Diphtheria antitoxin was discovered in 1894 and was widely adopted.

Thus, from 1875 on through the next fifty years, the chief efforts of health departments related to control of communicable disease. The cause of typhoid fever was discovered and the relationship of spread of disease to community water supplies was made clear. The respiratory infections, particularly pneumonia, were not reduced by public health measures. The infant death rate remained high. Various cities built communicable disease hospitals.

Attempt to Establish a National Board of Health.   The national government had no health services except for hospitals for American seamen. A National Board of Health was organized in 1879 but had a short life. It was sponsored by men who organized the American Public Health Association. It was poorly conceived and doomed to failure from the start. The Army, Navy, and Marine Health Services were anxious to control the National Board of Health, but it was set up as a separate body with twelve members. Its destruction was attributed to the political machinations of a Dr. John B. Hamilton, but it failed because the country was not yet ready for a nationwide health protection and promotion service.

The Twentieth Century

About 1900, a new trend toward individual health was initiated. Infant hygiene, maternal health promotion, school health administration, industrial health promotion, and health education are outgrowths of this period of research in public health administration. Voluntary health agencies began to interest themselves in public health affairs about 1900.

Visiting nursing associations had been active chiefly in the field of care of the sick-poor in their homes, but the leaders began to interest themselves in preventive measures. The Red Cross was founded and took a very active part in preventive measures in times of disaster. The Antituberculosis League was formed and became a tremendous force in the prevention and treatment of the disease.

Formal efforts in health education were instituted. The old school textbooks, relating chiefly to anatomy and physiology were discarded and modern programs of teaching were instituted. V. C. Vaughan's report of the shocking sanitary conditions of the Spanish-American concentration camps in Florida, due to carelessness in disposal of human feces, and the spread of typhoid fever through flies, educated the whole nation as to the modes of spread of typhoid fever.

Application lagged far behind the acquisition of new knowledge because of antiquated health machinery, untrained public health personnel, and lack of general public understanding and support. Gradually, health officers abandoned such measures as "swat the fly" campaigns and gave up garbage collection and street cleaning because they bore little direct relationship to disease prevention.

The Beginnings of Professional Training in Public Health

In the early 1900's, William T. Sedgwick was firing the imagination of a brilliant group of students at the Massachusetts Institute of Technology. George C. Whipple was beginning his eventful career at Harvard, specializing in the field of biostatistics. Charles V. Chapin was founding the basic principles of municipal health administration at Providence. William A. Evans introduced compulsory pasteurization of milk in Chicago, following a series of devastating community epidemics that were spread through raw milk. In 1909, under the aegis of President Charles W. Eliot, the first department of preventive medicine in a medical college was established at Harvard, and Dr. M. J. Rosenau was selected to head the department. It was a most fortunate choice. Dr. Rosenau's textbook *Preventive Medicine and Hygiene* had a profound effect on the teaching of medical students throughout the land. In 1913, Sedgwick, Whipple, and Rosenau founded a School of Public Health for training public health personnel. Later this became the School of Public Health at Harvard. A new school of public health was established at Johns Hopkins, with a superb faculty, and Toronto also developed a fine school of public health. Later a school was established at Yale. Michigan developed a well-financed school with excellent facilities. Minnesota established a good school with Dr. Gaylord Anderson as its director. Schools were established in California and in southern California, at Los Angeles.

Another factor with tremendous influence on public health training was the establishment during the first quarter of the century of the private foundation. Notable were the Rockefeller and Kellogg foundations. These foundations gave generously to the various schools of public health, aiding in the development of buildings, facilities, and excellent teaching personnel. Their funds made possible the development of the experimental method in public health administration and also enabled state and local public health officials to promote preventive measures rapidly and effectively.

The next fifty years will see a more comprehensive development in public health procedures than has occurred during the past hundred years. The whole concept of the functions of government in relation to protection and promotion of public health will be modified radically, and an entirely new philosophy will be developed concerning the proper place of public health in the organization and administration of government in relation to public health procedures.

The United States Public Health Service*

In America, the state is the power. Each state is autonomous in all matters relating to public health within its borders. The federal government possesses only those functions and powers that are specifically designated to it by the states. The Constitution does not specifically designate any public health powers to the federal government. Those public health laws that have been exacted have been passed under general provisions that relate to:

1. The regulation of commerce with foreign nations and among the several states.
2. The levying of taxes and promotion of the general welfare.
3. The power of the President to make treaties with foreign powers.

The major part of federal health activities is conducted under the supervision of the Federal Security Agency.

* See also Chapter 13.

The Federal Security Agency.   The health activities of the Federal government were rearranged and consolidated in 1946. The agency was reconstituted under four main operating branches:

1. Social Security Administration.
2. Education.
3. Public Health.
4. Special Services.

The Social Security Agency supervises three important activities: (a) old-age insurance, (b) unemployment assistance, (c) the Children's Bureau. The U.S. Public Health Service was assigned to the Public Health Division, Vital Statistics was transferred from the Department of Commerce to the U.S. Public Health Service. The Division of Food and Drugs was assigned to Special Services as was Vocational Rehabilitation. **The Children's Bureau.**   The Children's Bureau was transferred from the Department of Labor to the Federal Security Agency in 1946. The activities of the Bureau were not modified basically, but the reorganization did serve to bring important public health activities of the federal government into closer coordination and better working relationships with states and local communities. **The Social Security Act of 1935.**   The Social Security Act of 1935 set the pattern for the major activities of the Children's Bureau. This Act provides for grants-in-aid to states by the federal government for the development of states and local services in:

1. Maternal and child health.
2. Crippled children.
3. Child welfare.

All grants have been made to official state agencies. The Children's Bureau has required certain standards of training for personnel and asked that suitable administrative procedures, such as periodic reports of activity and achievements, budgetary supervision, and so forth be set up. These requirements were made in order that the Children's Bureau may be assured of satisfactory development of the program through federal grants-in-aid. **History of the U.S. Public Health Service.**   The United States Public Health Service originated in the Marine Hospital Service in 1798. Its function was medical and hospital care of American sailors. It was administered in the Treasury Department. In 1878, this service was given authority to impose quarantine at various ports to prevent entry of disease from abroad. This was a natural development because the Marine Hospital physicians were the first to see cases of cholera, smallpox, yellow fever, or plague. Shortly thereafter the medical examination of arriving aliens was made the duty of the Marine Hospital Service. In 1912, the Federal Health Service name was changed to the United States Public Health Service. The first research laboratory was established in the Staten Island Marine Hospital, in 1887. The Hygienic Laboratory was established in Washington in 1901. Its functions were largely epidemiological, and it soon became the center of a final series of epidemiologic investigations. Power to regulate and standardize biologic products was given to this laboratory in 1902. The Division of Venereal Disease Control was established in Carville, Louisiana, under USPH Service auspices in 1917.

The Social Security Act of 1935 greatly extended the scope and strength of the Service. The National Cancer Act of 1937 authorized the National Cancer Institute, and in 1939 the National Institute buildings were constructed in Bethesda, Maryland. In 1939, after 141 years of jurisdiction by the Department of the Treasury, the USPH Service was transferred to the Federal Security Agency, newly created by President Franklin D. Roosevelt to consolidate health education and welfare functions of the federal government.

The USPH Service was directed by its Surgeon General, who was chosen by the President of the United States. The Surgeon General had a National Advisory Council of fourteen members. Ten were chosen by the Surgeon General, each for a five-year term. The Director of the National Institutes of Health, and one member of the Army, Navy, and Bureau of Animal Industry were ex-officio members. The function of this command was purely advisory.

The major functions of the USPH service were assigned to four divisions (see Chapter 13 for present organizational structure):

1. Office of the Surgeon General.
2. National Institutes of Health.
3. Bureau of Medical Services.
4. Bureau of State Services.

Office of the Surgeon General. The Office of the Surgeon General was concerned with the administrative activities of the Service, including the Division of Public Health Methods and the Division of Sanitary Engineering.

The National Institute of Health. Located in Bethesda, Maryland, the National Institute of Health concerned itself largely with research. It had nine major divisions— (1) The National Cancer Institute, (2) Division of Infectious Diseases, (3) Division of Physiology, (4) Pathological Laboratory, (5) Biologic Control Laboratory, (6) Chemical Laboratory, (7) Zoological Laboratory, (8) Industrial Hygiene Research Laboratory, and (9) Division of Research Grants.

Bureau of Medical Services. The Bureau of Medical Services had three functions:

1. Hospital Division.
2. Mental Hygiene Division.
3. Foreign Quarantine Division.

The Hospital Division had 26 hospitals at important shipping centers, and care was provided for sailors in 150 ports. In addition, there was an outpatient service with over 400,000 patient visits per year. The Mental Hygiene Division conducted the operation of United States Narcotic Farms. The farm at Lexington, Kentucky, had a bed capacity for 1,000 males and a similar farm was located in Fort Worth, Texas, in 1937. The Division made studies on drug addiction, its treatment and rehabilitation. It also cooperated with states in administrative matters relating to supervision and treatment of drug addicts.

The Foreign Quarantine Division was concerned with the prevention of entrance of disease from foreign countries. It also conducted medical inspection of aliens who emigrated to the United States.

The diseases under Federal Quarantine jurisdiction were cholera, yellow fever, typhus fever, smallpox, leprosy, plague, and anthrax. Three lines of defense were followed:

1. Medical officers were stationed abroad to prevent diseased persons from entering ships that were bound for the United States.
2. A system of inspection was carried out of all ships from any foreign port, at port of entry. Both passengers and crew were inspected and ship quarantine imposed if necessary.
3. A system of cooperation was initiated with state and municipal health officials, at ports of entry, relating to diseases that are nonquarantinable by Federal authorities. Examples are, diphtheria, poliomyelitis, and cerebrospinal meningitis. Airplanes have added a new hazard particularly in relation to yellow fever and malaria.

A new system of national protection was required, namely: deinsectization of airplanes from South American and African ports; examination at port of entry of all passengers from South America and determination of their itinerary for nine days after arrival; vaccination against yellow fever of all airplane personnel that travel through South American countries.

The Public Health Service makes a medical inspection of all prospective immigrants. Formerly, this was made at port of entry, but in 1925, a new system was established whereby medical officers of the Service were assigned to work abroad at American Consulates in principal emigration centers.

Bureau of State Services.   The work of the Bureau of State Services is divided into five parts—States Relations Division; Venereal Disease Division; Tuberculosis Control Division; Industrial Hygiene Division; Hospital Facilities Division. Each of these divisions cooperates with state and local health departments in research, and in development of administrative procedures and control measures in each of their respective fields.

A profound change occurred in the activities of the Federal Services with the advent of Medicare and Medicaid. These matters are discussed in Chapter 14 of this text.

Public Health Nursing

In pioneer days, the families helped each other. The whole neighborhood shared in nursing care of the sick family. In case of childbirth, many of the women developed skill in care of mothers and became excellent community midwives.

Nurses were required for large municipal hospitals after the Revolutionary War. They were from the lower classes and often were drunken and disreputable. The first elementary training of nurses began in 1798 at The New York Hospital in a course with twenty-four lectures.

Home nursing care of the sick-poor began in 1839; "pious and prudent" women in

Philadelphia were trained by Dr. Joseph Warrington. Physicians supervised these activities.

Florence Nightingale was the patron saint of nurses' training. She organized nursing care of British wounded during the Crimean War. She then founded the Nightingale Training School in London.

This school attracted the attention of both physicians and social workers in America. The Civil War created an imperative need for skilled nursing in the care of wounded and sick sailors. Miss Nightingale aided in the formation of a nursing service. The program provided for the training and outlined the functions of the nurse in a military service.

President Lincoln made a mistake in appointing Dorothea Dix as superintendent of female nurses for the Army. She was over 60 years of age and debilitated by tuberculosis and malaria. She was a propagandist but no administrator. She was rigid in her concepts, i.e., *nurses must be over 30 years of age. They must be very plain-looking women. Their dresses must be brown or black with no bows, no curls, no jewelry, and no hoop skirts.*

Nurses came from all classes of society. Some were wealthy and socially prominent. From this group, outstanding women were to emerge. Clara Barton had worked in Switzerland where the Red Cross had just been formed. She proposed the Red Cross to Congress but was rebuffed. She then took her petition to President Garfield, who agreed that a National Red Cross should be formed and affiliated with the International Red Cross.

Louisa Schuyler, who was another socially prominent woman, organized the New York State Charities' Aid Association. This organization is still an important voluntary state health service in New York.

In 1862, a formal course for nurses' training was organized at the New England Hospital for Women, in Boston. Philanthropic organizations in Philadelphia and Boston, in 1866, formulated a plan for health teaching as an integral part of home nursing, and thus the modern concept of public health nursing was born.

Miss Lillian Wald, a young woman of good family and education, opened the Henry Street District Nursing Service in New York in 1892. In 1902, Miss Wald loaned a Henry Street nurse to serve in the New York City school system. The plan proved successful—twelve nurses were soon appointed to the system.

In 1903, Miss Wald loaned a nurse trained in infant hygiene to the New York City Health Department. She was officially appointed to the Department that same year. Thus, officially, school health nursing and maternal and child health nursing were born.

Public Health Nursing grew rapidly in all health departments from 1905 on. The U.S. Public Health Service eventually established a nursing division, and in 1912 the National Organization of Public Health Nursing was organized. Nurses' training was at first for one year, then two, then three. A four-year course of collegiate nurses' training was established. These nurses became supervisors and superintendents. The necessity for practical nurse training arose, and a one-year course of training for high school graduates was widely adopted. In many areas, practical nurses give most of the hospital bedside care.

The Schools of Public Health

As already noted, schools of public health were established in America, beginning about 1914. These facilities were very expensive—perhaps more than any other form of university graduate training. These schools have had a profound influence on the quality of public health care that is now given the American people. Graduates of Schools of Public Health now administer practically all public health departments, and the specialities such as biostatistics, epidemiology, sanitary engineering, child health promotion, health education, and the like are in the capable hands of the graduates of Schools of Public Health. The large philanthropic foundations have been generous in their financial support of these schools and their building facilities and in the recruiting of faculty of high quality.

Summary and Prospectus

This chapter has been concerned only with the *beginnings* of the development of public health in the United States. No attempt has been made to present a detailed history, but rather the origin of the different problems and approaches to their solutions have been traced—largely prior to World War I. The beginnings of the international era in public health—originating in the efforts of The Rockefeller Foundation, The Pan American Sanitary Bureau, and The World Health Organization are another, later and important development, but the same basic approaches and principles obtain in the field of international health.

The evolution of public health as a social force parallels the growth of an appreciation by the public that each individual has a responsibility to the community. Thus, each person and each family must contribute to the welfare of the whole, and thereby further his own personal and family welfare.

It follows, then, that public health is an index of the development not only of medical knowledge, but of personal idealism and maturity and a sense of social responsibility. The advances of public health in America have been an accurate index of our advancing civilization in all its aspects. Thus, it is axiomatic that the stage of development of public health service as an established and effective community function is a good measure of the stage of civilization of a nation.

From our observation of the past we can project the trends of the future. It seems likely that a sense of personal responsibility for the community will continue to develop in America and elsewhere, and that public health eventually will become even more widely applied and more effective, even as new problems continue to emerge.

REFERENCES

SMILLIE, W. G.: *Public Health Administration in the United States*, 3rd ed. The Macmillan Company, New York, 1947.

————: *Public Health: Its Promise for the Future*. The Macmillan Company, New York, 1955.

SECTION II

The Methods and Techniques of Public Health

6

Epidemiology

Kenneth G. Johnson

Definitions and Concepts

Epidemiology is that branch of the medical sciences that treats of epidemics. The word *epidemic* came into the written English language about 1575 and was defined in the Sydenham Society Lexicon of 1881 as (a disease or condition) "prevalent among a people or a community at a special time and produced by some special causes not generally present in the affected locality." The APHA definition of 1960 is almost identical: "the occurrence in a community or region, of a group of illnesses of similar nature, clearly in excess of normal expectancy and derived from a common or propagated source" (American Public Health Association, 1960).

Clearly, both definitions and the history of medicine refer to epidemics of infectious disease, but with the containment or eradication of the infectious diseases that regularly ravaged populations, the scope of epidemiologic interest has widened to include chronic, noninfectious diseases that contribute heavily to mortality. The epidemiologist, by studying groups of people and their environment, seeks a point of entry into the disease cycle at a step that is tractable to some kind of manipulation. Thus, in the modern sense, we define epidemiology more inclusively as *the study of the distribution of disease in the community, and the factors that influence or determine that distribution.*

Epidemiologic methodology is designed to detect an association between the disease and a characteristic of the person who has the disease or a factor in his environment. Epidemiology differs from other medical disciplines in one important respect, e.g., the patient is studied in his natural habitat, as a member of a community, and in reference to the patient's inherent (genetically determined) susceptibility and to the influences of the ecologic environment and the artificial environment that man has created.

It follows from this concept that *disease* is the resultant of a disadvantageous set of interactions among these several factors (Figure 6-1). For example, gastric cancer has been noted to occur more frequently in persons with blood group A than in persons with blood group O, and this observation suggests that having the blood group phenotype A confers risk. However, during the past two decades, the rate of gastric

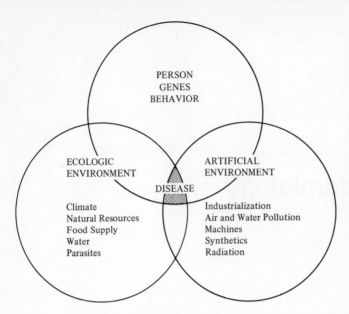

FIGURE 6-1. Diagram representing disease as a disadvantageous set of interactions between the environment (natural and artificial) and man. Ameliorative forces decrease the subtended "disease" area (e.g. sickle cell trait or the use of synthetic antimalarial prophylactic drugs in the presence of *P. falciparum* in the environment). Disadvantageous forces increase the subtended area (e.g. poor rather than abundant food supply, the use of nuclear energy as a weapon rather than as a source of harnessed energy). Quantitative relationships will vary with the major determinant of the disease.

cancer in the United States has shown a great decline, whereas in Japan the extremely high incidence of this disease remains unchanged. But Japanese born in Hawaii or mainland United States have gastric cancer rates that approach the United States rates. These observations suggest that some change in the environment, as yet undefined, rather than a change in the gene pool, would best explain the secular trend of gastric cancer in the United States, and that the presence of an environmental factor is apparently necessary to promote gastric cancer in genetically susceptible individuals.

Multiple factors may be causally related to a single disease. For example, exposure to cigarette smoking, chromates, asbestos, ionizing radiation, or the refining of nickel can be related to an increased risk of lung cancer. Conversely, *the effect of a single factor may become manifest in several diseases.* Heavy cigarette smoking is associated with cancer of the oropharynx, lung, and urinary bladder, a not unreasonable distribution of a toxic inhalant, whose products are excreted in urine (Table 6-1). The combination of Down's syndrome (mongolism) and leukemia, of Bloom's syndrome and lymphoma, rare and apparently different diseases, suggests a common etiologic factor.

So far, a concept of disease as the proper fit of genes and environment has been proposed. Although human bioengineering of the future may manipulate genetic

TABLE 6-1

Mortality Ratios* for Causes of Death by Smoking

	Smoking Category			
	Cigarettes/Day		Pipe/Cigar	Ex-cigarette
	10–20	21–30		
CA lung	9.05	16.93	1.67	4.71
CA larynx	8.33	13.26	7.28	7.22
CA bladder	2.29	3.15	1.09	1.60
Bronchitis	4.34	4.01	0.48	3.06
CHD	1.64	1.82	1.05	1.21

Adapted from Kahn, H. A.: Dorn Study of Smoking & Mortality, *Nat Cancer Inst Monogr* 19, January 1966.
* Mortality ratio = mortality rate among persons in a smoking category/mortality rate among persons who never smoked.

material to man's advantage, the present activities of epidemiology stress the role of the environment and the natural history of disease. Chronic diseases, like infectious diseases, have incubation periods, which are called latent periods, viz., the time which elapses between initiation of the disease process and the moment of clinical recognition (by first symptom or diagnosis). For example, leukemia followed exposure to radiation after a latent period of 5–9 years in two populations, in English patients following radiotherapy for rheumatoid spondylitis (Court-Brown and Doll, 1959), and in survivors of the atomic bombings of Hiroshima and Nagasaki (Bizzozero *et al.*, 1966) (Figure 6-2). In the absence of a known date of first exposure, the latent period cannot

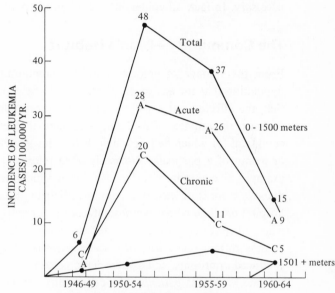

FIGURE 6-2. The relationship of peak incidence of leukemia in atomic bomb survivors to age and time following irradiation. (Adapted from Bizzozero, O. J., Jr., Johnson, K. G., and Ciocco, A. : *New Eng J Med*, **274** :1095, 1966.)

Average Period of Latency for Leukemia
Among Persons Exposed within 1500 Meters of Hypocenter,
Hiroshima and Nagasaki

Leukemia Type	Age in 1945	Latent Period (years)	No. Cases	Variance
Acute	0-14	8.6	38	19.9
	15-29	9.4	40	22.1
	30+	13.0	26	14.3
Chronic	0-29	8.1	30	17.3
	30+	7.2	26	10.5

be sharply defined, but enough evidence exists in the form of precursors of disease to mitigate the despair of biologic predeterminism. This is borne out in studies that show a form of protection against lung cancer for persons who quit smoking, and partial protection against coronary heart disease for persons who follow a prudent diet. In other words, in addition to the period of latency, the duration of exposure to an environmental factor is an important consideration.

Finally, clinical epidemiology deals with human beings who can resist successfully those health measures that are unpleasant, as those that require quitting smoking or foregoing dietary items that are enjoyed.

The social structure and behavioral norms of the community bear an important relationship to the genesis of disease or its control. Animals in overcrowded environments develop herd disease; all living organisms readily adapt their behavior to a new milieu. For man such conditions as malnutrition, inadequate housing, and low levels of education exist in parallel with a high degree of estrangement from the dominant society. Within a particular subculture one type of consumer preference may override a recommendation for health. For example, in several countries attempts to control population growth by contraceptive techniques have foundered on the society's conception of the reproductive process. In order to understand these cultural factors, epidemiologic investigation utilizing the techniques of the behavioral sciences is necessary. In fact, all epidemiologic inquiry is multidisciplinary in nature.

The Community—Man's Habitat

From the vantage of epidemiology, the community is that portion of the human population that for any given disease would be expected to include the disabled and sick, the affected but asymptomatic, the susceptible, and the relatively immune. By contrast, the practice of medicine is concerned chiefly with the individual who has a complaint for which he has sought help. This symptomatic portion of the total array or gamut of a particular disease is often referred to as the top of the iceberg. For example, all community surveys for diabetes mellitus have found that for every known diabetic there is at least one unknown diabetic in the community. In contrast to the hospital or clinic where symptomatic *patients* report, the community contains *persons* who will never develop certain disease symptoms, who are apparently well but who possess certain precursors of disease, persons whose disease process has not as yet produced symptoms, and symptomatic persons who for a variety of reasons have not become known as *patients*. The community can be expected to describe the natural history of disease if, by the use of appropriate markers, persons at great risk and in progressive stages of disease can be identified.

The community is never homogenous, but is a mix of men, women, and children of several ethnic, racial, or religious groups, of varying degrees of affluence and levels of education (and health awareness), and of different occupations. The community is dynamic, changing over time, adapting to political, social, and economic influence. The demographic characteristics of the community have been considered in Chapter 1. Here it suffices to state that this type of information is useful in the formulation and interpretation of epidemiologic studies.

The community's pattern of disease is influenced greatly by its economy. Industrialization and economic depression have wrought impressive changes in the birth rate and in infant mortality without the assistance of modern biomedical technology.

The community, in addition to being a mix of persons, is turbulent. People move in and out. Immigrants carry over the effects of a different environment and are a selected group of persons whose health status permitted uprooting and, generally, whose socioeconomic status in the mother country required improvement.

The main point is that each community is likely to differ from another community, often to an important extent. It is thus important to describe the community in which an epidemiologic study is planned in the greatest detail possible so that the separate and independent effects of certain variables *that are not shared by all segments of the community* can be identified. For example, suppose that *A*, a sample of urban residents, is compared to *B*, a sample of rural residents. The prevalence of rheumatoid arthritis (RA) is found to be greater in *A* than in *B*. Even in the absence of the knowledge that the incidence of RA is three-fold greater in women (Wood *et al.*, 1967) and increases with age, ordinary scientific methodology would dictate an adjustment for the effect of age and sex in each sample before ascribing the observed difference in the prevalence of RA to some rural or urban characteristic. The same kind of adjustment (standardization, cf. Glossary) can be made for secular differences (different time periods), for ethnic, occupational, and other socioeconomic variables.

The community is the human population laboratory of the epidemiologist. He recognizes the community as a dynamic, complex organism in which certain variables among segments of the community must be controlled in the experimental design so that the effects of others can be studied. A wealth of scientific knowledge derived from epidemiologic studies attests to the feasibility of studying large populations systematically, i.e., exercising controls. Each person believes himself unique, but given the same factors in the environment, be they dietary or microbial, the distribution of disease among separate samples of the world's population is monotonously similar.

Sources of Information

Information about the community is derived from several sources, which include census data, vital statistics, various municipal listings, utility company subscriber listings, and the results of previous surveys in the community.

Census data provide by aggregates of the unit *census tract* an estimate of area population size by the enumeration every ten years of every man, woman, and child in the United States. In the process of census taking, various demographic data are also obtained, such as information relating to race, age, length of residence, median income, and occupation. Census data provide the denominator for the estimate of birth rates, mortality rates, and, of course, population growth. The demographic data provided are of great value in describing the gross characteristics of the community, but of little value in providing an association between these data and particular diseases because one cannot relate individual instances of mortality, for example, to the mean value of a community.

Vital statistics provide a rich source of information about the community. Registration of live births, fetal deaths, deaths, marriages, divorces, and annulments in the United States is maintained by an interstate cooperative system. These statistics were generated originally for ecclesiastic and legal purposes. In addition, they serve the important function of health surveillance of the community. The birth and death certificates have been revised through the years to provide important information for research and health planning.

The birth certificate provides information about the infant (birth date, sex, birth order, place of birth, birth weight, and presence of congenital anomalies), the father (name, age, birthplace, race, and years of education completed) and the mother (as for the father, but in addition, parity, length of gestation, length of prenatal care, and complications of pregnancy).

The death certificate contains information relating to the deceased person's age, race, nativity, usual residence and occupation, social security number; immediate and underlying cause of death, other significant diseases, whether death was due to suicide, homicide, or injury; the name of the physician or coroner certifying death, and the burial place.

Because ascertainment of births and deaths through compulsory registration is considered essentially complete, these data in any year, or for any period, can be and are used effectively to answer a multitude of research questions. However, in order to obtain the information about a particular person it is necessary to know the place and date of the event, be it birth or death. The information could be put to far greater use if a national system of record linkage were adopted, using a single identifying number, such as social security, for each person. Loss of information due to migration would then be less, and it would be possible through the cooperation of hospitals to piece together the health experience of an individual from birth to death.

The quality of death certificate information is not considered to be very high by most physicians. Its accuracy is limited by the specificity of the medical diagnoses, by the ability of the physician to recognize specific diseases, and by the knowledge of the patient and his illness prior to death. For example, in the diagnosis of cancer of a specific site, a fair degree of accuracy would be expected. However, certain underlying diseases such as diabetes mellitus and chronic bronchitis are underreported. Sudden death in the United States is commonly ascribed to coronary heart disease. Fortunately, it is possible to establish a level of credibility for the cause-of-death information. For example, Moriyama and his associates (1966) investigated a national sample of 1,362 deaths ascribed to cardiovascular-renal disease, occurring in July and August 1960, and after reviewing clinical information for each case, concluded that from 70 to 75 per cent of deaths classified as cardiovascular disease in the United States may be considered as reasonable inference. Court-Brown and Doll's observations of the leukemogenic (1957) and carcinogenic effects (1965) of radiation in rheumatoid spondylitic patients were based on death certificate information; these observations were completely supported by similar observations in A-bomb survivors, which were based on histologic and autopsy information (Bizzozero et al., 1966; Wanebo et al., 1968). Information at the level of the death certificate is useful, and its limitations can be estimated scientifically.

Information relating to the prevalence of illness (morbidity) and disability in a community is not easily obtained. Getting this kind of information involves interviews and/or physical examination of a representative sample of the community. Admissions to hospital, biased by the progression of a given disease and by socio-economic factors, are not likely to furnish a fair representation of morbidity in a community. Ideally the collective experience of all physicians in a community, isolated from other competing medical services, would furnish excellent estimates of morbidity, but with few exceptions this situation remains Utopian. Information relating to morbidity in several large geographic regions of the United States has become available through the efforts of the U.S. National Health Survey. The activities of this survey are (1) household interviews of a national sample, (2) physical examination of selected samples of United States residents, and (3) survey of samples of health information provided by selected health caring institutions. Local health agencies, public and private, do from time to time conduct morbidity surveys, but in general there is little direct information about morbidity in a community. Stated alternatively, there is a lack of information for the prevalence of even the common diseases; the incidence of a chronic disease that is not rapidly fatal is virtually unknown.

The situation is somewhat better for those infectious diseases that are required by law to be reported to local health authorities. The list of reportable conditions and diseases is formidable but easily understood in terms of the purposes of reporting certain specific diseases, e.g., to limit the spread of infectious disease and to alert the community to the presence of unusual diseases or conditions likely to affect others. Venereal disease (syphilis, gonorrhea, chancroid, lymphogranuloma venereum, granuloma inguinale) and tuberculosis (active primary disease, unexplained pleural effusion, evidence of soft pulmonary infiltrate or cavity, extra pulmonary tuberculosis of meninges, bone, kidney) are clearly reportable diseases. The occurrence of such diseases as anthrax, botulism, brucellosis, cholera, dengue, diphtheria, encephalitis, smallpox, trichinosis, tularemia, and yellow fever is dramatic and suggests quite easily a report to the local health officer. Rubella has serious teratogenic effects and knowledge of its presence in a community is important. Reporting of cases of hepatitis (infectious or homologous serum jaundice) and salmonellosis will call attention to inadequacies in the community's control of food handling, and, in the case of serum hepatitis, focus attention on the practices of blood banks. Diseases, ordinarily unreportable, such as diarrhea and candidiasis, become reportable when they occur in a hospital nursery.

Although not every physician is a diligent reporter, a quantity of information is collected from cooperative physicians and laboratories (serology and microbiology), which is useful in detecting local and national epidemics.

Sources of morbidity data for cancer are the central tumor registries of the states of Connecticut, California, Massachusetts, and upstate New York, and several surveys conducted by the National Cancer Institute. The continuing survey of the residents of Tecumseh, Michigan, which includes household interviews, physical examination, and surveillance, is an ideal mechanism for gaining morbidity data for a community.

Sampling the Community. Sampling is a technique for obtaining information about the community, described in sampling terms, as the sampling frame or universe. Sampling eliminates the need to study the entire community provided that the process of selection of the sample has afforded some guarantee of representativeness and freedom from selection bias. It allows more intensive study of a smaller group of individuals.

Depending on the nature of the information being sought, certain sampling techniques are used. A simple random sample is one in which the selection process gives every individual in the universe the chance of being selected by using a chance mechanism, for example, the tables of random numbers. (Random means with equal chance although the term is often misused to describe a haphazard, unguided process.) These tables of random numbers were generated by a process similar to a fair lottery of selecting one of ten cards bearing a number 0 to 9, noting the number, recording the number, replacing the card, repeating the lottery.

To illustrate, for some bizarre purpose a member of the faculty was interested in the fasting blood glucose level of the 18 medical students in his 8:00 A.M. seminar. The cost of obtaining a glucose determination is five dollars. He obtained with permission samples from all 18 students, paid $90.00 and received the following results:

Student	mg per cent	Student	mg per cent	Student	mg per cent	
01	92	07	72	13	82	
02	80	08	82	14	74	
03	86	09	88	15	90	$\bar{x} = 83$ mg%
04	88	10	84	16	70	
05	100	11	78	17	94	
06	86	12	74	18	76	

Instead, by using the table of random numbers, he could have selected from the total sample of 18 a sample of 6 and for $30.00 have received the following results:

Random Sampling Numbers—1

1 2	3 4	5 6	7 8	9 10 11 12	13 14 15 16
0 6	2 8	3 5	7 6	4 9 0 7	6 6 8 0
3 4	2 5	2 0	3 0	5 1 5 1	3 5 7 1
3 4	7 4	1 5	8 8	9 9 4 0	3 4 3 6
4 7	5 0	4 8	3 3	0 5 7 4	8 4 5 9
9 3	5 6	8 1	1 7	2 0 7 8	3 5 8 6
8 6	1 5	7 5	3 7	6 6 4 9	5 0 7 1
2 2	2 3	2 7	1 2	4 4 3 6	2 6 5 0
2 3	3 4	7 5	8 2	0 2 8 7	4 4 1 8
2 0	4 2	6 0	5 7	9 4 8 5	4 6 0 3
6 5	3 3	1 1	0 3	6 9 0 2	7 3 1 7

Student
06   86 mg%
15   90
11   78 $\bar{x} = 84.7$ mg%
17   94
12   74
03   86

The sample mean or average is quite close to the actual mean for all 18 students.

A sample may also be formed on the basis of some population parameter that is known, for example, ethnic and age-sex proportions. For the design of a study to estimate the prevalence of coronary heart disease in men 40–59, the simple random technique would be quite inappropriate. Instead one can licitly construct a stratified random sample with each stratum defined by a homogeneous characteristic, such as men by 5-year age groups, 40–44, 45–49, and so on. The process of selection within each stratum is accomplished by a chance or random mechanism. The proportion of each stratum sampled need not be equal because it is possible to adjust for unequal proportions among strata by using a weighting factor, e.g., multiplying by the inverse of the sampling proportion.

Another method of sampling is cluster sampling, a method used in surveys. Neighborhoods, postal zone areas, and census tracts in the community to be studied are selected at random in the first stage. These selected clusters should contain as varied a mixture of persons as is possible, thereby increasing the chance that each cluster will be similar to another. However, in practice, some clusters are not mixed but relatively homogenous, and for this reason sampling by clustering will provide a less precise estimate of a population parameter than simple random or stratified random technique. It is used because it is more economical to concentrate manpower in selected geographic areas. Sampling by clusters is usually done in two stages: first the random selection of the primary clusters, and then the formation of the elementary sampling unit by selecting randomly a subsample of the cluster.

Systematic sampling is used when lists of names are available. For example to select systematically 100 names from a list of 1,000, one would select *by random means* a number (n) between one and ten. This number would then be used to select the name occupying every nth position on the list.

These brief and superficial descriptions of sampling are intended to remove a portion of the mystique surrounding the sampling process and to stress the qualities of a proper sample—representativeness and freedom from selection bias. Whichever technique is employed, selection bias has been eliminated by randomization, and if the distribution of some characteristic in the sample resembles closely the known distribution of the corresponding parameter in the population, representativeness has been achieved.

The sampling procedures touched upon in this section apply directly to surveys and to cohort or prospective studies. The sampling method for the retrospective study is one of matching a disease group with one or several groups of similar but unaffected persons, with other, unrelated diseases or, in the case of nonhospitalized patients, with fellow workers or family members.

The Use of Volunteers

Underlying the sampling procedure is the assumption that the population, the universe to be sampled, is itself free from selection bias *with respect to the important variables in the study*. If the universe is so biased, then one cannot expect sampling procedures to remove the bias, for processed garbage is still garbage. *With respect to important variables in the study* is the key phrase, because most epidemiologic studies do not deal with master lists of the community but depend on the cooperation of persons who then become subjects; they are volunteers for the study. The main point is that to apply inferences or conclusions to the community the sampling frame must be representative of the community. For example, one investigator noted that over a period of one year shipments of rats of known genetic strain and age were becoming larger and heavier. A well-meaning caretaker was breeding rats whose progeny seemed healthier, i.e., larger and aggressive. One need not emphasize that the investigator's sample of rats was unrepresentative of the community from which they were drawn.

If the important variable was prior exposure to tubercle bacillus, because the experiments involved testing tuberculin sensitivity, then the caretaker's selection process presents no difficulty. But if the investigator, being a rat demographer, wishes to obtain the *average* values of length, weight, organ size, and so on, for this particular strain of rat, then the caretaker has done him in. Translated into studies involving people, studies to determine the prevalence or the incidence of a disease in a community, or to evaluate the effect of applying some control measure to the entire community, have as a basic requirement that the community be fairly represented and that sources of possible bias be indentifiable.

Studies whose inferences are not to be applied to the community as a whole can properly use volunteers. In these studies (drug or vaccine trials) the important controls are artificial, i.e., imposed by the investigator, and include such measures as "live" and "dummy" vaccine, active agent and placebo, treatment category unknown to patient (single blind), unknown to both patient and physician (double blind). The forces that prompted persons to volunteer are likely to have been distributed equally among the study groups by the process of randomization.

Direction of Epidemiologic Inquiry

In general it is the task of epidemiology to define the burden of disease in the population, to identify individuals at great risk, and to generate knowledge of those factors that, if manipulated, might reasonably be expected to modify or prevent disease.

The first steps in an epidemiologic study are to formulate as clearly as possible the research hypothesis and to design methods of study that will permit testing the hypothesis.

Formulation of the Hypothesis.   Vital statistics demonstrate secular (changes over time) differences in the patterns of disease of populations of various countries, states, and groups and thus afford basic material for the formulation of hypotheses. For example, the increasing rate of mortality from lung cancer in British men prompted Hill and Doll in 1947 to test the hypothesis that lung cancer was causally related to cigarette smoking. The high frequency of anencephaly and spina bifida in Ireland (8.7 per 1,000 births) suggested to Naggan and MacMahon (1967) that if these congenital defects are altered by environmental differences, they may have a different frequency in children born to Boston mothers of Irish nativity. Clues from demographic data are gained from intergroup differences and from the concomitant variation of one factor and a disease (for example, international variations in fat consumption and coronary heart disease).

Epidemiologic hypotheses may be based on experimental data. The observations of Jacobson (1949) that shielding the spleen of rats increased their tolerance to radiation were the basis of the hypothesis by Gregory *et al.* (1968) that a relative paucity of A-bomb survivors would be found who were irradiated in a position offering poor spleen-shielding. Neel (1963) on the basis of experimental data in Drosophila that radiation induced x-linked lethal mutations, examined the sex ratio of progeny born to A-bomb survivors.

The hypothesis is simply a statement, based on knowledge of a disease or condition, that a relationship may exist between the disease and some factor to be investigated. There is no formula for arriving at a hypothesis because such is clearly the interaction of knowledge and the imaginative, perceptive mind. In the formulation of the hypothesis, however, careful consideration must be given to the number of reasonable alternative hypotheses that would serve as well, and to the terms of the hypothesis-statement, which should be precise, because it is the hypothesis that determines the specificity of the methods used to test it. Broad general hypotheses lead to questionnaires several feet in length and a large proportion of wasteful data processing—and represent an illusion that somewhere in the subsequent avalanche of data an important relationship will show itself. The broad approach may be practicable in certain clinical situations where opportunity exists for repeating and expanding studies on individual patients (for example, the "FUO [fever of unknown origin] work-up"), but it is much too expensive in epidemiologic research. As in all other disciplines, the research problem and the conditions of the experiment are designed to furnish a "yes-or-no" answer, i.e., to generate a quantity of data sufficient for testing the hypothesis.

Design of the Study. The epidemiologic study is designed to put the hypothesis into a testable form. If the goal of the study is descriptive, for example, to study the frequency of postneonatal death in a ghetto to determine whether measures to prevent it should be taken, then a survey of postneonatal deaths without a control or comparison group is sufficient. If, on the other hand, the hypothesis states a relationship between a factor, cigarette smoking, and infant mortality, it becomes necessary to know not only how often smoking mothers experienced deaths of their infants, but also how often did nonsmoking mothers have this same experience? Mothers who do not smoke cigarettes, but who are similar in other respects (age, parity, health status, and so on) form the control group. Further, both groups must be studied by identical methods. The second study will furnish an estimate of the probability of infant death by the relative frequency of smoking. To determine a more quantitative relationship between smoking and infant mortality, the study would be designed to include a large group of pregnant women who were heavy smokers, light smokers, occasional smokers, ex-smokers, and nonsmokers, and to follow the outcome of their pregnancies. These examples serve to introduce the three types of epidemiologic studies: survey, retrospective, and prospective.

Surveys. Performing a survey is synonymous with asking questions. Questions are asked by means of a questionnaire, self-administered or given by an interviewer, or by a clinical examination, which is designed to answer specific questions (e.g., blood-pressure level, serum cholesterol). Careful attention should be given to individual questions to insure that the information they generate will be useful, that the questions are clear and intelligible to the subject, and are stated in unambiguous, culturally sensitive terms (for example, in the Bahamas vomiting is known as cascading). Questionnaires should be pretested in the study area with persons who are obviously not members of the study sample. Provision should be made for every question to have some type of answer. Those administering questionnaires should have a uniform approach to the subject, and the emphasis with which particular questions are asked should be agreed upon. In short, the process of questioning should operate under control measures.

Procedures of clinical examination in a survey must also be controlled. Quality control in the laboratory needs no emphasis (although the actual magnitude of change from day-to-day in the same laboratory is seldom appreciated). It does make a difference if different makes of ECG machines are used (varying RS amplitude) or if patients are weighed or blood pressure measured without attention to preset standards. In general, all personnel, whatever their jobs, should have access to a written protocol. A limited number of highly skilled personnel can be used more effectively by introducing a screening technique (see Chapter 8), for example, a standardized phonocardiogram to screen subjects for the presence of heart murmurs in a survey to detect the prevalence of rheumatic heart disease.

Aside from human sources of error, the limitations of the testing device must be evaluated, e.g., its sensitivity and specificity. *Sensitivity* in this context is the ability to detect a disease or condition when it is truly present, and *specificity* is the ability of the testing device to exclude a condition when it is indeed absent. A *fasting* level of blood glucose set at a lower limit of 130 mg per cent in diabetes screening would catch none but the overt diabetics in the community, and thus would be a test of low sensitivity. Because it would exclude all members in the nondiabetic group, the test would have a high degree of specificity. Sensitivity and specificity are estimated in the following manner.

Disease*	Test Positive	Negative	Total
Present	a	b	$a + b$
Not present	c	d	$c + d$
	$a + c$	$b + d$	

Sensitivity $= a/(a + b)$
Specificity $= d/(c + d)$
False positives $= c/(a + c)$
False negatives $= b/(b + d)$

* Judged to be present by means other than the test.

The same method can also be applied to the answers of questions asked at interview. For example, the question "Do you regularly take any drug or medicine?" is ambiguous (aside from raising a further question about the interpretation of "regularly"); most of the aspirin eaters in the community would answer "no" since aspirin is considered neither a drug nor a medicine. Any inquiry into emotional responses is best done with the assistance of the behavioral scientists and with thoroughly tested questionnaires appropriate to the culture.

The survey performs admirably the function of detecting the burden of disease in the community only if proper preparation has preceded knocking on doors.

Retrospective Study.   The retrospective, or case history, study furnishes a great deal of information inexpensively. One starts with a group of affected individuals and tests the hypothesis that some characteristic or exposure is more common in persons with the disease than in unaffected persons, or persons with other unrelated diseases. An unrelated disease, in this context, is one that does not share a causal relationship to the characteristic being investigated. For example, comparison groups of patients with chronic pulmonary disease, oropharyngeal cancer, and bladder cancer would not be suitable for a lung cancer study since cigarette smoking, a risk factor for lung cancer, has also been shown to increase the risk of these other three diseases (Table 6-1, Kahn, H. A., 1966). The retrospective study differs from the prospective study cited in Table 6-1 in that it furnishes *indirect* estimates of risk, e.g., the frequency of a characteristic in the affected group compared to the frequency in the comparison group, or the proportion of affected individuals having the characteristic to the proportion found in the control group, and not the rate of new cases per year in persons with the characteristic.

The main disadvantage of this type of study is its dependence on the patient or his family for memory recall. The stress of illness, and feelings of guilt or despair may produce biased responses, which may be misleading. It is known that people tend to report diminutively on their use of alcohol; they also respond to the social or authority status of the interviewer. The reliability of information gathered retrospectively is improved by measures that include the use of other substantiating or corroborative sources of information, or that blind the interviewer by providing no identification of the subject as a case or control by duplicate interviews and the use of "dummy" questions that bear no relation to the disease and would be expected to be answered similarly by both case and comparison groups.

Prospective Study. The prospective study looks forward at the events of the groups comprising the sample strata, which differ from each other by the level of exposure to an agent (for example, consumption of cigarettes) or the level of a characteristic (for example, serum cholesterol levels). It is also called a cohort study and, unlike the retrospective or case history method study, starts with *unaffected* individuals.

The main advantage of the prospective study are the relative freedom from sampling selection bias and the opportunity provided to collect and record information on individuals *before* the clinical recognition of disease. It permits the prior establishment of procedures for surveillance, the control measures that increase the reliability of historical, clinical, and laboratory data and the rules and conditions that guide decisions about the inclusion or exclusion of a case or event. In a prospective study of cerebral vascular disease in the Japanese residents of Hiroshima, it was possible to relate the presence of antecedent diastolic hypertension to a subsequent increased incidence of cerebral vascular disease (Figure 6-3), a 2–4 fold increase for men and 3–4 fold increase for women having this characteristic was found. Further, in this study it was possible to measure the association of other factors, i.e., the level of serum cholesterol, proteinuria and left ventricular hypertrophy, to the subsequent occurrence of cerebral vascular disease. As shown in Figure 6-4, these three factors alone had little influence on the risk of developing CVD and were important *only* when associated with hypertension.

These examples illustrate the ability of the prospective study to furnish direct estimates of incidence (i.e., the number of *new* cases per unit of population within a defined time period) for groups that differ from one another by one characteristic or

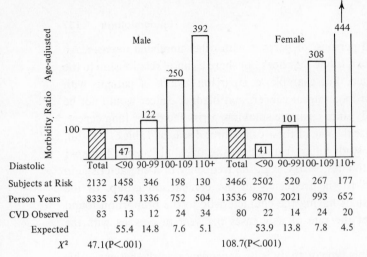

Morbidity Ratio — Age-adjusted

Male ... 392, 250, 122, 47 (100 line)
Female ... 444, 308, 101, 41

Diastolic	Total	<90	90-99	100-109	110+	Total	<90	90-99	100-109	110+
Subjects at Risk	2132	1458	346	198	130	3466	2502	520	267	177
Person Years	8335	5743	1336	752	504	13536	9870	2021	993	652
CVD Observed	83	13	12	24	34	80	22	14	24	20
Expected		55.4	14.8	7.6	5.1		53.9	13.8	7.8	4.5
X^2	47.1(P<.001)					108.7(P<.001)				

FIGURE 6-3. Initial levels of diastolic blood pressure and risk of subsequent CVD (age 40 and over). (Reproduced from Johnson, K. G., Yano, K., and Kato, H.: Cerebral vascular disease in Hiroshima, Japan, *J Chronic Dis*, **20**:545–49, 1967.)

gradations in exposure to an agent. In turn, the intergroup ratio differences in incidence furnish a direct estimate of risk.

The main disadvantages of the cohort study are the great expenditures of time and money required in the surveillance of the study sample in order to obtain relatively little information. In order to demonstrate statistically significant differences among various groups in the prospective study, extraordinarily large groups are necessary if the expected difference is small.

Another disadvantage of the cohort study is presented by those persons who were selected from the sampling frame but who do not participate in the study for a number of reasons, predominantly personal rather than medical. These persons are the non-respondents. Another source of loss is migration. To illustrate the problem of non-respondency, in the Japanese study cited previously (Johnson *et al.*, 1967), the mortality rate from CVD of the nonrespondents was 1.4 times higher than the rate in respondents. This information suggested that the incidence of CVD in respondents may underestimate the true incidence by a factor of 10 per cent.

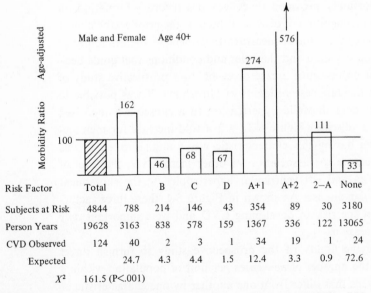

Morbidity Ratio — Age-adjusted

Male and Female   Age 40+ ... 576, 274, 162, 111, 68, 67, 46, 33 (100 line)

Risk Factor	Total	A	B	C	D	A+1	A+2	2–A	None
Subjects at Risk	4844	788	214	146	43	354	89	30	3180
Person Years	19628	3163	838	578	159	1367	336	122	13065
CVD Observed	124	40	2	3	1	34	19	1	24
Expected		24.7	4.3	4.4	1.5	12.4	3.3	0.9	72.6
X^2	161.5 (P<.001)								

FIGURE 6-4. Risk of subsequent CVD in relation to four risk factors initially present (age 40 and over). (Reproduced from Johnson, K. G., Yano, K., and Kato, H.: Cerebral vascular disease in Hiroshima, Japan, *J Chronic Dis*, **20**:545–59, 1967.)

A Hypertension (≥ 160/95), *B High Cholesterol* (≥ 220), *C Proteinuria*, *D LVH by ECG*

Interpretation of the Results of Epidemiologic Studies

The questions that are addressed to epidemiologic data are the following:

1. How large is the difference between or among groups?
2. Is there a dose-response relationship, i.e., a gradient between groups with varying levels of the characteristic?
3. Is there any other evidence gained from previous studies that supports observed differences; alternatively, are the results reproducible?
4. Can another hypothesis explain equally well the observed differences?

How Large Is the Difference. Differences between disease and comparison groups are evaluated by the use of statistical testing. The common types of statistical tests employed are presented in summary form in a subsequent section. The statistical analysis of observed results defines the contributions of chance and other disturbing influences and sets a credibility limit for conclusions. A statement is derived that gives the strength of the relationship between the characteristic and the disease. This kind of statement is shown in Figure 6-3. The probability that the effect of antecedent diastolic hypertension was not truly associated with subsequent CVD but was due to a chance occurrence is less than 1 in 1,000 ($x^2 = p < 0.001$). It must be remembered, however, that the level of blood pressure was selected as a variable *prior* to the knowledge of statistical results. In other words, the use of statistics is not a case of searching every possible relationship to find one of statistical significance, a prevalent misconception, but represents a means of expressing in precise terms the strength of associations and the limitations of the data.

The strength of the relationship is usually expressed in the form of a ratio, the numerator being the observed number of cases in a defined category and the denominator the expected number derived without reference to the characteristic, from the age-specific rates for the entire sample, or from the age-specific rates for the general population. For example, in Table 6-2, the observed number of cases of breast cancer in a sample of Japanese women who were exposed to varying doses of ionizing radiation and their matched controls is compared to the expected number. Note that the strength of the association of breast cancer and radiation is greatest in those women who received > 90 rad. The strength of the association, the difference between the irradiated and the controls, is small compared to the incidence of leukemia following radiation (Figure 6-2). Clearly the larger leukemogenic effect of radiation is more impressive than its effect for breast cancer, but not nearly as much when it is appreciated that breast cancer is uncommon in Japanese women and that the breast being a superficial structure received a fair portion of the total body radiation dose. Stated alternatively, in addition to the *size* of the observed differences, the difference must make biological sense before a reasonable statement of the strength of the association between a disease and a characteristic can be made.

To borrow from Sir Austin Bradford Hill, the glitter of the *t* tables must not disguise the poor quality of the fare. To make biologic sense does not imply that the relationship found is already known, but that the new finding is not unreasonable. For

TABLE 6-2

Observed and Expected Cases of Breast Cancer in Women Examined 1958–1966, by Estimated Total Radiation Dose

Total Dose (rad)	Number of Examined Women	Women with Breast Cancer			
		Definite Only		Definite + Possible	
		Obs	Exp	Obs	Exp
Not in City					
ATB	2458	2	5.4	2	6.1
0–9	3082	3	6.5	3	7.3
10–39	1262	4	2.7	5	3.0
40–89	857	2	1.8	2	2.0
90–199	802	4	1.7	5	2.0
200+	841	5	2.0	8	2.3
Not Estimated					
Unknown	840	2	1.9	2	2.3
Total	10142	22	22.0	25	25.0

A Comparison of the Observed Number of Breast Cancer Cases Found after First Examination and the Expected Number of Cases in the Examined-More-Than-Once Population Assuming Miyagi Prefecture Incidence Rates

Rad	90+	0–89	Unknown
Observed	6	9	1
Expected	1.53	10.36	0.61

* Adapted from Wanebo, C. K., et al.: Breast cancer after exposure to the atomic bombings of Hiroshima and Nagasaki. New Eng J Med, **279**:667–71, 1968.

example, relating the prevalence of coronary heart disease (CHD) to the frequency of subscriptions to private telephones may indicate a higher degree of affluence in CHD patients but the relationship is clearly of a tertiary order at best. In contrast, the clustering of cases of deafness and blindness in Australian patients by particular years of birth suggested that these defects were related to exposure at or near birth to an infectious disease appearing in the community in epidemic form; the infectious disease was identified subsequently as rubella.

To recapitulate, statistical methods are applied to quantitative data in order to express with precision an association between a disease and a characteristic in the population. The greater the difference that exists between groups of persons having or not having the characteristic, the stronger is the association. The association must have biologic significance.

Is There a Dose-Response Relation? Differences in the amount of exposure to an agent would be expected to produce corresponding variation in the total effect of the agent. Gradations in the strength of the stimulus ought to be followed by gradation in response. In many biological systems a critical or threshold value for the stimulus must be attained before any response is apparent, and doses of the stimulus beyond the capacity of the organism to respond appropriately results in obscuration of the linearity of the dose-response relationship.

The prospective or cohort study is ideally suited to demonstrate a possible dose-response relationship. The number of new cases in a given time period, for groups differing by levels of exposure to an agent, can be estimated and compared. For example, variations in the use of cigarettes in Dorn's study of ex-servicemen correspond to differences in mortality rates for lung cancer, expressed as mortality ratios in Table 6-1. All current cigarette smokers had mortality rates approximately 11 times higher than nonsmokers and those who smoked less than 10 cigarettes per day. The relative risk was 9-fold in men smoking 10–20 cigarettes per day, and almost 17-fold in men smoking over 20 cigarettes per day. The ratio for pipe or cigar smokers was close to that for nonsmokers or light smokers (1.67). Ex-cigarette smokers, who had stopped smoking voluntarily and without physician's order, had a relative risk 4.71 times that of nonsmokers, but nevertheless an appreciably lower risk than experienced by persons who continued to smoke cigarettes. A consistent dose-response relation is seen in these data. In this study the specificity of the relationship of cigarette smoking and cancer was supported by the experience of ex-smokers, and by the lack of an association between cigarette smoking and other diseases such as rectal cancer for which there is no reason to expect an association with cigarette smoking.

In the case of lung cancer, the threshold level may be less than ten cigarettes per day. However, in other situations a relatively small dose at any point may suffice to initiate a pathogenic process, a point mutation, and detection of a dose response may be difficult.

Perhaps the greatest value in considering the dose-response concept is the suspicion generated when one sees the greatest effect in intermediate exposure groups, producing a hump in the dose-response curve. The correlation between dose and effect in this situation becomes so poor as to cast a serious doubt on the existence of any association. However, before reaching this conclusion, the duration of time after exposure and age at time of exposure must be considered. A gross example follows: if the detection of leukemia in A-bomb survivors commenced in 1965 (Figure 6-2), the proportion of heavily irradiated persons is so weighted with persons who have successfully withstood the leukemogenic effect of radiation received 20 years earlier, that a dose-response relationship would be extremely difficult to detect. The confounding effect of the bias introduced by survivors can be controlled by standardizing incidence rates for age and time elapsed since exposure. In the Dorn study of smoking and mortality, cited previously, it was noted that for heavy smokers and for the same duration of smoking, persons who started smoking before age 20 were at substantially greater risk than those who started smoking later.

In summary, demonstration of a dose-response relationship adds great weight to the strength of the association between a disease and exposure in the population. Human data do not always provide the opportunity to make such an association. However, poor correlation between dose and effect weakens the strength of an association.

The Existence of Other Epidemiologic Evidence.   Seeking confirmation of one's own observations in the observations of others is common scientific practice. Take for example the remarkable similarity of results in the studies of Court-Brown and Doll, and the Atomic Bomb Casualty commission (Bizzozero *et al.*, 1966; Wanebo *et al.*, 1968), both concerned with the late effects of irradiation, by employing distinctly different approaches. Observations of thromboembolism in women taking contraceptive pills are strengthened by studies that demonstrate increased blood coagulability in subjects taking this hormone. The significance of increased rates of lung cancer in persons exposed to asbestos is enhanced by the histologic studies of these neoplasms that show a larger than expected number of a relatively rare type of lung cancer, mesothelioma.

To the extent that results do not fit other epidemiologic evidence, an explanation must be sought in sampling and other methodologic differences.

Can Another Hypothesis Serve Equally Well?   The search for alternative hypotheses is the keystone of advances in epidemiology. Mention was made earlier, in the example of lung cancer, of the association of a *single* disease with *multiple factors*, and of the coexistence of two rare and different diseases in the same person, unexplainable by chance, which suggests a common etiology. It follows that although a characteristic is strongly related to a disease, both may be related to a characteristic whose effect is greater than either. High levels of serum cholesterol, triglycerides, and blood glucose are associated with greater risk for CHD. Glucose intolerance, whether it be florid diabetes or the defect in insulin transport seen in obese patients, favors lipogenesis. It may be that the essential characteristic of persons who are prone to coronary heart disease is a genetically determined polymorphic defect in carbohydrate metabolism. As in all scientific disciplines, one study begets another; each contributes a small portion to the ultimate discovery of the cause of a disease.

The Uses of Epidemiology

Epidemiological techniques are used to place the health of the community under surveillance, to plan for its health needs and to evaluate the efficacy of disease control measures. They are also used to identify groups of individuals who have characteristics that are associated with increased risk of disease and, after identification of the characteristics, to plan experiments which will demonstrate their relative importance in the causation of disease. They are valuable in the study of the natural history of disease in the community and in extending the range of clinical knowledge beyond the sick or symptomatic patient. Thus, they provide a rational basis for programs designed to prevent disease.

The epidemiologist is concerned with the health of the community. Faced with the burden of diseases such as coronary heart disease and cancer in the population, and awaiting the ultimate knowledge of the basic pathologic process, the epidemiologist is justified on the basis of associations, in proceeding with recommendations directed toward the prevention of disease. As Doll points out, although carcinogenesis is still poorly understood, preventive medicine measures based on epidemiologic evidence have virtually eliminated certain types of cancers related to occupation (Doll, 1967).

CHOOSING AN APPROPRIATE STATISTICAL TEST

Isabel M. Mountain

In planning an investigation, or in evaluating observations already made, statistical aid can provide a powerful ally. Statistical planning can lead to the most efficient experimental design, which gives the highest yield in results; or it may reveal that the experiment as planned would require a sample so large as to be exorbitantly expensive. (See Tables 6-3, 6-4, and 6-5.)

TABLE 6-3
Summary of Some Commonly Used Statistical Tests

Statistic	Test for significance	Degrees of freedom
mean of the sample	Student's t-test for significance of difference between means	
$\bar{x}$	$t = \dfrac{(\bar{x}_1 - \bar{x}_2)}{\sqrt{\text{pooled } S^2\left(\dfrac{1}{n_1} + \dfrac{1}{n_2}\right)}}$	$(n_1 - 1) + (n_2 - 1)$
binomial $p = x/n$	Test for significance of difference between proportions	for large samples, assume ∞
$q = 1 - p$ (p_o, for entire population)	$z = \dfrac{(p_1 - p_2)}{\sqrt{p_o q_o\left(\dfrac{1}{n_1} + \dfrac{1}{n_2}\right)}}$	
variance S^2 or SD^2	Test whether variance$_1$ (numerator) is greater than variance$_2$ (denominator)	
	$F = \dfrac{\text{variance}_1}{\text{variance}_2}$	$(n_1 - 1)$ for numerator $(n_2 - 1)$ for denominator
distribution	Test for distribution of frequencies into K categories	
	$\chi^2 = \sum^{K} \dfrac{(O - E)^2}{E}$	K minus the number of linear restrictions

At the outset, an investigator wants to know whether the study proposed has a reasonable chance of yielding a definite answer, positive or negative. Suppose that an observer, whether laboratory investigator or epidemiologist, notices a difference in some measurable characteristic between two groups of individuals which he wants to compare. If he claims that this difference is valid, he may be challenged. But his position is fortified if, as a result of statistical analysis, he can state the degree of confidence of his claim. Furthermore, his claim enforced by such a probability statement, can be compared with other related findings on a common standardized basis.

The types of questions suitably addressed to statistical analysis are basically few, with many ramifications. The nature of the characteristics that are amenable to statistical analysis can be called central tendency, variation, and distribution. Only a few commonly used statistical tests will be discussed here.

Central Tendency.   Central tendency is measured as the mean (average), the median, or the mode. Student's t-test for comparison of means is appropriate when samples are relatively small.

TABLE 6-4
Short Glossary of Symbols

Symbols

x	the value of a variable, x, for an individual
f	the frequency of occurrence, or number of times that same value of x occurs
Σ	sum (sigma, cap. letter)
df	degrees of freedom
P	probability of occurrence (usually a capital letter) such as $P = 0.01 = 1\% = 1$ out of 100, or $P = 0.05 = 5\% = 5$ out of 100
p	a proportion (usually a small letter) such as $36/1200 = .030 = 3\%$
$\|n\|$	vertical lines mean the absolute value of n, without $+$ or $-$ sign

Parameters of a Population			Statistics of a Sample from a Population	
μ	mu	the true arithmetic mean of all values of the variable, x, in the entire population	$\bar{x}$, x bar	the arithmetic mean of the N values in a sample from the population
			SD^2 or S^2	the standard deviation squared = the variance of the values of x in the sample
σ^2	sigma^2	the true variance of the variable, x, in a population		
σ	sigma	the true standard deviation of the variable, x, in a population	SD	the standard deviation of the values of x in the sample
			$(x - \bar{x})$	the deviation of the value of each x to the mean of the sample
$(x - \mu)$		the deviation of the value of each x to the true mean of the population		
			$S_{\bar{x}}$ or $SE_{\bar{x}}$	standard error of the mean, $\bar{x}$, of the sample
			SS	sum of squares; $SS/df = SD^2$

TABLE 6-5
Definitions and Examples of Statistical Terms

Definitions

Population refers to the total collection of individual entities that are available (or potentially available) for study—the group about which we want to make inferences.

Sample is some subset of the population. Usually it is selected so that the probability of inclusion of any individual from the population can be specified. The sample is then called a probability sample. The goal in sampling is to achieve representativeness.

Random means "with equal chance." It is usually misused to apply to a situation where no particular selection process has been followed.

The (arithmetic) *mean* of a group of numbers is simply their numerical average. It is used as a measure of the central value of the group of numbers.

The *variance* of a group of numbers is an average of the squares of the amount by which the individual numbers deviate from the mean of the group. It is used as a measure of the degree of spread among the group of numbers.

A *parameter* is a numerical constant in a mathematical expression and refers to a characteristic of the population. For example, in the linear equation $y = a + bx$, the letters a and b represent parameters, x and y usually representing the independent and dependent (response) variables, respectively.

Usually, the values of population parameters are not known, and one of the purposes of studying a sample from the population is to derive estimates of the population parameters.

A *statistic* is a number calculated from sample data. The sample mean, sample variance, standard deviation, and so on are all statistics.

TABLE 6-5 *(Continued)*
Definitions and Examples of Statistical Terms

An *estimate* is a numerical value obtained from a statistical sample and assigned to a population parameter. For example, the sample mean is usually (though not always) taken as the estimate of the population mean. An estimate is considered to have an associated distribution in the following sense. For concreteness, consider the sample mean. If we were to draw repeated, independent samples of a fixed size from some population, and calculate the mean for each sample, we would have a distribution of values. This is frequently referred to as "the distribution of the sample mean." In general, a statistician may talk about "the distribution of the estimate," for whatever estimate he happens to be referring to.

Expected number is the average value which is derived from a known distribution frequency for an entire sample or population. If the incidence of myocardial infarction in men 40–59 is 1 per 100 (1%) per year, in a group of 1000 such men, 10 new events per year would be expected. To illustrate further, in a controlled study, 500 such men were treated with some control measure (ex. clofibrate) and 500 were not. In the entire group of 1,000, 8 new events occurred one year after the study was begun. In performing a chi square test, 4 new cases would be the *expected* number (500 × 0.8%) in the experimental group. Actually the *observed* number in this group after the first year was 3.

Risk

The chance of a person developing a disease, having an accident, undergoing some event, is derived from the incidence of the given event in large appropriate samples of the population. It is a derived *average*.

One can estimate risk directly by summing up the incidence rates in each 1-year age group. For example if the sum of the incidence rates of coronary heart disease for men 35–49 equals 200 per 1,000 then the average risk of CHD in men of this age group is 1 in 5. Risk can be derived more accurately by using actuary life-table methods.

More often we speak of relative risk, which is a comparison of rates (mortality or incidence) between persons having a certain habit or characteristic and persons who do not, expressed by a ratio. (Refer to Table 6-1.)

Sensitivity is a commonly used index of the efficacy of a test and refers to the proportion of affected individuals in the population that the test will correctly diagnose as affected.

Specificity refers to the proportion of unaffected persons in a population that the test will correctly classify as unaffected.

False positive refers to the proportion of unaffected persons in a sample that the test will incorrectly classify as affected.

False negative refers to the proportion of affected persons that the test will incorrectly classify as unaffected.

Rates

Death rate
Over-all crude death rate, per year =

$$\frac{\text{Number of deaths per year}}{\text{Total population}} \times 1,000 = \text{Death rate (per 1,000 persons per year)}.$$

For a specific disease, a larger denominator is usually reported (for convenience of the size of the numbers):

$$\frac{\text{Number of deaths from a specific cause per year}}{\text{Total population}} \times 100,000 = \text{Specific disease death rate}$$

The annual death rate for the United States in 1965 was 9.4 per 1,000 for the year.

Morbidity rate
As an example, if 100 persons developed Klebsiella pneumonia in one year in a city with a population of 10 million persons,

$$\text{Morbidity rate} = \frac{100 \text{ cases per year}}{10 \text{ million persons}} = 10 \text{ cases per million persons per year}.$$

Case fatality rate
If 60 of the 100 affected persons died,

$$\text{Case fatality rate} = \frac{60 \text{ persons died}}{100 \text{ affected persons}} = 60\%.$$

TABLE 6-5   (Continued)

Definitions and Examples of Statistical Terms

The mortality rate *specific for Klebsiella pneumonia* is

$$\frac{60 \text{ deaths per year}}{10 \text{ million persons}} = 6 \text{ deaths per year per million persons.}$$

Birth rate

$$\frac{\text{Number of live births per year}}{\text{Total population}} \times 1{,}000 = \text{birth rate per 1,000 persons per year.}$$

The annual birth rate for the United States for the year 1966 was 18.5.

Infant mortality deals with deaths of children under 1 year of age. (Neonatal period, 1–28 days.)

$$\text{Infant mortality rate} = \frac{\text{Number of deaths of infants per year}^*}{\text{Number of live births in that year}} \times 1{,}000 = \frac{\text{Number of deaths per}}{1{,}000 \text{ live births per year.}}$$

In the United States the annual infant mortality rate in 1965 was 24.7 per 1,000 live births. This rate is higher than rates for the Scandinavian countries, the Netherlands, England, Wales, Australia, and New Zealand.

In developed countries the usual figures for the annual birth rate are around 20 per 1,000; the overall crude death rate in the population is around 10 per 1,000. In underdeveloped countries the annual birth rate is around 40 per 1,000; the death rate around 20 per 1,000.

Rate vs. ratio

A population consisting of persons with characteristics of *a* or *b*, for example, *a* with diabetes or *b* without diabetes,

$$\text{the } \textit{prevalence rate} \text{ of diabetes} = \frac{a}{a + b};$$

$$\text{the } \textit{ratio} \text{ of diabetics to non-diabetics} = \frac{a}{b}.$$

Incidence rate (usually referred to as "Incidence") implies a time base and describes the frequency of occurrence of some event in a group, sample or population *in a specified period of time* (the number per unit of population per unit of time). We refer to incidence as the number of *new* cases, and the calculation of an incidence rate necessarily requires knowledge of the disease status of members of the group of interest for at least two times. One must know who is free of the disease at the beginning of the time period and how many cases of the disease developed among this group during the period of study.

Prevalence rate refers to the proportion of persons studied who are shown to have a given condition, usually at a given point in time. For example, one might talk about the prevalence of balding in second year medical students, or the prevalence of lung cancer in the 1967 New York Hospital autopsy series.

Adjustment of rates

When comparing morbidity or mortality rates between different populations adjustments must be made for differences in racial, age, and sex composition. To illustrate, surveys for rheumatoid arthritis in an urban and rural area show the prevalence of R.A. to be 4.6 per 1,000 among women in the urban area and 10.6 per 1,000 among women in the rural area. The survey data show:

Rheumatoid Arthritis	Urban				Rural			
Age	40	40–59	60+	Total	40	40–59	60+	Total
No. cases	0	21	16	37	0	10	75	85
Population	3000	4000	1000	8000	1000	2000	5000	8000
Prevalence/1,000	—	5.2	16	4.6	—	5.0	15	10.6

By inspection of each age category it is clear that the age-specific rates are almost identical. To obtain a single comparable value for each area the age specific rates for each area can be applied to some standard population as the WHO standard population of 100,000, which is used for international comparisons.

---

* excluding fetal deaths and stillborns

As an example, we might compare the average serum cholesterol levels ($\bar{x}_1$, $\bar{x}_2$) of two groups of men (within a certain range of age): (1) who have had demonstrable coronary heart disease, and (2) who have not had symptoms. The question is, "Is the level in group 1 greater than that in group 2?"

The test is based simply on the magnitude of the difference as compared to the standard error of the difference. The question is whether the ratio exceeds a critical point at a stated level of significance, as found in a table of critical values for Student's t-test. If the observed t value exceeds the table value, the difference can be declared significant at the given level. The outcome of the test is expressed as a probability, P, that a difference as great as, or greater than, the observed difference might be attributable to chance alone. Thus, the smaller the value of P, the safer the claim that the difference was real.

Thus observed

$$t = \frac{(\bar{x}_1 - \bar{x}_2)}{\sqrt{\text{pooled } S^2 \left(\frac{1 + 1}{n_1 + n_2}\right)}}$$

where

$$\text{pooled } S^2 = \frac{(n_1 - 1)S^2 + (n_2 - 1)S^2}{(n_1 - 1) + (n_2 - 1)}$$

If, in our example,

$$\bar{x}_1 = 195.0 \text{ mg}\%; \; n_1 = 30; \; S^2 = 2164.20$$

and

$$\bar{x}_2 = 146.0 \text{ mg}\%; \; n_2 = 30; \; S^2 = 1585.20$$

$$t = \frac{(195.0 - 146.0)}{\sqrt{\frac{29(2164.20) + 29(1585.20)}{29 + 29} \left(\frac{1}{30} + \frac{1}{30}\right)}} = \frac{49.0}{\sqrt{124.98}} = \frac{49.0}{11.2} = 4.7$$

Next we need to consider the size of the samples, because the critical value of t increases as the sample size decreases. When testing for significance of difference between two samples, $df = (n_1 - 1) + (n_2 - 1)$. The critical value of t corresponds, in this case, to $df = (30 - 1) + (30 - 1) = 58$. Choosing $\alpha = 0.01$ level of significance for a one-tail test, we have asked a one-sided question: Is the mean of 1 greater than the mean of 2? From the table, the critical value of $t_{58,0.01}$ is 2.39. Since our observed $t = 4.7$ is greater than the critical value, we can declare significance at the 0.01 level, expressed as $P < 0.01$.

In testing hypotheses, the most familiar consideration is whether an observed difference can be declared significant, at a stated α level of significance. For testing, we started with the assumption that there was in fact no real difference; that is, the null hypothesis. However, there is another consideration. Suppose that under an alternative hypothesis, the two samples were drawn from populations with distinctly different means. In this case we would like to recognize this difference. If our test failed to detect the difference which in fact existed, we would incur a false negative result. This outcome is called the β error.

As an example, suppose that a new drug is given an initial trial, by testing its efficacy compared to a placebo control. There are four possible outcomes.

1. The drug is in fact not effective (null hypothesis)
    a. The test indicates that it is not effective: true.
    b. The test indicates that the drug is effective: a false positive, α error.
2. The drug is really effective (alternative hypothesis)
    a. The test indicates that it is effective: true.
    b. The test fails to detect its efficacy: a false negative, β error.

Having chosen a test statistic and selected an α level, the probability of a β error can be reduced by increasing the sample size, when this is feasible.

Comparative variability of Samples. The comparative variability of samples is measured as the ratio of two variances. An F test is invoked to answer the question, Is the variance of a certain sample significantly greater than that of another? In this test, $F = \text{variance}_1/\text{variance}_2$. Thus, the F test has two sets of degrees of freedom, one for the numerator, the other for the denominator.

In the example given under central tendency,

$$F_{(n_1-1),(n_2-1)} = \frac{S_1^2}{S_1^2} = \frac{2164.20}{1585.20} = 1.37$$

An appropriate table value for comparison is $F_{29,29,.05} = 1.85$. Because the observed F did not exceed the table value, the variance of x_1 is not significantly greater than that of x_2.

Ramifications of such F ratios lead to the powerful analysis of variance by which the variation among many mean values can be compared to background variability. The investigator is usually fully aware of the question that defines the numerator; for example, do the mean values of the blood pressures for men, subdivided into age brackets, vary significantly from each other? He selects as denominator the appropriate measure of background variability, pooled from within each group. Answers to a host of important (as well as not important) questions can be derived from well-planned experiments. The importance of the question is a matter of judgment not of statistics.

Distribution. A third basic phenomenon subject to statistical evaluation is the question of arrangement of values of a variable, that is, their *distribution*, or how frequently individuals fall into subdivisions of the entire population. Gauss described a distribution so commonly observed in nature that it is called the normal distribution. Data can be analyzed to test whether the values fit this distribution. Furthermore, categories can be set up appropriate to the question under study.

Another distribution is the binomial, in which the population is dichotomous. For example, patients who had influenza are now either "dead" or "still living." For example, the case fatality rate for influenza:

$$p = \frac{\text{number of deaths observed}}{\text{number of cases of influenza}}.$$

A group of physicians wanted to determine whether administration of penicillin affected the fatal outcome from influenza, in either direction. Available were 16 patients randomly selected into two groups, distributed nearly equally by age and sex. Penicillin was given to individuals in one group, a placebo to the other.

The outcome was

Group 1	Group 2	Over-all
$p_1 = \dfrac{5}{58} = 0.086$	$p_2 = \dfrac{7}{58} = 0.121$	$p_0 = \dfrac{5+7}{58+58} = 0.103$ $q_0 = 1 - p_0$

The standard error of the difference is $\sqrt{p_0 q_0(1/n_1 + 1/n_2)}$.

Test for significance of difference:

(Vertical lines mean the absolute value; that is, the larger minus the smaller p.)

$$z = \frac{|p_1 - p_2|}{\sqrt{p_0 q_0\left(\dfrac{1}{n_1} + \dfrac{1}{n_2}\right)}} \qquad df = \text{assume } \infty$$

$$= \frac{0.121 - 0.086}{\sqrt{(0.103)(0.897)\left(\dfrac{1}{58} + \dfrac{1}{58}\right)}} = \frac{0.035}{0.56} = 0.6.$$

Suppose a level of significance of 0.05 was chosen and the observed $z = 0.6$ did not exceed the critical $z = 1.96$. (A two-tail test was used because we asked about the difference "in either direction.")

The conclusion is that, based on these two samples, in which penicillin or a placebo was given to influenza patients, the difference in fatality was not significant, $P > 0.05$.

A most useful test for detection of differences of distribution is the chi square (χ^2) test. Its proper application does not depend on the nature of the distribution under question. It is said to be distribution-free, or a nonparametric, test. It depends on a comparison of the observed distribution with an expected distribution based on some reasonable hypothesis.

$\chi^2 = (O - E)^2/E$, the sum for each category, where O = observed frequency and E = expected frequency. Frequency is used in the sense of number of events.

As an example, the association between serum cholesterol level and coronary heart disease (CHD) in males was (Johnson *et al.* 1968)—

Serum cholesterol	<180	180–219	220 +	Total
Subjects at risk	1631	401	96	2128
Person years	6677	1559	370	8606
CHD Observed	20	11	5	36
CHD Expected	27.7	6.8	1.5	

$$\chi^2 = \frac{(20 - 27.7)^2}{27.7} + \frac{(11 - 6.8)^2}{6.8} + \frac{(5 - 1.5)^2}{1.5} = 2.1 + 2.6 + 8.2 = 13.$$

This shows the χ^2 test in its simplest form; in practice, it is appropriate to apply a correction for small numbers. The degrees of freedom is $k - 1$, where k is the number of categories. The table value for $\chi^2_{2,.01} = 9.2$, and because the observed value was greater than the table value, the distribution can be declared significantly different from a random (or chance) distribution.

χ^2 value does not tell the direction of the association; nor where was the greatest effect. These can be found by looking at the data. Note that the greatest contribution to the χ^2 was made by the category of serum cholesterol (mg%) of 220 and above. Here, more than three times as many cases were observed as expected.

REFERENCES

American Public Health Association: *The Control of Communicable Disease in Man*, 9th ed. American Public Health Association, New York, 1960.

BIZZOZERO, O. J., JR., JOHNSON, K. G., and CIOCCO, A.: Radiation-related leukemia in Hiroshima and Nagasaki, 1946–1964, I. Distribution, incidence and appearance time. *New Eng J Med*, **274**:1095–1101, 1966.

COURT-BROWN, W. M., and DOLL, R.: *Leukaemia and Aplastic Anemia in Patients Irradiated for Ankylosing Spondylitis*. Med Res Counc Spec Rep Ser, no. 295, Her Majesty's Stationery Office, London, 1957.

———, and ———: Mortality from cancer and other causes after radiotherapy for anykylosing spondylitis. *Brit Med J*, **2**:1327–32, 1965.

DOLL, R.: *Prevention of Cancer, Pointers from Epidemiology*. The Rock Carling Fellowship, 1967, the Nuffield Provincial Hospitals Trust Publisher, London, 1967.

———, and HILL, A. B.: Smoking and carcinoma of the lung. *Brit Med J*, **2**:739, 1950.

DUNN, O. J.: *Basic Statistics: A Primer for the Biomedical Sciences*. John Wiley & Sons, Inc., New York, 1964.

GREGORY, P. B., MILTON, R. C., JOHNSON, M-L. T., and TAURA, T.: Spleen shielding in survivors of the atomic bomb. *Radiat Res*, **33**:204–15, 1968.

JACOBSON, L. O., MARKS, E. K., ROBSON, M. J., GASTON, E. O., and ZIRKLE, R. E.: The effect of spleen protection on mortality following x-irradiation. *J Lab Clin Med*, **34**:1538–43, 1949.

JOHNSON, K. G., YANO, K., and KATO, H.: Cerebral vascular disease in Hiroshima, Japan, *J Chronic Dis*, **20**:545–59, 1967.

KAHN, H. A.: The Dorn study of smoking and mortality among U.S. veterans: Report on eight and one half years of observation. National Cancer Institute Monograph no. 19: *Epidemiological Study of Cancer and Other Chronic Diseases*. U.S. Government Printing Office, Washington, D.C., 1966, 125 pp.

MORIYAMA, I. M., DAWBER, T. R., and KANNEL, W. B.: Evaluation of diagnostic information supporting medical certification of deaths from cardiovascular disease. National Cancer Institute Monograph no. 19: *Epidemiologic Approaches to the Study of Cancer and other Chronic Diseases*. U.S. Government Printing Office, Washington, D.C., 405–30, 1966.

NAGGAN, L., and MACMAHON, B.: Ethnic differences in the prevalence of anencephaly and spina bifida in Boston, Massachusetts. *New Eng J Med*, **277**:1119–23, 1967.

NEEL, J. V.: *Changing Perspectives on the Genetic Effects of Radiation*. Charles C. Thomas Publisher, Springfield, Ill., 1963.

WANEBO, C. K., JOHNSON, K. G., SATO, K., and THORSLUND, T. W.: Breast cancer after exposure to the atomic bombings of Hiroshima and Nagasaki. *New Eng J Med*, **279**:667–71, 1968.

WOOD, J. W., KATO, H., JOHNSON, K. G., UDA, Y., RUSSELL, W. J., and DUFF, I. F.: Rheumatoid arthritis in Hiroshima and Nagasaki: prevalence, incidence and clinical characteristics. *Arthritis Rheum*, **10**:21–31, 1967.

7

Experimental Epidemiology

Jerome L. Schulman

GENERAL CONSIDERATIONS

Definition

Experimental epidemiology may be defined as the laboratory study of disease patterns in subjects under circumstances in which factors affecting the relationship of the host, the environment, and microbial parasites may be manipulated by design. This definition, although arbitrary, is necessary to distinguish experimental epidemiology as originally conceived and defined by Topley from any investigation of epidemic disease in which experimental methods are employed. Controlled experiments in which one variable is manipulated, as when part of a susceptible population is given a vaccine or when fluoride is added to the water supply of one of two comparable communities, are essential to our understanding of epidemic disease and could readily be termed experimental epidemiology, but for the purposes of this discussion only laboratory models will be considered.

History

The concept of experimental epidemiology was first introduced by W. W. C. Topley at the London School of Hygiene following the influenza pandemic of 1918–19. Topley proposed that there were controlling principles common to all epidemics that might best be investigated by controlled experimental studies of naturally occurring epidemic disease in populations of small laboratory animals. Epidemics of mouse typhoid, ectromelia, and Pasturella muriseptica were initiated in herds of mice, which were replenished by the introduction of "immigrant" mice at regular intervals. Varying the size of the herd and the rate of introduction of new susceptibles, and studying the effects of immunization of portions of the herd, Topley, Greenwood and their colleagues (Greenwood *et al.*, 1936) were able to follow the changing course of epidemics subsequent to these experimental manipulations. Particular emphasis was given to the

151

role of immunity, and from these elegant studies emerged one of the earliest experimental demonstrations of the potential effectiveness of herd immunity (particularly in the case of ectromelia) in protecting susceptibles within the population from infection.

At about the same time, Leslie T. Webster and his colleagues at the Rockefeller Institute were engaging in similar studies of experimentally perpetuated epidemics in mice. By inbreeding and selection of tested litters, they were able to select two strains of mice markedly different in their innate susceptibility to mouse typhoid. When mixtures of varying proportions of mice from the two strains were exposed to mouse typhoid introduced by infected immigrant mice, it was possible to demonstrate not only that the resistant mice survived whereas mice of the susceptible strain succumbed, but also that the progress of the epidemic was greatly influenced by the numbers of susceptible and resistant mice remaining in the population. Furthermore, Webster and his colleagues established that genetic resistance to mouse typhoid was specific and operated separately from genetic resistance to St. Louis B encephalitis virus, and therefore was not simply an expression of selection of mice for "pan-resistance" (Webster, 1946).

Potential Value of Studies in Experimental Epidemiology

Topley's hypothesis that the spread of epidemic disease within a population is largely determined by factors common to all epidemics has not been supported by the scientific evidence gathered over the last 40 years. There are, however, important areas of knowledge concerning specific epidemic diseases that can most effectively be elucidated by experiments appropriately designed to study the expression of epidemic disease in controlled populations of laboratory subjects.

Independent Evaluation of Multiple Variables.   In their original experiments, Topley and Webster attempted to determine whether the fluctuating or intermittent nature of epidemic infection was a consequence of changing virulence of the infecting parasite or whether it reflected changes in the susceptibility of the exposed population. This concern exemplifies one of the most troubling aspects of the study of most epidemic diseases of man. The complex interrelationships of factors operating on the host, the environment, and the parasite, make it difficult to assess the relative importance of any single factor influencing the course of the epidemic. At times it is possible, retrospectively, to compare epidemics that arise naturally in isolated populations under specific circumstances, but the systematic study of single variables under controlled experimental conditions frequently provides essential additional information. One example of the difficulty of evaluating the significance of multiple variables in human epidemics is seen in the seasonal variation in the incidence of respiratory infection. The "winter factor" has been attributed to the opening of schools in the fall, indoor crowding with low rates of ventilation, effects of the environment on survival of respiratory viruses, decreased resistance of the host due to chilling and to reactivation of latent infection. The use of appropriate, controlled experimental models provides a potential opportunity to assess the degree to which each of these hypothetical explanations is operative.

Observation of Epidemic Disease Over a Period of Time.   The use of laboratory animals to study microbial disease is of course, commonplace. The specific value of experiments in experimental epidemiology is in the opportunity they provide to examine epidemic disease in a fixed population over a period of time, and to determine how the progress of the epidemics is affected by experimental manipulation.

Inferences Referable to Naturally Occurring Human Epidemic Disease

Caution is always necessary in applying the results of experiments on laboratory animals to human disease because of the obvious differences in susceptibility and behavior patterns that are associated with species differences. Infectious agents that are transmitted by one route or are influenced by certain environmental factors in rodents might readily be spread by an entirely different route and be influenced by other environmental factors in the human host. Nevertheless, these experiments do provide conceptual generalizations concerning the kinds of interrelationships that influence specific epidemic agents. The applicability of these generalizations to human disease subsequently can be tested by appropriate experimental design.

An additional source of contention is raised by the question of whether it is more appropriate to study infectious agents natural to the species of laboratory animal employed or to investigate agents alien to the laboratory host that cause epidemic disease in man. Both kinds of experiments have advantages in their applicability to human disease, and accordingly, both types of investigations will be referred to in the discussion that follows. Furthermore, the behavior of a specific pathogenic agent in laboratory animals may be much more relevant to understanding the behavior of the same agent in man than the generalizations derived from studies of another parasite in the human host. Transmission of influenza in mice for example, may provide more pertinent information about human influenza than can be obtained from comparisons of adenovirus infection in man and influenza in man.

EXAMPLES OF TYPES OF PROBLEMS THAT CAN BE INVESTIGATED

No attempt is intended in this section to provide a comprehensive review of all experimental epidemiology. Instead, some examples of the kinds of problems that have been studied by these methods will be discussed.

Mode of Transmission

Many human parasites can produce disease in human volunteers when inoculated by a variety of routes, e.g., aerosol, oral ingestion, parenteral inoculation, etc. Such experiments provide information about what is *possible* under artificial conditions, but they do not help to determine what is the *usual* or natural method of transmission. **Influenza.**   Alternative hypotheses have been offered to explain the method of transmission in influenza. One theory postulates that the virus is contained in large droplets expelled from the respiratory tract of infected individuals and is transmitted to the upper respiratory tract of a susceptible host in close proximity. The second theory postulates that the virus emerges in very small droplets, which evaporate very rapidly leaving small residues or droplet nuclei capable of remaining airborne for prolonged periods. These are distributed by air currents throughout the room into which they are introduced. According to the second theory, infection is acquired when the airborne virus is inhaled and the infectious particles are deposited in the lower respiratory tract. Results with an experimental model designed to study transmission of influenza virus infection in mice have demonstrated that:

1. Transmission is inversely related to ventilation.
2. Transmission is not reduced by physical separation of infectors and contacts.

These results could be explained most readily by airborne transmission of influenza virus infection in mice (Schulman and Kilbourne, 1962). According to expectation, transmission by large droplets would not be influenced by the rate of air flow through the experimental chamber and would be reduced by physical separation of infectors and contacts. These results were supported by later experiments in which infectious virus was recovered from the air surrounding infector mice during the period of their infectiousness (Schulman, 1967a), and by the earlier observation of a lower incidence of influenza in patients housed in a hospital wing equipped with ultraviolet irradiation compared to a similar wing not equipped with ultraviolet lights (McLean, 1961). However, in studies of the transmission of Newcastle Disease Virus (an influenza-like myxovirus infection of chickens), Andrewes and Allison (1961) found that proximity of the chicks did influence transmission and that infection could not be carried over or under a glass partition separating infectors and contacts.

Tuberculosis.   The experiments of Riley and O'Grady (1961) have provided considerable support to the theory that human tuberculosis is transmitted primarily by the airborne route. These investigators placed guinea pigs in compartments above hospital units housing patients with active tuberculosis. By means of specially designed ventilating and duct systems air from the patients' rooms was directed into the guinea pig chambers and the rate at which the guinea pigs became infected was observed. From their results they could calculate a mean concentration of airborne tubercle bacilli in the air within the patients' rooms. They then calculated the approximate exposure of student nurses inhaling the infected air during their routine activities and found that the values they obtained correlated remarkably well with the observed rate of tuberculin conversion among the nurses. These experiments have very broad implications. If tuberculosis is spread primarily by airborne droplet nuclei, many of the isolation procedures used in treating tuberculosis patients need to be re-evaluated, and new precautions substituted.

Rabies.   When animals inside wire mesh cages were placed in caves known to contain rabid bats, they proceeded to develop rabies although protected from bites or other direct contact (Constantine, 1962). These observations confirmed the hypothesis that bats could transmit rabies by aerosols of infectious virus as well as by bites. Airborne transmission of rabies by other species has not been demonstrated.

Common Cold Viruses. As with influenza virus the method of transmission of the viruses responsible for the common cold is a subject of great controversy. Unfortunately, convenient animal models are not available, and experiments with human volunteers have provided conflicting results. Buckland *et al.* (1965) inoculated human volunteers with Coxsackie A21 virus and induced them to sneeze. Airborne virus was recovered rarely, and in low titers, compared to the quantity of virus expelled as droplets (4–20 μ in diameter). Conversely, Couch *et al.* (1966) using somewhat different methods with the same virus found that infected volunteers expelled appreciable quantities of virus as airborne droplet nuclei. Furthermore, in a transmission experiment they found that contacts separated by a double-mesh wire screen from infected volunteers readily acquired infection, indicating that airborne transmission can occur.

Mouse-pox. Ectromelia has been studied in a series of experiments by Fenner (1949) as a model for an investigation of the epidemiology and pathogenesis of pox diseases. Fenner found that although mice could be infected by intradermal, intraperitoneal, intracerebral, or intranasal inoculation of virus, the naturally occurring disease was most closely reproduced by intradermal inoculation with scarification. The naturally occurring infection was found to be introduced through minute abrasions of the skin and to spread from the primary or secondary skin lesions that subsequently developed. Although this mode of transmission obviously has little bearing on the spread of poxvirus infections in humans, the circumscribed period of infectiousness, limited to the period of skin eruption, is similar to what is thought to occur in human variola and varicella virus infections.

Effect of Immunity on Transmission – Herd Immunity

The resistance conferred by artificially or naturally acquired immunity may be expressed in the form of decreased susceptibility to the disease-producing potential of an infectious agent, as an increased resistance to the initiation of infection following exposure to the parasite, or as a combination of both of these effects. The term "herd immunity" is used to characterize the indirect protection conferred on the nonimmune segment of a population by a large segment of immune individuals who are less susceptible to infection and therefore less likely to serve as reservoirs for the spread of infection to others. The extent to which herd immunity influences the epidemic spread of an infectious agent through a population depends not only on the proportion of immune and nonimmune individuals in the population but on the degree to which immunity reduces susceptibility to the initiation of infection. Furthermore, it is essential to distinguish the effects produced by specific immunity acquired by previous infection from the kinds of effects engendered by vaccines.

Influenza. Observations of epidemic influenza in man have shown that immunity derived either from previous infection or by immunization against one of the subtypes of influenza virus provides protection against manifestations of disease following subsequent exposure to virus of the same subtype, and subjects possessing specific serum antibody are less likely to acquire infection (as shown by a rise in antibody titer) than nonimmune subjects under the same conditions of exposure (Francis, 1953; Davenport, 1961). However, infection with a subsequent rise in antibody titer has been clearly and repeatedly shown to occur in individuals with pre-existing antibody to the infecting influenza virus (Francis *et al.*, 1944; Bell *et al.*, 1961; Sigel *et al.*, 1950). It has been much more difficult to determine in the human host whether partially immune but infectable individuals can transmit infection to others. This problem has been investigated with an experimental model designed to study transmission of influenza virus infection in mice (Schulman, 1967b). Table 7-1 summarizes

TABLE 7-1

Effects of Immunity Induced by Prior Homotypic Infection or Injection with Inactivated Homotypic Virus on Transmission of Influenza A$_2$ Virus Infection in Mice

Immunization Procedure		Per cent of Contacts Infected
Infectors	Contacts	
1) A$_2$ infection		0
2)	A$_2$ infection	0
3) A$_2$ vaccine		50
4)	A$_2$ vaccine	6.4
5)		47.5

a series of experiments in which mice immunized by prior infection or injection of inactivated influenza A$_2$ virus were either exposed to aerosols of homotypic virus and used as infectors to transmit infection to other mice, or were used as contacts to assess their susceptibility to transmitted infection. Mice immunized by prior infection with live virus were completely refractory to reinfection on exposure to either artificial aerosols of virus or to "normal" infector mice, and therefore could not participate in transmission of infection either as infectors (line 1) or as contacts (line 2). In contrast, although mice immunized by injection with inactivated virus were as contacts less susceptible to the acquisition of transmitted infection (line 4), they were infectable by aerosols of virus, and following infection were fully capable of transmitting infection to normal contacts (line 3). If immunity against influenza operates in a similar fashion in men, the current practice of immunization with subcutaneously administered formalin inactivated vaccine would not be expected to exert an appreciable effect on herd immunity. There is very little doubt that immunization protects the recipients against disease caused by viruses antigenically similar to those in the vaccine, or that immunized subjects are less likely than unimmunized individuals to acquire infection under the same conditions of exposure. However, the likelihood of infection of immune individuals increases with repeated exposures during an epidemic, and if prior immunization with inactivated virus has no effect on the subsequent ability to shed virus and spread infection, then the unimmunized segment of the population would derive little secondary benefit.

Foot-and-Mouth Disease Virus Infection. Principles similar to those discussed in relation to influenza appear to be operative in infection of cattle with foot-and-mouth disease virus. Active or passive immunization by parenteral inoculation prevents the development of vesicles following challenge by the intramuscular, pharyngeal, or intranasal routes. Nevertheless, virus can readily be recovered from the esophageal-pharyngeal fluids of immunized animals challenged by the pharyngeal or intranasal

route (Sutmoller *et al.*, 1968). Parenteral immunization thus protects cattle against the development of subsequent disease, but it does not prevent infection of the animals or reduce the likelihood that they will become carriers capable of infecting other animals.
Poliovirus Infection. Some of the early observations of spread of infection with live attenuated poliovirus among immune and nonimmune individuals have been characterized as examples of experimental epidemiology in human subjects (Paul *et al.*, 1959). In these experiments, the duration and magnitude of virus shedding, the susceptibility to gastrointestinal infection and the spread of infection to contacts was studied in antibody-free subjects, and in subjects possessing serum antibody derived either by previous infection with wild-type virus or as a result of prior parenteral inoculation with inactivated poliovirus vaccine. The following conclusions summarize the results of several such studies:

1. Prior parenteral immunization with inactivated poliovirus does not reduce susceptibility to gastrointestinal infection with attenuated poliovirus administered orally or acquired as a result of contact infection (Sabin, 1959; Paul *et al.*, 1957, 1959).
2. Following infection with orally administered attenuated poliovirus, persons previously immunized with inactivated vaccine excrete virus in the stool for as long a period and in as high titer as nonimmune individuals, and are therefore a fully effective source for the spread of infection (Fox, 1959).
3. Naturally immune subjects are less readily infected than nonimmune or artificially immune subjects and when infected they excrete virus in lower titer and for a shorter period of time (Paul *et al.*, 1959).

The implications of these observations for the control of poliomyelitis are of great importance: Immunization with attenuated live virus vaccine not only protects the individual from viremia and paralytic poliomyelitis, but reduces the likelihood of gastrointestinal infection and subsequent spread of infection to nonimmune persons. However, in making comparisons of the effects on herd immunity induced by immunization with live and inactivated virus a note of caution must be introduced. There is evidence that circulation of wild-type virus has been suppressed in populations immunized exclusively with inactivated virus. The explanation that has been offered is that immunization with killed vaccine inhibits poliovirus replication in the oropharynx, and that in highly developed urban populations pharyngeal spread of infection is an important means of transmission (Gard, 1961).

Effects of Other Host Factors on Transmission of Infection

Other Infections. The interrelationships of one infection on susceptibility to a second infection have been a subject of extensive study over a considerable period of time. Such phenomena as the increased susceptibility to bacterial pneumonia associated with viral respiratory disease and the capacity of one virus to interfere with the initiation of infection with another are well-established biologic events. However, the specific effects on *transmission* of one infection mediated by simultaneous infection with another parasite have been more difficult to determine, and as a consequence, significant epidemiologic questions have remained unanswered. In a few instances, experiments in experimental epidemiology have provided models that have pointed to possible modes of interaction between human pathogens and their effects on transmission.

SIMULTANEOUS RESPIRATORY INFECTION WITH INFLUENZA VIRUS AND BACTERIAL PATHOGENS.   Glover (1941) infected ferrets by the respiratory route with both influenza virus and Group C streptococci, and compared the frequency of transmission of infection with each pathogen to uninfected contacts, with the results obtained with ferrets infected with either the bacterial or viral agent alone. The capacity to transmit streptococcal infection was enhanced in the doubly infected animals, but transmission of influenza virus was reduced. In another study, Schulman and Kilbourne (unpublished data) found that mice previously infected with *Bordetella bronchiseptica* (a pathogen commonly encountered in the lungs of mice) were less able to transmit influenza virus infection than mice infected with the virus alone, although pulmonary virus titers were similar in the two groups. Thus, in experimental animals, the pathologic response to bacterial infection of the respiratory tract reduces the release and transmission of influenza virus.

DISSEMINATION OF STAPHYLOCOCCI BY INFANTS INFECTED WITH ADENOVIRUS.   Eichenwald *et al.* (1961) observed that newborn infants infected with adenovirus were better disseminators of airborne staphylococci than other infants free of the upper respiratory virus infection. It was postulated that the nasal secretions produced by the adenovirus infection favored release and dispersion of staphylococci into the surrounding air.

"Bacterial Interference."   Shinefield *et al.* (1966) found that when infants were deliberately colonized with nonpathogenic strains of staphylococci soon after birth infection with more virulent strains was prevented and the pathogenic strain was eliminated from the nursery. This method has been successfully employed to prevent and to terminate epidemics of staphylococcal disease in newborn nurseries.

The Dangerous Transmitter.   Instances in which the source of infection of a number of people has been traced to a single individual have been common with a variety of infectious diseases other than the obvious examples such as typhoid or food poisoning where the carrier state or breaks in sanitary technique are critical factors. As a result of these observations the concept of the dangerous transmitter has evolved, which assumes that (1) some individuals have a far greater capacity to transmit infection than others, (2) these variations in the ability to transmit are not necessarily related to the severity of infection, and (3) in some instances the epidemic spread of infection may be more closely related to the number of good transmitters than to the total number of potential infectors in a population.

TUBERCULOSIS.   In their study of the airborne infection of guinea pigs with tubercle bacilli derived from tuberculosis wards, Riley and O'Grady (1961) observed that some patients disseminated more airborne tubercle bacilli, and infected exposed guinea pigs more quickly, than other patients with similar clinical findings.

INFLUENZA.   Similar variations in the capacity to transmit infection have been observed with influenza virus infection of mice. In each of a series of small cages three contact mice were exposed to a single infector for a 24-hour period. The contact animals then were removed, quarantined in separate cages and subsequently tested for infection. As shown in Table 7-2, contact mice exposed to the same infector tended

TABLE 7-2

**Expected and Observed Frequency of Infection Among Groups
of Three Contact Mice Exposed to Transmitted Influenza
Virus Infection**

	*Expected		Observed	
	No.	Per cent	No.	Per cent
3/3 contacts infected	3.0	15.9	7	36.8
2/3 contacts infected	7.7	40.5	4	21.1
1/3 contacts infected	6.5	34.2	2	10.5
0/3 contacts infected	1.8	9.4	6	31.6

19 cages (57 contact mice) 3 contacts and 1 infector in each cage; 31/57 infected; $p < 0.001$.

* $p^3 + 3p^2q + 3pq^2 + q^3 = 1$.

to have a similar likelihood of acquiring infection; more cages were found in which all or none of the contact mice were infected than would be expected by chance. In those cages where the infector mouse was an effective transmitter there was a tendency for all the contacts to acquire infection. In cages where the infector was a less effective transmitter, all the contacts tended to remain uninfected. When titers of pulmonary virus and extent of pneumonia in good and poor transmitters were compared, no differences were found (Schulman and Kilbourne, 1963).

The impact of such differences in the capacity to transmit infection on the epidemiology of human influenza could be profound. Exposure to a dangerous transmitter might be an important factor in explaining why persons with partial or heterotypic immunity, though less susceptible to the initiation of infection, frequently do become infected. Repeated exposure increases the likelihood of such an encounter and of eventual exposure to a large enough concentration of virus to overcome the increased resistance.

Variations in Transmissibility Among Different Strains of the Same Organism

The terms transmissibility, infectiousness, and virulence are sometimes used almost interchangeably to assess the propensity of an organism to initiate infection, replicate, and produce disease. However, these attributes are frequently unrelated and the terms used to describe them should be distinguished accordingly. *Transmissibility* refers to the contagiousness of a pathogen, e.g., its capacity to be disseminated from an infected host, to survive physical-chemical stresses in the environment and initiate infection in a new host. *Infectiousness* refers simply to the infective dose when administered by a particular route, e.g., the number of organisms required to initiate infection. *Virulence* relates to the capacity of an infecting organism to overcome host defenses and to produce disease. Studies in experimental epidemiology have shown clearly that these attributes are separable among different strains of the same organism.

Streptococci.   Coburn *et al.* (1957) found that streptococci isolated from naval recruits during epidemics were more infectious for mice by the respiratory route than other Group A streptococci, isolated during nonepidemic periods. No differences among the two varieties of streptococci were demonstrable in their infectiousness or virulence when given by the intraperitoneal route, indicating that only the capacity to initiate infection and produce disease in the respiratory tract of mice was related to the period of isolation.

Ectromelia.   Fenner (1948, 1949) found that the properties of virulence and trans-missibility were dissociable among different strains of ectromelia virus. When one strain (Moscow) was introduced into a mouse colony it spread very rapidly and was associated with a high mortality rate. The spread of a second strain (Hampstead) was slower, and resulted in a lower morbidity and mortality in the population into which it was introduced (Figure 7-1). Although the infectivity titers (ID/50) of the two strains by foot pad or intraperitoneal inoculation were identical, the lethality (LD/50) of the Moscow strain was much greater by both routes (less virus was required to kill mice). When mice were exposed to equal quantities of the two strains of virus sprayed on the bottom of equal amounts of sawdust in clean cages, nine times as many mice were infected with the Moscow strain as with the Hampstead strain (Fenner, 1949). There-fore, the Moscow strain though no more infectious by direct inoculation was not only more virulent for mice than the Hampstead strain, but was also more transmissible; i.e., more infectious when introduced into the environment. In a further dissociation of

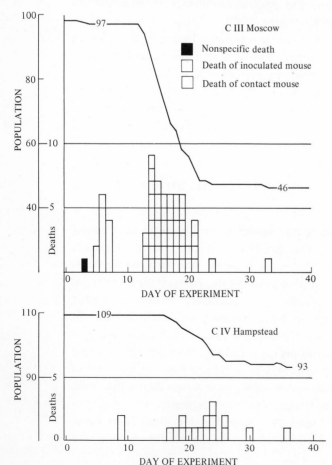

FIGURE 7-1. Mortality in epidemics of "Moscow" and "Hampstead" mouse-pox among normal adult male mice. Each block indicates the death of one mouse. (Reproduced from Schulman, J. L.: *J Exp Med*, **125**:484, 1967.)

virulence and transmissibility, Fenner (1949) demonstrated that an egg-passaged line of the Hampstead strain was as readily transmitted from mouse to mouse as the mouse-passaged strain, although its capacity to produce lesions and mortality was considerably reduced.

Influenza. The transmissibility of a variety of strains of influenza virus have been compared in an experimental model using mice (Schulman, 1967a, 1968). As indicated in Table 7-3, some strains of virus, notably the A_2 strains, were found to be more

TABLE 7-3

Comparison of Transmissibility of Different Strains of Influenza Virus

Virus	Infector Mice		Contact Mice	
	Pulmonary Virus Titer 48 hr.*	Lung Lesions day 7†	No. Infected	Total Per cent
S-15 (Swine)	7.8	45	2/20	(10)
NWS (A_0)	7.6	65	3/40	(7.5)
FM-1 (A_1)	8.7	65	2/20	(10)
Lee (B)	6.9	20	1/20	(15)
Jap. 305 (A_2)	7.6	60	25/40	(62.5)
A/A_2/60 (A_2)	7.1	20	11/20	(55)

* EID/50, $\log_{10}$.
† Extent of lung lesions (per cent).

readily transmitted than other strains that replicated to higher titer and produced more pneumonia in the lungs of infector mice. Detailed comparisons of two of these strains, the NWS strain of influenza A_0 (poorly transmitted) and the Jap.305 strain of influenza A_2 (well transmitted) produced the following results:

1. The Jap.305 strain was not better adapted to entering or surviving in the airborne state following aerosolization from a nebulizer.
2. Aerosols of the Jap.305 strain were no more infectious for mice than aerosols of similar quantities of NWS virus as shown in Figure 7-2.
3. Airborne virus could be recovered from the environment of infector mice infected with Jap.305 virus but not from the environment of NWS infected mice. Therefore, although the Jap.305 virus is no more virulent and no more infectious for mice, it is more transmissible, presumably because it possesses some property that facilitates release from the respiratory epithelium and enhances shedding into the environment.

Environmental Factors

The potent and varied effects of environmental influences on the incidence and severity of most epidemic infections of man are universally appreciated although not always precisely defined. The variations of disease related to seasonal and geographic factors are only the most obvious expressions of the crucial effects exerted by the environment.

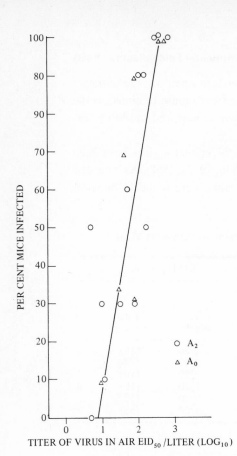

100

80

90

70

60

50

40

30

20

10

0

PER CENT MICE INFECTED

○ A$_2$

△ A$_0$

0   1   2   3

TITER OF VIRUS IN AIR EID$_{50}$/LITER (LOG$_{10}$)

FIGURE 7-2. Per cent of mice infected when exposed to varying airborne titers of influenza A$_0$ (NWS) and influenza A$_2$ (Jap.305) viruses. (Reproduced from Fenner, F.: *Brit J Exp Path*, **29**: 75, 1948.)

This section is not intended to provide a comprehensive review of such influences, but only to provide a few examples of the ways in which environmental influences have been elucidated by models in experimental epidemiology.

Relative Humidity and Transmission of Influenza. In some of the early studies with the previously described experimental model used to examine transmission of influenza virus infection in mice, it was found that virtually no transmission of infection occurred during the summer months, although virus replication and pneumonia in infector mice was identical to that observed during the winter. When the animal quarters were equipped to maintain constant conditions of temperature and relative humidity, most, but not all of this seasonal variation in transmission was eliminated, as seen in Table 7-4. In subsequent transmission experiments, conducted within a closed chamber with a regulated air flow, the profound effect of relative humidity was demonstrated more directly. At relative humidities above 50 per cent less transmission of infection occurred than at lower relative humidities (Schulman and Kilbourne, 1966). These observations were in accord with earlier studies (Hemmes, 1960; Harper, 1961), which showed that aerosolized influenza virus survived progressively less well as the relative humidity was increased above 30 per cent. In temperate areas the relative humidity tends to be lower during the winter months when the peak incidence of influenza is observed. However, other respiratory viruses, such as rhinoviruses, which also cause a higher incidence of infection during the winter months, are better adapted to survive at higher relative humidity (Buckland *et al.*, 1964).

Chilling. The physical stress on the host resulting from exposure to cold has also been suggested as a possible explanation for the higher incidence of respiratory

162

TABLE 7-4

Seasonal Variations in the Frequency of Transmitted Influenza Virus Infection in Mice*

Environmental Controls	Season	Number of Contact Mice Infected[†]
Room air conditioner and steam heat	July–October December–January	1/120 (0.8%) 48/216 (22.2%)
Year round controls 72 °F 50% R.H.	May–October November–April	109/320 (34.1%) 192/320 (58.2%)

* Reproduced from Schulman, J. L., and Kilbourne, E. D.: *Biometeorology*, **2**:83–84, 1966.

† Exposure to transmitted infection in small cages, two infected mice and two contact mice in each cage.

infections during the winter. Experiments were conducted at the Common Cold Research Unit at Salisbury to evaluate the effect of chilling on the susceptibility of volunteers to colds induced by rhinoviruses. No evidence was obtained to suggest that the frequency or severity of colds was increased in the chilled volunteers (Andrewes, 1965; Tyrrell, 1965). On the other hand, in similar studies, Dowling *et al.* (1957) found that chilling increased susceptibility to colds, but only in women in the middle third of the menstrual cycle.

Diet. Continuing the work initiated by Webster with *Salmonella typhimurium* infections in genetically resistant, genetically susceptible, and randomly bred strains of mice, Schneider (1967) has defined other variables that influence the pathogenesis of infection. Among these factors are the virulence of the organism and the presence or absence of a specific dietary substance (Salmonella resistance factor) that increases the resistance of mice to salmonella infection. In contrast to synthetically constituted diets, which lack the resistance factor (SRF), natural foodstuffs, particularly whole wheat, are rich sources of this substance, which has undergone extensive chemical analysis (Schneider, 1967). The complex relationships among diet and genetic attributes of the host and of the parasite are summarized schematically in Figure 7-3. Genetically resistant mice survive infection with virulent or avirulent strains of salmonella whether they are fed synthetic diets or natural foodstuffs. Similarly, dietary factors

FIGURE 7-3. The effect of a natural (N) and a synthetic (S) diet on survivorship following infection in nine different genetic circumstances. (Reproduced from Schneider, H. A.: *Science*, **158**: 597, 1967.)

		Host-Genotype		
		Inbred, selected, resistant	Random-bred, (outbred) nonselected	Inbred selected, susceptible
Pathogen-Genotype	Uniformly virulent	N - Died S - Died	N - Died S - Died	N - Died S - Died
	Mixed virulent and avirulent	N - Survived S - Survived	N - Survived ↑ Dietary effect ↓ S - Died	N - Died S - Died
	Uniformly avirulent	N - Survived S - Survived	N - Survived S - Survived	N - Survived S - Survived

do not influence the outcome in genetically susceptible mice infected with virulent salmonella or with mixtures of virulent and avirulent organisms. The effects of the dietary resistance factor can be seen only in randomly bred mice infected with mixtures of virulent and avirulent organisms. These experiments are an excellent example of the subtlety with which environmental factors may sometimes affect the pathogenesis of infection. It may be that some factors are demonstrable only when other variables have been properly manipulated so that they do not mask the expression of an effect attributable to the environment.

Ecologic Factors

The importance of animal reservoirs in the perpetuation and transmission of infectious pathogens of man may be far from fully appreciated. Although there are innumerable examples of the vital role played by animal reservoirs in some infections, there is a strong possibility that other epidemic human infections currently thought to be transmitted from man to man may also be influenced by animal reservoirs (Shope, 1965). For example, there is speculation that animal reservoirs may harbor influenza virus during interepidemic periods and may be an important source for the reintroduction of virus into the human population.

Swine Influenza.   The extensive studies of Shope on the ecology of swine influenza provide an excellent example of the complex mechanisms by which animal reservoirs interacting with pathogens and environmental influences may profoundly affect the epidemiology of infection. Shope's experiments have suggested that swine influenza is perpetuated by the following series of events:

1. While residing in the lungs of swine, the hog lung worm becomes an intermediate host to swine influenza virus, harboring the virus in a "masked" form.
2. Lung worm larvae excreted onto the soil are ingested by earth worms which in turn are ingested by pigs.
3. The lung worm larvae migrate from the gastrointestinal tract to the lungs still hardoring the hidden swine influenza virus.
4. Under suitable conditions of provocation, such as exposure of the pigs to cold weather, the virus begins to multiply and to produce influenza in the swine.
5. Once activated the swine influenza virus infection can be transmitted directly from one pig to another.

According to this hypothesis, the masked infection of the lung worm provides a mechanism to maintain the swine influenza virus in the pig population between epidemics (Shope, 1954).

Experimental Models with Tumor Viruses

One of the most active areas of virus research in recent years has been concerned with attempts to define the role played by virus infections in cancer. Although numerous examples of virus induced neoplasms have been clearly demonstrated in animals, the evidence for virus-induced human cancers has been far less conclusive. Animal models designed to study the epidemiologic relationships between viruses, animal hosts of different ages and genetic background, and the incidence of cancer have the potentiality of providing valuable information concerning the kinds of interactions which also may be operative in human cancer. Two such models will be discussed as examples.

Bittner's Mouse Mammary Carcinoma.   Bittner (1936) demonstrated that the differences among strains of mice in their susceptibility to mammary cancer was not exclusively a reflection of genetic attributes characteristic of different strains of mice as had previously been believed. He found that if newborn progeny of low-incidence strains were separated from their mothers after birth and were suckled by females from strains with a high incidence, strains of mice with a high incidence of mammary cancer developed. Conversely, high-incidence strains could be converted into low-incidence strains if the newborn mice were nursed by females from a low-incidence strain (Bittner, 1936). Subsequently the transmissible milk agent was shown to be a virus that could remain in the tissues of mice for long periods even skipping generations without producing disease.

Gross Mouse Leukemia Virus.   The interrelationships between genetic factors in inbred strains of mice, and selected strains of Gross mouse leukemia virus are more complex than those observed with mouse mammary cancer virus. Leukemia occurs spontaneously in high incidence (> 85 per cent) in the AKR strain of inbred mice which were specifically bred for this susceptibility, whereas the C3H strain has a very low incidence of spontaneous leukemia. When cell-free extracts from leukemic AKR mice were inoculated into newborn C3H mice only a few animals developed leukemia, but by serial passage of virus from selected mice a more virulent strain of virus was isolated capable of causing leukemia in over 95 per cent of suckling C3H mice inoculated in the neo-natal period. Infected females were capable of transmitting infection to their progeny through the milk. However, newborn C3H mice born of infected mothers but nursed by uninfected females had a low incidence of leukemia, proving that congenital transmission did not occur. In contrast, transmission of infection in AKR mice occurs regularly, even when newborn mice are nursed by low-incidence females, indicating that transmission in the AKR strain occurs *in utero*. (Gross, 1961)

At present, no equivalent relationships between tumor viruses, their mode of transmission, and the incidence of tumors have been established for man, but models such as these provide fundamental knowledge concerning methods for appropriate investigation directed at elucidating the relationships between viruses and human cancer.

CONCLUSIONS

All the examples cited in this chapter have dealt with infectious diseases, but experimental epidemiology also has the potentiality of providing information relevant to other types of diseases. Social and reproductive patterns have been studied in groups of laboratory animals subjected to a variety of environmental manipulations such as crowding, changes in diet, and chronic infection. Other experimental models have been designed to investigate the effects of long-term exposure to air pollutants on bronchopulmonary tissues of laboratory animals, and incidences of spontaneously occurring diseases like coronary artery disease and peptic ulcer have been observed in laboratory animals subjected to stress or dietary manipulations.

Therefore, properly designed models of experimental epidemiology can provide invaluable data concerning the relationships of a number of variables influencing the epidemic nature of disease and in conjunction with other types of investigations can help to formulate a rational basis for the prevention of these diseases.

REFERENCES

ANDREWES, C. H.: *The Common Cold*. Weidenfeld and Nicolson, London, 1965.
———, and ALLISON, A. C.: Newcastle disease as a model for studies of experimental epidemiology. *J Hyg (Camb.)* **59**:285–93, 1961.

BELL, J. A., CRAIGHEAD, J. E., JAMES, R. G., and WONG, D.: Epidemiologic observations on 2 outbreaks of Asian influenza in a children's institution. *Amer J Hyg*, **73**:84–89, 1961.

BITTNER, J. J.: Some possible effects of nursing on the mammary gland tumor incidence in mice. *Science*, **84**:162, 1936.

BUCKLAND, F. E., and TYRRELL, D. A.: Experiments on the spread of colds. 1. Laboratory studies on the dispersal of nasal secretion. *J Hyg (Camb.)*, **62**:365–67, 1964.

———, BYNOE, M. L., and TYRRELL, D. A. J.: Experiments on the spread of colds. II. Studies in volunteers with coxsackievirus A21. *Ibid.*, **63**:327–43, 1965.

COBURN, A. F., FRANK, P. F., and NOLAN, J.: Studies on the pathogenesis of streptococcus pyogenes. IV. The relationship between the capacity to induce fatal respiratory infections in mice and epidemic respiratory disease in man. *Brit J Exp Path*, **38**:256–67, 1957.

CONSTANTINE, D. G.: Rabies transmission by non bite route. *Public Health Rep*, **77**:287–89, 1962.

COUCH, R. B., CATE, T. R., DOUGLAS, R. G., GERONE, P. J., and KNIGHT, V.: Effect of route of inoculation on experimental respiratory viral disease in volunteers and evidence for airborne transmission. *Bact Rev*, **30**:517–29, 1966.

DOWLING, H. F., JACKSON, G. G., and INOUYE, T.: Transmission of the experimental common cold in volunteers. II. The effects of certain host facts upon susceptibility. *J Lab Clin Med*, **50**:516–25, 1957.

EICHENWALD, H. F., KOTSEVALOV, O., and FASSO, L. A.: Some effects of viral infection on aerial dissemination of staphylococci and on susceptibility to bacterial colonization. *Bact Rev*, **25**:274–81, 1961.

FENNER, F.: The epizootic behavior of mouse-pox (infectious ectromelia). *Brit J Exp Path*, **29**:69–91, 1948.

———: Mouse-pox (infectious ectromelia of mice): A review. *J Immun*, **63**:341–73, 1949.

FOX, J. P.: The influence of artificial immunization against poliomyelitis upon virus dissemination. In Najjai, V. A. (ed.): *Immunity and Virus Infection*. John Arley and Sons, New York, 1959.

FRANCIS, T., Jr., PEARSON, H. E., SALK, J. E., and BROWN, P. N.: Immunity in human subjects artificially infected with influenza virus, Type B. *Amer J Public Health*, **34**:317–34, 1944.

GARD, S.: Exit Poliomyelitis—what next? *Yale J Biol Med*, **34**:277–88, 1961–62.

GLOVER, R. E.: Spread of infection from the respiratory tract of the ferret. II. Association of influenza A virus and streptococci group C. *Brit J Exp Path*, **22**:98–107, 1941.

GREENWOOD, M., HILL, A. B., TOPLEY, W. W. C., and WILSON, J.: Experimental epidemiology. *Med Res Counc Spec Rep (London)*, Ser 209. 1936.

GROSS, L.: *Oncogenic Viruses*. Pergamon Press, New York, 1961.

HARPER, G. J.: Airborne micro-organisms: survival tests with 4 viruses. *J Hyg (Camb.)*, **59**:479–86, 1961.

HEMMES, J. C., WINKLER, K. C., and KOOL, S. M.: Virus survival as a seasonal factor in influenza and poliomyelitis. *Nature (London)*, **188**:430–31, 1960.

MCLEAN, R. L.: In *International Conference on Asian Influenza*. *Amer Rev Resp Dis*, **83** Part 2: 36–38, 1961.

PAUL, J. R., HORSTMANN, D. M., MELNICK, J. L., NIEDERMAN, J. C., and DEUTCH, J.: Immunization against poliomyelitis: Killed vaccine followed by induced infection with live virus. *Spec Pub NY Acad Sci*, **5**:141–47, 1957.

———, ———, and NIEDERMAN, J. C.: Immunity in poliomyelitis infection: Observations in experimental epidemiology. In Najjar, V. A. (ed.): *Immunity and Virus Infection*. John Wiley and Sons, New York, 1959.

RILEY, R. L., and O'GRADY, F.: *Airborne Infection: Transmission and Control*. The Macmillan Company, New York, 1961.

SABIN, A. B.: Present position of immunization against poliomyelitis with live virus vaccine. *Brit Med J*, **1**:663–80, 1959.

SCHNEIDER, H. A.: Ecological ectocrines in experimental epidemiology. *Science*, **158**:597–603, 1967.

SCHULMAN, J. L.: Experimental transmission of influenza virus infection in mice. IV. Relationship of transmissibility of different strains and recovery of airborne virus in the environment of infector mice. *J Exp Med*, **125**:479–88, 1967a.

———: Experimental transmission of influenza virus infection in mice. III. Differing effects of immunity induced by infection and by inactivated influenza virus vaccine on transmission of infection. *Ibid*, **125**:467–78, 1967b.

———: The use of an experimental model to study transmission of influenza virus infection in mice. *Amer J Public Health*, **58**:2092–96, 1968.

———, and KILBOURNE, E. D.: Airborne transmission of influenza virus infection in mice. *Nature (London)*, **195**:1129–30, 1962.

———, and ———: Experimental transmission of influenza virus infection in mice. II. Some factors affecting the incidence of transmitted infection. *J Exp Med*, **118**:267–75, 1963.

———, and ———: Seasonal variations in the transmission of influenza virus infection in mice. *Biometeorology*, **2**:83–87, 1966.

SHINEFELD, H. R., WILSEY, J. D., RIBBLE, J. C., BORIS, M., EICHENWALD, H. F., and DITTMAR, C. J.: Interaction of staphylococcal colonization. *Amer J Dis Child*, **111**:11–21, 1966.

SHOPE, R. E.: Ecology and virus reservoirs. In Hartman, F. W., Horsfall, F. L., Jr., and Kidd, J. G. (eds.): *The Dynamics of Virus and Rickettsial Infections*. Blakiston, New York, 1954.

———: Transmission of viruses and epidemiology of viral infections. In Horsfall, F. L., Jr., and Tamm, I. (eds.): *Viral and Rickettsial Infections of Man*, 4th ed. Lippincott, Philadelphia, 1965.

SIGEL, M. M., KITH, A. W., LIGHT, A. B., and HENLE, W.: The recurrence of influenza A prime in a boarding school after 2 years. *J Immun*, **64**:33–38, 1950.

SUTMOLLER, P., MCVICAR, J. W., and COTTRAL, G. E.: The epizootiological importance of foot-and-mouth disease carriers. I. Experimentally produced foot-and-mouth disease carriers in susceptible and immune cattle. *Arch Ges Virusforsch*, **23**:227–35, 1968.

TYRRELL, D. A. J.: *Common Colds and Related Diseases*. Arnold, London, 1965.

WEBSTER, L. T.: Experimental epidemiology. *Medicine (Balt.)*, **25**:77–109, 1946.

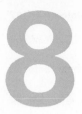

Screening
and
Mass Surveys

Jerome L. Schulman

With the growing importance of chronic degenerative neoplastic, and congenital diseases as the major health problems in highly industrialized societies, increasing attention has been given in recent years to finding methods to control these diseases by early diagnosis. This interest has resulted in a number of projects, supported privately and by local, state, and federal agencies, designed to survey large numbers of asymptomatic individuals in the population for the presence of previously undetected disease. These attempts at mass screening should be distinguished from the procedures employed by individual physicians and by clinics providing periodic routine examinations to patients under their care. There are several examination procedures that are an integral part of the routine practice of physicians delivering a high standard of medical care that obviously are not suited to the examination of large groups of people over a relatively short period of time (see Chapter 15).

PURPOSES

Epidemiologic Survey

Mass screening procedures provide the opportunity to obtain data that will permit a more accurate assessment of the prevalence of certain diseases in our society. Such information about the patterns of disease in turn may be useful in providing hints about factors that contribute to these disease processes.

Obtaining Data Concerning the Pathogenesis of Specific Diseases

Confirmation of the presence of specific diseases in appreciable numbers of asymptomatic people provides the opportunity to enhance our understanding of the natural history and pathogenesis of these diseases.

Early Diagnosis

The most important practical purpose served by mass screening procedures is to detect the disease early in its course in order to prevent the expression of its full pathogenic potential. In the case of infectious diseases such as tuberculosis there are obviously additional advantages to early detection of asymptomatic cases. Not only may the spread of disease to other individuals be prevented by treatment of infectious cases, but detection of infection in the index case may lead to the discovery of previously unsuspected disease in close family members.

Health Education

Mass screening procedures also provide an opportunity to educate the public about prevention of certain diseases and to create a constructive awareness of the useful function served by periodic health examinations.

CRITERIA USED TO ASSESS THE SUITABILITY OF SPECIFIC EXAMINATIONS PROCEDURES FOR USE IN A MASS SCREENING PROGRAM

In evaluating a particular procedure for use in a mass screening program, attributes of the procedure itself, and of the disease it is designed to detect, must both be considered. Neither a simple reliable test for an unimportant disease, nor a difficult, inaccurate test for a disease with high morbidity and mortality is appropriate for a mass screening program.

Sensitivity

Diagnostic procedures that result in a high frequency of false negative results are undesirable for use on a mass basis because of their obvious inefficiency.

Specificity

A high frequency of false positive results is also undesirable and requires a disproportionate effort in following up the initial diagnostic results to disprove their validity. With some screening procedures the requirements for sensitivity and specificity conflict with one another, sometimes making it difficult to determine at what values the results of a particular test should be considered abnormal. There may be a range of values in which both false positive and false negative results are encountered, requiring that sensitivity or specificity be sacrificed. For example, in glaucoma screening some cases are missed if the normal limits for ocular tension are set at 25.8 mm Hg, but if the limits are lowered to 23.7 mm Hg the number of false positives increases appreciably. Such difficulties are much more likely to be encountered when the diagnostic procedure measures an attribute distributed normally in the population than when the values it measures are distributed in a bimodal fashion.

Safety and Ease

Obviously only those diagnostic procedures that are simple and convenient to perform and that are associated with virtually no complications or discomfort are acceptable for use as mass screening procedures. Ideally, physicians or other highly trained personnel should not be required to perform the procedures or to interpret the results because such a requirement increases the cost and limits the number of tests that can be made.

Expense

The cost of the procedure is also of crucial importance. With only limited funds available for mass screening purposes it would be wasteful to allocate a disproportionate amount of money for any single test. In considering expense however, an evaluation of the cost to society of not performing the test on a mass basis also has to be made. The burden placed upon society, economic or social, that results from failing to detect the particular disease in a reversible stage may justify a greater initial effort at mass screening. Thus, relative to the number of confirmed diagnoses that are made, the cost of performing routine tests on all newborn infants for phenylketonuria (see Chapter 2) may be great, but the cost to society, to say nothing of the human suffering, that results from failing to prevent the mental retardation associated with this inborn error is appreciably greater.

Prevalence and Pathogenic Potential of Disease

Whenever possible it is desirable to employ procedures designed to detect those diseases that are most prevalent and that produce the most morbidity and mortality in the population being tested. The yield from attempts to diagnose rare or relatively innocuous diseases may not be great enough to justify the effort.

Capability of Reversing or Preventing the Pathogenic Potential of the Disease for Which the Test Is Designed

To be effective as a mass screening procedure, a diagnostic test must have the capability of detecting disease early enough in its course to prevent the severe complications and mortality that otherwise would result. Therefore, it is appropriate to demand that treatment measures are more effective when they are initiated in an asymptomatic stage of the disease than when therapy is begun after the appearance of symptoms. It would be foolish, for example, to suggest mass screening for systemic lupus erythematosis, not only because it is a relatively uncommon disease, but because there is no evidence to suggest that the normal pathogenesis of the disease can be reversed by therapy begun before symptoms appear.

Facilities for Follow-up

One of the most important requirements for screening programs in general and for any specific screening procedure to be effective is that results can be integrated into the activities of existing health services. Unless new cases are reported and verified and appropriate therapy instituted, the potential therapeutic benefits of a screening program will be dissipated.

SCREENING FOR SPECIFIC DISEASES

Cancer Detection

In theory at least, neoplastic diseases seem ideally suited to some degree of control by early detection through mass screening programs. Cancers originating in a single primary focus presumably pass through a stage when they are localized to the tissues in which they originate. If they can be detected during this stage, they can be surgically removed or destroyed by irradiation before they invade other tissues and metastasize. Unfortunately, not all cancers can be discovered during this stage because techniques are not available for early detection and because some highly malignant forms of cancer appear to spread extremely early in the course of their growth. Although several cancer detection clinics have organized a routine series of examinations and laboratory measurements designed to detect a wide variety of asymptomatic malignancies, no general statement can be made concerning the usefulness of currently available techniques for the early detection of cancer. Each form of cancer and the procedures available for its detection must be evaluated separately.

Carcinoma of the Cervix.   Probably the most universally accepted and proved screening test for cancer is the use of exfoliative cytology for the detection of cancerous and precancerous lesions of the cervix. The sensitivity of this technique in detecting preinvasive cervical cancer and the extremely low mortality following treatment during this stage has been demonstrated in numerous studies. In fact, the results from appropriate use of this technique has led to the conjecture that death from cancer of the cervix is 100 per cent preventable (Day, 1964). The requirement for a physician to obtain the cervical scrape specimen has prompted trials of a substitute procedure in which the patient obtains the specimen herself by vaginal irrigation, then mails the specimen to a central laboratory for diagnosis. Evaluations of this technique have suggested that it is only slightly less sensitive than the older method and that it has the distinct potential advantage of being accessible to segments of the population that are not now routinely examined for cancer of the cervix.

Carcinoma of the Breast.   According to estimates of the American Cancer Society, cancer of the breast is the most common fatal cancer in women in the United States, accounting for 20 per cent of all cancer deaths in women. The vast majority of these cancers are discovered only after the patient herself has noticed a gross abnormality, unfortunately, at a time when many of these tumors have spread to adjacent lymph nodes. The five-year survival rate for such patients in many studies has been around 50 per cent. In contrast, follow-up of patients who had their breast cancer detected by breast palpation during a routine examination at the Cancer Detection Center of the University of Minnesota has shown a 92 per cent five-year survival, indicating considerable improvement in prognosis resulting from early diagnosis of breast cancer in asymptomatic women (Gilbertsen, 1967). In recent years, attempts have been made to utilize mammography and infrared thermography to facilitate the diagnosis of small cancerous lesions of the breast. Mammography is capable of detecting cancers of the breast that were not evident on physical examination, but conversely, mammography failed to detect some microscopically proved cases of breast cancer initially diagnosed by breast palpation (Shapiro et al., 1966). Thermography has not had as extensive an evaluation, but preliminary findings indicate that thermography is abnormal in 94 per cent of proven cases of breast cancer. However, 25 per cent of women with normal breasts or with benign dysplasia also had abnormal findings on thermography. (Gershon-Cohen et al., 1965). Thermography although associated with a 25 per cent incidence of false positive results appears to be a highly sensitive technique to detect very early asymptomatic breast cancers, and has the distinct advantage of requiring far less participation of highly trained physicians to perform or interpret the test than is necessary for breast palpation or mammography. It may be that thermography will be useful as a preliminary mass screening device, directing the attention of physicians to those women who require careful palpation of the breast and mammography.

Carcinoma of the Colon.   According to figures of the American Cancer Society, cancer of the colon is the most common internal cancer in the United States, and ranks second only to cancer of the lung as a cause of death from cancer. The five-year survival rate for localized cancers of the colon is 68 per cent but the five-year survival rate for patients with cancers that have spread regionally is only 34 per cent, emphasizing the value of early diagnosis. Furthermore, approximately 70 per cent of all tumors are within reach of the sigmoidoscope and therefore are potentially recognizable in an early asymptomatic stage. However, sigmoidoscopy is not a simple procedure; it is time-consuming for the physician and unacceptable to many patients. Routine sigmoidoscopy is desirable in patients over 40 years of age and is a feasible practice for many private practitioners and clinics, but facilities and personnel are presently not available to employ sigmoidoscopy as a mass screening procedure.

Bronchogenic Carcinoma.   Cancer of the lung is presently the leading cause of death from cancer. Unfortunately attempts at early diagnosis by periodic routine chest x-ray examination have not produced impressive results in terms of increased 5-year survival. Asymptomatic patients who have had their lung cancer diagnosed by participation in such a screening program have only a slightly higher survival rate than the over-all 5-year survival of 5–8 per cent observed in most medical centers (Lilienfeld et al., 1966). It would appear that many of these tumors have already spread regionally or metastasized by the time they are detectable by x-ray. Therefore, unless new techniques such as cytologic examination of sputum prove to be more sensitive in detecting bronchogenic carcinoma at a very early stage, it would appear that continued public education about the relationship of lung cancer to cigarette smoking is a more promising approach to the reduction of morbidity and mortality from lung cancer. However, x-ray examination of the chest is such a simple and relatively inexpensive procedure that is capable of detecting abnormalities other than lung cancer that it would be difficult to justify not including it in a mass screening program.

Cancer of the Prostate.   Although its importance is often not appreciated, cancer of the prostate accounts for approximately 10 per cent of the cancer deaths in men.

According to data collected at the National Cancer Institute the 5-year survival of men with this form of cancer is only 40 per cent of that seen in men of the same age without prostatic cancer. In contrast, the relative 5-year survival of men who had their prostatic cancers diagnosed at the University of Minnesota Cancer Detection Center was 95 per cent (Gilbertsen, 1967).

Cancer of the Oropharynx, Larynx, and Neck.   Cancer of the oropharynx, larynx, and neck accounts for approximately 11,000 deaths/years in the United States, and according to Day (1964) 50 per cent of these deaths could be prevented by early diagnosis. Adequate examination requires inspection and palpation of the tissues of the oropharynx and neck and indirect laryngoscopy with adequate light.

Skin Cancer.   Although cancer of the skin is the most commonly occurring cancer, it is the cause of only 1.5 per cent of all cancer deaths in the United States. With the exception of melanoma, however, deaths from skin cancer are thought to be nearly 100 per cent preventable (Day, 1964) by early detection and treatment.

Cancer of the Stomach.   Although the incidence of cancer of the stomach in the United States has been steadily decreasing in recent years, it was still responsible for the deaths of over 17,000 Americans in 1967, many of which could have been prevented if early diagnosis were possible. It is obvious that routine x-ray examination of the upper gastrointestinal tract is neither feasible nor desirable on a mass basis. An alternative approach based on the observation that patients with gastric carcinoma frequently are achlorhydric has been to measure gastric acidity with and without histamine stimulation. Unfortunately this test results in an incidence of 40–75 per cent false positives depending on the age distribution of the population being tested (Gilbertsen and Knatterud, 1967). In addition, the 5-year survival rate was only 9 per cent in patients with stomach cancer associated with achlorhydria, in contrast to a 20 per cent survival rate in patients with gastric carcinoma and normal gastric acidity. Gastric analysis therefore is not a sensitive method to detect early potentially curable cases of stomach cancer.

Cancer Detection Programs

In the past 20 years several clinics have been established for the sole purpose of screening relatively large numbers of asymptomatic people for cancer. These clinics obtain a pertinent history and perform thorough physical examinations including gynecologic examination and sigmoidoscopy. Laboratory tests include blood counts, urinalysis, chest x-ray, and usually stool guaiac. Although these centers have been able to detect 10–20 cancers for every 1,000 patients they have examined (Day, 1964; Gilbertsen, 1967), it is evident that such clinics can screen only a small segment of the population, and their value thus far has been primarily to demonstrate the lifesaving potentialities of screening programs specifically for cancer.

Screening for Cardiovascular Disease

Elevated Blood Pressure.   Ignoring for the moment the controversial question of defining what is an abnormal blood pressure, there is very little doubt that hypertension is one of the most prevalent conditions in the United States. According to data from the National Health Survey, U.S. Public Health Service (1964) there are over 11,000,000 adult Americans with diastolic blood pressures of 95 mm Hg or greater. There is also very little doubt that although many individuals survive long-standing hypertension without complications, the increased morbidity and mortality consequent to hypertension in some segments of the population is appreciable. The association of hypertension with cerebral vascular accidents, coronary artery disease, hypertensive heart disease, and renal insufficiency is well known. There is still considerable controversy over the interpretation of results of long-term follow-up of treated hypertensive individuals in terms of the degree to which risks of complications of hypertension are reduced. Some investigators found that cerebral vascular accidents, heart disease, and renal insufficiency were encountered less frequently in subjects whose blood pressures were well controlled by treatment, (Lee *et al.*, 1963; Moyer and Brest, 1961; Perry *et al.*, 1966; Sokolow and Perloff, 1965), but others argue that the meager benefit for most patients does not justify the risk of complications of therapy (Goldring and Chasis, 1966). However, there is abundant evidence that treatment of malignant hypertension results in a considerably improved prognosis. Furthermore, an appreciable proportion of individuals with elevated blood pressure suffer from disorders that are potentially correctable. These conditions, which are reviewed elsewhere in this text (see Chapter 15), include pheochromocytoma, hyperaldosteronism, Cushing's disease, coarctation of the aorta, and renal vascular disease. Mass screening for hypertension can be justified therefore because (1) it is such a simple rapid examination procedure, (2) a significant proportion of hypertensive individuals have underlying disorders that can be altered by therapy, and (3) early onset of therapy may reduce the risks of complications.

Screening for Coronary Artery Disease

Although at present there is no sensitive technique available to detect asymptomatic coronary disease at a time when its further pathogenesis can be interrupted, it is possible to screen large numbers of people for the presence of factors associated with an increased risk of developing coronary artery disease. These risk factors, which include hypertension, hyperlipidemia, obesity, diabetes, family history of coronary artery disease, and history of smoking are discussed more fully in Chapter 15. For the purposes of the present discussion, the pertinent question is whether mass screening of appropriate segments of the population is a potentially effective approach to the prevention of coronary artery disease. Considered from this standpoint it is not sufficient merely to identify the presence of one or more risk factors in screened individuals; it is essential that appropriate treatment or change of habit patterns results in a decreased risk of subsequently developing coronary artery disease. United States Public Health Service statistics indicate clearly that the discontinuance of smoking is associated with a decreased mortality from coronary artery disease, but it is still not clear whether the treatment of obesity, hypertension, diabetes, and hypercholesterolemia result in similar reductions of risk.

Screening for Diabetes

Estimates of the prevalence of diabetes in the United States place the number of un-diagnosed diabetics at more than 2 million (McDonald *et al.*, 1965). Efforts to detect these unsuspected cases have been increasing in recent years especially with the advent of the Auto Analyzer and its capacity to inexpensively determine blood glucose levels in a number of specimens simultaneously. The yield from such screening programs varies with the population being tested, the percentage of new cases being highest in obese individuals over 40 years of age with a family history of diabetes. Most of these unsuspected cases of diabetes are relatively mild and are less likely to be associated with subsequent acidosis or coma. Nevertheless, this form of diabetes is associated with a significantly increased risk of coronary artery disease, renal disease, and neu-ropathy and the need to detect the disease very early in its course would be urgent if early detection decreased the risk of developing one or more of these complications. Unfortunately evidence for such a clearly demonstrable beneficial effect is not avail-able. In a 10-year follow-up of patients at the Joslin Clinic in Boston the death rate from heart disease and cerebral vascular accident was more than two times greater and the death rate from renal vascular disease 17 times greater in diabetics than in normal individuals of the same ages (Entmacher *et al.*, 1964). However, the presence of diabetes in these patients was not detected by mass screening procedures, and diagnosis and initiation of treatment in an earlier stage might have resulted in lower mortality from these complications. There is no doubt that with the advances in treatment of diabetes the life expectancy of diabetics has been increased. Furthermore, in recent years the concept of prediabetes has been introduced (Camerini, 1965) to define "the state of those individuals who will eventually develop diabetes but in whom no abnormality of carbohydrate metabolism is demonstrable." Prediabetics are considered to be those individuals with a strong genetic or constitutional (obesity, history of delivering large babies, etc.) disposition to develop overt diabetes in the future, and as a group they demonstrate several subtle abnormalities (higher rates of bound/free insulin, etc.). Studies are in progress to determine whether treatment of these individuals with oral hypoglycemic agents will prevent the onset of frank diabetes.

Screening for Glaucoma

It is estimated that glaucoma which is the second leading cause of blindness in the United States is present in over one million people in an undiagnosed form. As there is abundant evidence that treatment of this disease in an early stage can prevent blindness, the need for early detection is clear, and in consequence a number of mass screening programs for glaucoma have been conducted in recent years. In some of these surveys nurses have been trained to make the actual determinations of intra-ocular pressure with a Schütz tonometer under the supervision of opthalmologists (Frydman *et al.*, 1966). This technique is safe, simple, rapid, and inexpensive, but one difficulty has been in assigning limits for normal values. In one study (Frydman *et al.*,

1966) lowering the value from 25.8 mm Hg to 23.7 resulted in an increase of 8.6 per cent in the number of cases found, but 91 per cent of those referred for additional examination were found to be normal, and it was found to be more efficient to rescreen individuals with borderline measurements than to refer them to opthalmologists directly.

Screening for Phenylketonuria

The genetically determined inability to convert phenylalanine to tyrosine is a rare disorder, but one with profound consequences. Lack of treatment of infants results in severe mental retardation (see Chapter 2). The development of suitable screening tests such as the Guthrie inhibition assay method has led to the adoption of legislation in many states making it mandatory to screen newborn infants for this disorder. With wide applications of these tests several difficulties have become evident. Conditions other than phenylketonuria can produce elevated blood levels of phenylalanine in the neonatal period, requiring careful chemical analysis of serum and urinary amino acids before a definitive diagnosis is made. The fact that overtreatment in the form of too severe a restriction of phenylalanine has resulted in mental retardation, anemia, growth failure, and rachitic bone formation only serves to emphasize the need for accurate differential diagnoses. Furthermore, it is now evident that non phenyl-ketonuric children born of mothers in whom the metabolic deficiency is present in an asymptomatic form may suffer mental retardation as a consequence of exposure to elevated levels of phenylalanine *in utero* (Mabry *et al.*, 1966). The problem of mental retardation resulting from maternal phenylketonuria could become magnified as treated phenylketonuric female infants reach childbearing age unless phenylalanine restriction is reinstituted during gestation.

Screening of Infants and School-age Children

The value of periodic health examinations during infancy and childhood is so generally accepted as an integral part of good pediatric practice that it does not require defending. An outline and some examples of the most essential examinations are given below.

A. Neonatal Period
   1. Congenital defects, e.g., cardiac defects, omphacele, meningocele cleft palate, pyloric stenosis, etc.
   2. Disorders arising during the neonatal period, e.g., sepsis, respiratory distress syndrome, etc.

B. Post neonatal period
   1. Growth and development—including height, weight, motor coordination.
   2. Congenital disorders not evident at birth.
   3. Nutritional status.

C. Childhood
   1. Growth and development.
   2. Intellectual development.

3. Sensory development.
   a. Visual acuity and eye-muscle balance.
   b. Audiometric tests.
4. Congenital disorders—especially cardiac.
5. Other abnormalities, e.g., orthopedic, hernia, undescended testes, and so on.

In many communities, examination of school-age children is mandatory and physicians are often provided to examine children in the schools. Nevertheless many children in the United States still do not have periodic health examinations, and the need to extend these services to those segments of the population, particularly in the lowest socioeconomic classes is urgent.

Screening for Tuberculosis

Although the incidence of tuberculosis has declined steadily in the United States in recent years, there are still groups within our population that have 10–15 times as much active tuberculosis as the national average. Screening tests for unsuspected tuberculosis is usually advised for the following groups:

1. Contacts of known active cases.
2. High-risk groups.
   a. Institutionalized populations.
   b. Alcoholics.
   c. Immigrants from areas of high prevalence of tuberculosis.
   d. People residing in close contact in poorly ventilated areas, e.g., naval personnel.
3. Residents of area in the United States with a high incidence of tuberculosis, particularly slum dwellers.
4. Medical personnel.

The type of screening test performed depends on the group being tested. Thus, the tuberculin skin test is particularly useful in testing school children. Not only can positive reactors be treated as potential new cases of tuberculosis, but family contacts can be examined to find the source of the infection. In segments of the population where the rate of positive skin reaction to tuberculin is higher, such as in alcoholics or institutionalized populations, periodic chest x-ray examination is the most useful procedure.

Screening for Chronic Pulmonary Disease

With the growing importance of chronic bronchitis and emphysema as a major health problem in the United States, convenient methods have been sought to detect loss of pulmonary function in its earliest stages, with the view of preventing further loss of respiratory reserve. Most commonly, the method used is to measure a 1- or 2-second timed vital capacity and to compare the value with standards for persons of the same age and height. In a single examination this technique is prone to false positive results because it requires the complete understanding and cooperation of the patient. Furthermore, with the exception of avoidance of bronchial irritants, particularly cigarette smoke and known allergens, specific methods of treatment have not been conclusively shown to alter the usual course of the disease. Nevertheless, it seems prudent to include such examinations of respiratory function in any mass screening program partiçularly of men over 40 years of age and of habitual cigarette smokers.

AUTOMATED MULTIPLE SCREENING PROGRAMS

One of the greatest handicaps to establishing mass screening programs is the difficulty in procuring sufficient trained personnel to operate the program, and even when such personnel are available, the cost may be prohibitive. One answer to this problem has been the use of automated procedures operated by paramedical personnel to handle as much of the examination procedure as is possible. In one such system (Collen, 1966) the automated laboratory provides electrocardiography chest and breast x-rays, tests of visual acuity, tonometry, retinal photography, audiometry, and a 1 sec. vital capacity measurement. Gynecologic examination on female patients and sigmoidoscopy are performed routinely on all patients over 40 years of age. Blood pressure, resting pulse, and anthropometric measurements, blood counts, and urinalysis are obtained routinely. From a single blood sample eight blood chemistry measurements are determined simultaneously in a multichannel chemical analyzer. In addition, the patient is given a health questionaire in the form of a series of prepunched cards. A diagram of the system is shown in Figure 8-1. All the data are fed into a computer, which prints out a summary report including recommendations for further tests. Only then does the patient see a physician, who can then explore more fully those areas that require further investigation.

Although the mechanical, assembly line nature of such a system seems contrary to long-cherished values of privacy and individuality in medical care, these automated systems could potentially increase the efficiency and reduce the cost of mass screening programs, and could provide a realistic basis by which systematic periodic examinations could be provided for the large portion of our population for which they are not now available.

ROLE OF THE INDIVIDUAL PHYSICIAN

Mass screening programs have not been designed to compete with the activities of the individual private practitioner. In most instances, the screening programs do not provide treatment. Instead they refer suspicious cases to the patient's physician for further evaluation and treatment. It is mandatory therefore that the individual practitioner be familiar with these programs, and further that he be equipped to evaluate the reliability and provide adequate follow-up to the reports furnished to him.

FUTURE POSSIBILITIES

As technologic advances are made, the value of mass screening programs may expand dramatically in the future. New techniques may become available that will permit

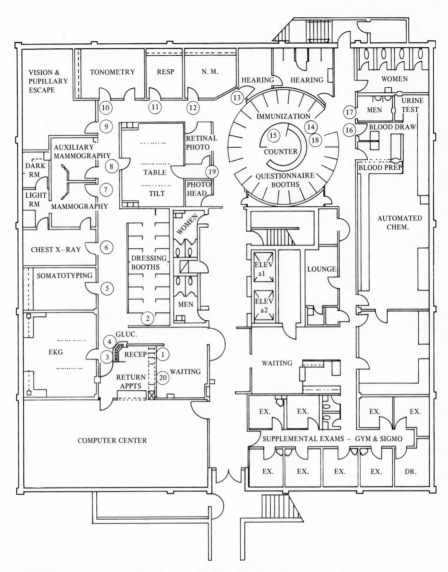

FIGURE 8-1. Design of facility for automated multitest laboratory. (Reproduced from Collen, M. F.: *JAMA*, **195**:831, 1966.)

screening for diseases for which accurate detection methods do not presently exist. For example, a reliable screening method for serum hepatitis could appreciably affect the incidence of this disease by excluding currently unrecognizable infected individuals from serving as blood donors. Another future function of mass screening may be as an adjunct to genetic counseling (see Chapter 2). Convenient methods may become available to detect heterozygous carriers of disease traits (e.g., persons heterozygous for phenylketonuria). This detection would provide a basis for assessing the risks of genetic abnormalities developing from specific matings.

REFERENCES

CAMERINI-DAVALOS, R. A.: Prevention of diabetes mellitus. *Med Clin N Amer*, **49**:865–79, 1965.

COLLEN, M. F.: Periodic health examinations using an automated multitest laboratory. *JAMA*, **195**:830–33, 1966.

DAY, E.: A critique on cancer detection program. *New York J Med*, **64**:365–75, 1964.

ENTMACHER, P. S., ROOT, H. F., and MARKS, H. H.: Longevity of diabetic patients in recent years. *Diabetes*, **13**:373–77, 1964.

FRYDMAN, J. E., CLOWER, J. W., FULGHUM, J. E., and HESTER, M. W.: Glaucoma detection in Florida. *JAMA*, **198**:1237–40, 1966.

GERSHON-COHEN, J., HABERMAN-BRUESHKE, J. D., and BRUESHKE, E. E.: Medical thermography: A summary of current status. *Radiol Clin N Amer*, **3**:403–31, 1965.

GILBERTSEN, V. A.: The case for periodic cancer detection examination. *CA*, **17**:219–25, 1967.

———, and KNATTERUD, G. L.: Gastric analysis as a screening method for cancer of the stomach. *Cancer*, **20**:127–33, 1967.

GOLDRING, W., and CHASIS, H.: Antihypertensive drug therapy: An appraisal. In Ingelfinger, F. J., Relman, A. S., and Finland, M. (eds.): *Controversy in Internal Medicine*, W. B. Saunders Co., Philadelphia, 1966.

LEE, R. E., SELIGMANN, A. W., CLARK, M. A., and ROUSSEAU, P. A.: Freedom from cerebral vascular accidents during drug-induced blood pressure reduction in "benign" hypertensive disease. *Amer J Cardiol*, **11**:738–42, 1963.

LILIENFELD, A. *et al.*: An evaluation of radiologic and cytologic screening for the early detection of lung cancer: a cooperative pilot study of the American Cancer Society and The Veterans Administration. *Cancer Res*, **26**:2083–2121, 1966.

MABRY, C. C., DENNISTON, J. C., and CALDWELL, J. G.: Mental retardation in children of phenylketonuric mothers. *New Eng J Med*, **275**:1331–36, 1966.

McDONALD, G. W., FISHER, G. F., and PENTZ, P. C.: Diabetes screening activities July 1958 to June 1963. *Public Health Rep*, **80**:163–72, 1965.

MOYER, J. H., and BREST, A. N.: Long-term effects of antihypertension therapy. In Brest, A. N., and Moyer, J. H. (eds.): *Hypertension, Recent Advances*. Lea and Febiger, Philadelphia, 1961.

PERRY, H. M., JR., SCHROEDER, H. A., CATANZARO, F. J., MOORE-JONES, D., and CAMEL, G. H.: Studies on the control of hypertension: VIII. Mortality, morbidity and remissions during twelve years of intensive therapy. *Circulation*, **33**:958–72, 1966.

SHAPIRO, S., STRAX, P., and VENET, L.: Evaluation of periodic breast cancer screening with mammography. *JAMA*, **195**:731–38, 1966.

SOKOLOW, M., and PERLOFF, D.: The choice of drugs and the management of essential hypertension. *Progr Cardiov Dis*, **8**:253–77, 1965.

9

Systems Approach to Public Health

Walter R. Lynn

INTRODUCTION

Since the turn of the twentieth century, the field of medicine has been concerned primarily with two interdependent classes of activity: clinical or personal medicine and managerial or impersonal medicine. The questions that arise under the rubric "public health" are clearly questions that relate to the managerial aspect of medicine.

PUBLIC HEALTH—ENVIRONMENTAL HEALTH

Man's struggle for survival with his surroundings is not new, and actions that man takes to modify the environment in turn force changes in his relationship with it. Response to new environmental stresses has taken the form of evolutionary adaptation. Modern man, through his increasing numbers and new technologies has accelerated the rate at which he modifies his environment to the point where the survival of modern society requires that actions be taken to control the environment.

The interrelationships between man and his environment, particularly as they influence his health, are in the domain of what is called public health or environmental health. Environmental health is concerned with "the control of all those factors in man's physical, biologic and social environment which exercise deleterious effects on his well-being."

René Dubos (1965) has proposed ". . . that states of health or disease are expressions of the success or failure experienced by the organism in its efforts to respond adaptively to environmental challenges." Medicine is dedicated to helping the *individual* adapt to environmental challenges. Managerial medicine or public health management is concerned with the control of the environment for the benefit of man.

181

Certain semantic difficulties are inherent in the term management because it connotes both an art and a science. The art of managing is concerned with the implementation of policies or decisions. The scientific aspect of public health management concerns the analysis and measurement necessary to make optimal public policy decisions pertaining to man's health.

The techniques of social decision-making required for effective management involve the development of methods of forecasting the probable effects of various innovations (both individual actions and public policy decisions) on man's environment and the effect of these changes upon man's health and welfare. With such information, public policy-makers should be able to make better management decisions that produce maximum beneficial effects for the members of the society. These concepts of *optimization* and *forecasting* are the keystones of the systems analysis approach to public health.

CONCEPTS OF WELFARE ECONOMICS

There is no doubt that the training of physicians is almost exclusively centered upon the clinical relationship between the attending physician and the patient. Such special emphasis requires no rationalization inasmuch as this appears to be the physician's primary role. However, it may not be as apparent that the relationship between the attending physician and the patient (which hopefully improves the patient's health) generates effects that are external to the direct patient-physician situation. For example, if a patient is correctly diagnosed and treated for a venereal disease, everyone with whom the patient may come in contact is made somewhat better off, because "curing" this individual reduces the likelihood (or probability) that he is able to transmit the disease (see Chapter 10). However, the fact that others benefit from his treatment was probably not involved in his making a decision to seek medical assistance. This is frequently referred to as an *external effect* or *external economic effect* in that as a result of the treatment the patient's "health" has improved and everyone else has benefited. On the other hand, there are situations in which the recipient of a medical action is made better off and everyone (or at least some individuals) are made worse off. These effects are frequently called *external diseconomies* or *negative external effects*. For example, one can argue that any action that results in prolonging a terminal illness presumably benefits the patient but may make his family worse off.

The concept of externalities is extremely helpful when considering many of the complex issues involved in public health.

Any viable economic system operates under the assumption that in the long term, the resources available to the system will be used efficiently. In the short run, there may be misallocation of resources, but the economic system must be self-correcting. Thus a *market economy*, to operate efficiently, must meet the following conditions (Weisbrod, 1961).

1. Individuals must be able to determine the variety and quantities of goods and services upon which to spend their money.
2. A means must exist to permit individuals to transmit these wants to those who can and will satisfy them.

3. The consumption and production of these goods and services must occasion no significant external economies or diseconomies.

When these conditions are not completely satisfied the market functions imperfectly
and it is not possible to achieve an optimal or most efficient allocation of resources. To
illustrate the significance of condition 1, let us look at the question of air pollution.
Assume that air pollutants result exclusively from the production of goods (and
services) for which a market exists. Because these pollutants are waste products
resulting from the production of manufacturing processes it is reasonable to assume
that they have zero (or negative) value to the producer. Further, let us assume that
we are concerned with the gross problem of air pollution that results from the cumulative, synergistic effect of the atmosphere receiving various kinds of pollutants from a
large number of producers. (The producers can be considered to be manufacturing
plants, automobiles, trucks, jet aircraft, household incinerators, municipal incinerators,
etc.) According to condition 2, a resident, living in the airshed into which these
pollutants flow, should be able to offer some *price* which would induce the producers
to change their *modus operandi* such as to reduce (or eliminate) the pollutants. Unfortunately, no successful market mechanism exists by which an *individual* consumer
can negotiate such a change for two reasons: (a) the consumer usually detects the
gross effects of the combination of all the pollutants and thus is unable to determine
which of the producers are causing him what fraction of his discomfiture (synergistic
effect); and (b) as an individual it is unlikely that he has the resources to offer a
sufficiently attractive price to each producer (or for that matter, even one producer).
It should also be obvious that the air pollutants in the above example generate external
effects. (In economic terms the effect can be quantified in terms of the price the consumer was willing to pay to the producer to have the pollutants removed.) Clearly
where the producers of pollutants (or individuals with infectious communicable
diseases) make decisions regarding their activities without considering the impact
or cost of their discharges, these decisions result in external effects.

Weisbrod (1961) has illustrated how these conditions are violated in terms of the
purchase of health services.

Improvement in the health of one person has an impact upon the state of health of each
of the rest of us in varying degree, when communicable diseases are involved. Each person,
then, has a financial stake in the preservation of the health of others. Many persons gain,
in terms of diminished chance of becoming ill, when the health of one person is improved.
But these external gains are generally not taken into account when people determine the
part of their income to allocate to health. When deciding how to utilize his income, a
utility-maximizer would equate the marginal utility of a dollar in all uses; but since he
ordinarily would gain no utility from the fact that his health expenditures increased the
level of utility of others (i.e., improved their health), he would spend less on his health than
would be socially desirable. Social and private benefits diverge.

In situations where the market no longer operates effectively it is reasonable to
place these kinds of activities in the hands of governmental agencies. (Thus, we have
state, Federal, and local agencies with various titles and responsibilities, such as:
Water Pollution Control Administration, State Board of Health, Air Pollution
Agency.) Usually these agencies take actions that require the producer of these
external effects to internalize them in their production processes. The most common

mechanism for achieving this end is to establish performance standards for the quality of waste materials discharged. (The question of how an agency develops these standards is in itself a very interesting and complex question we will discuss further. Obviously if the standards are erroneously applied the result is a further misallocation of resources.) Consequently public actions, such as pollution control, provision of health services, and vaccination programs, can be undertaken in behalf of a collection of individuals (i.e., a community, a government) with the costs of the action distributed through various forms of taxation and enforcement through the police power of the state.

In the sections that follow we shall be concerned primarily with some of the problems, issues, and techniques that are involved in policy decisions that pertain to public health. We shall give special emphasis to the techniques of systems analysis more in terms of its utility as a device for generating useful information than as a set of sophisticated analytical methods. The literature pertaining to the analytical and computational techniques is extensive and the interested reader is encouraged to explore this field. Little of this material, however, is immediately relevant to the medical student, especially if he has little interest in mathematics. Finally, we believe that this approach to problem solving is especially useful to the medical student in understanding and contributing to the solution of the complex problems of public health.

SYSTEMS ANALYSIS

The formalization of systems analysis (or operations research) as an aid to decision-making can be traced to the methods applied to a variety of tactical military problems of World War II. Following this period, there continued to be a great deal of effort given to questions involving the military and even greater emphasis to industrial operations in the private sector. Most recently these methods and approaches have been applied to a host of problems involving government managerial questions in the public sector. These efforts generally have been quite successful in providing quantitative information in situations that previously were not believed to be amenable to analysis.

Level of System

A system can be considered to be a collection of components (subsystems) which interact in some prescribed way to produce certain effects or results (outputs). Obviously one can *conceive* of systems at various *levels* of complexity. For example, the ECG is a system by which electrical impulses are detected in an individual through the electrode subsystem; transformed and amplified through a complex electronic subsystem; and recorded (output) on a graph or oscilloscope. The detailed operational characteristics of the electronic equipment that produces the output signal is of little interest to the physician, but there is no doubt that this apparatus is in itself a complex system. For the physicians' purposes the apparatus is a "black box" that must meet certain performance specifications. (An engineer concerned with the amplification system most likely would view the signal generator—the patient—as a black box. The physician's primary concern is the quality of the output signal.) The purpose of this illustration is to emphasize that one can study a system for various purposes at many levels of complexity. We deliberately define the limits of a system as well as its level and complexity in order to increase our understanding of how it operates.

As a more relevant illustration, compare the different levels of systems required for assessing public health programs for tuberculosis treatment and control on a national or regional basis with a similar program for an individual patient. Obviously, many clinical issues are subsumed in public health control programs that are necessarily made explicit when treating an individual. Conversely, numerous issues in managerial or public health medicine (i.e., budgeted funds available, equipment for detection; availability of medical and paramedical staff; availability of drugs for treatment; numbers of hospital beds available; and so on) usually are of minor concern when one is considering the diagnostic and therapeutic regime for an individual patient.

Evaluation Criteria

It is, perhaps, deceptively simple to develop criteria for evaluating health systems that are focused on an individual. These criteria could include the following measures: improvement of the health of the patient; extension of life; reduction of pain and suffering. In public health, the development of criteria for evaluating programs involves extremely complex and cloudy issues. It is apparent that *absolute criteria do not exist.* Since public health programs are supported by public funds they reflect a range of social, economic, and political conditions which exist at points in time. (Although we may speak of "optimal solutions" to these problems it is implicit that these are temporal solutions for situations at particular times and places.)

Because criteria for evaluating activities imply measurement, it is useful if one deals in quantities that are measurable. There is little value in asserting that a program is to be evaluated on the basis of "how effectively it improves health" unless we are able to be specific as to how we will measure health. If one quantifies measures of health then it is somewhat simpler to assess improvements as well as the effectiveness of the program. Although many measures of health leave much to be desired in terms of their precision, there is no doubt that certain measures are used by those who make decisions in public and individual health situations. Many gross measures such as morbidity and mortality are frequently useful in discussing and evaluating alternative public health programs.

Effectiveness

The concept of effectiveness provides us with an entree to the utility of the systems approach. Assuming that we can quantify health (albeit imperfectly) and that we have various *resources* (e.g., funds, time, manpower, technology) that can be committed to this objective, there is a sizeable problem in determining how these resources should be allocated. Thus, for instance, one could state the purpose of an inquiry as to ". . . determine the minimum budget required to reduce infant mortality from level

A to level *B*; given that there are *N* physicians and *M* paramedical personnel . . ." In this case we have presented a *target* (viz., infant mortality at level *B*) and we wish to determine the most efficient way to achieve this goal within existing real-world constraints that exist. To successfully analyze this problem we need to be able to state what effect the services of the physician and other medical personnel have on infant mortality. (This is one of those little black boxes discussed earlier, whereby we are mainly concerned with the general effect or output rather than with knowing in detail how a particular physician produces a particular reduction in mortality.)

Although it is conceivable that real world experiments could be conducted to evaluate various alternative ways of allocating these resources, such experimentation is wasteful, expensive, and disruptive. In managerial situations it is desirable to utilize ". . . a research approach that does not involve experimentation . . . entailing physical manipulation of the subject under study . . ." (Ackoff and Sasieni, 1968). Where experimental manipulation of the real world is untenable, it is useful to construct *representations* or *models* of the system that can be studied.

Ackoff and Sasieni (1968) describe the operations research-systems analysis approach as follows:

Models in OR (operations research) take the form of equations which—although they may be complicated from a mathematical point of view—have a very simple underlying structure:

$$U = f(X_i, Y_j)$$

where *U* is the utility of value of the system's performance.

X_i are the variables that can be controlled.
Y_j are variable (and constants) that are not controlled but do affect *U*.
f is the relationship between *U* and X_i and Y_j.

In addition, one or more equations or "inequations" are frequently required to express the fact that some or all of the controlled variables can only be manipulated within limits. For example, the amount of . . . (physicians' time allocated to providing service) . . . allocated to products cannot be less than zero or greater than the total time available; and the sum of the amounts of money budgeted to different departments . . . (of an organization) . . . cannot exceed the total amount available. The performance equation and the constraints together constitute a model of the system and of the problem we want to solve. Hence it is a *decision*, as well as a *system* model.

Once the model is constructed, it can be used to find, exactly or approximately, the optimal values of the controlled variables—values that produce the best performance of the system; that is, we can *derive a solution* to the problem from the model. How this can be done depends on the nature of the model.

A solution may be extracted from a model either by conducting experiments on it (i.e., by *simulation*) or by mathematical analysis. In some cases mathematical analysis can be conducted without any knowledge of the values of the variables (i.e., abstractly or symbolically), but in others the values of the variables must be known (i.e., concretely or numerically).

TUBERCULOSIS CONTROL—AN ILLUSTRATIVE CASE

In the following section we shall present a detailed illustration of a systems approach to the question of tuberculosis control. The model used in this illustration is largely taken from the work of ReVelle (1967) and ReVelle, Lynn, and Feldmann (1967).

This situation we wish to examine pertains to the question of how to best utilize available medical technology for the control of tuberculosis in a developing nation. (The developing nation covenant is not intended to be restrictive inasmuch as the incidence of tuberculosis in certain sections of United States metropolitan areas may be equivalent to those in India, for example.)

This system is conceived from the point of view of the public health manager who wishes to evaluate alternative tactics that can be employed to control the disease. Five control measures will be considered: (1) vaccination of newborn, (2) vaccination by mass campaign, (3) prophylaxis to two categories of individuals, and (5) curing infectives.

The first task is to describe the "tuberculosis system."

In this section a mathematical model of tuberculosis epidemiology is developed. This descriptive model can be used to project the trend of the disease with and without intervention.

Tuberculosis, Uncontrolled

Tuberculosis, uncontrolled, can be described with four categories*: susceptibles, nonactive cases, active cases, and recovered nonactive cases. Susceptibles, designated as group X, are individuals who have never been infected by the disease but could be if sufficiently exposed. Nonactive cases, indicated as group WA, have been infected but have not yet developed lung damage and are unable to communicate the disease. Members of this group only gradually develop lung damage and may consist of up to 25–35 per cent of the population of some developing nations (Waaler, 1962).

An individual who has developed lung damage is an active case or an infective and belongs to class Y. This group receives its primary inputs from group WA. Active cases can transmit the disease to susceptibles. The process of infection results in the shifting of an individual from the susceptible class X to the nonactive class WA. Recovered nonactive cases, designated as group WC are those who naturally recover from the active form of the disease; they are subject to relapse back to Y (Figure 9-1).

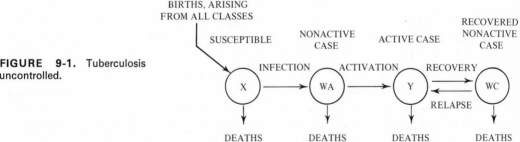

FIGURE   9-1.   Tuberculosis uncontrolled.

Deaths occur in all groups in proportion to the number in the groups. All death rate coefficients have the same value, except in class Y where a high rate is due to tuberculosis and its complications. All individuals are considered to be born susceptible and so enter group X initially; births arise from all classes.

* The words *category*, *group*, and *class* are used interchangeably.

Tuberculosis Controlled by Prophylaxis and Cures

Prophylaxis with isoniazid and supporting drugs to group WA creates an additional nonactive class, designated WD. The advantage of prophylaxis is that the rate coefficient for movement to class Y from the new class WD is roughly half that of group WA. Prophylaxis to the nonactive class WA is the first of the control variables to be considered. Isoniazid and supporting drugs will also cure an individual in class Y, transferring him to another new nonactive class WF. The relapse rate of those in WF is less than the relapse rate of those who naturally recovered. Cures of active cases via izoniazid constitute a second control variable (Figure 9-2).

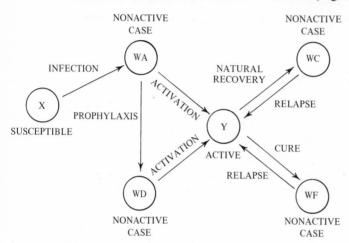

FIGURE 9-2. Tuberculosis controlled by prophylaxis and cures. (Births and deaths are not shown.)

Tuberculosis Controlled by Propyhlaxis, Cures, and Vaccinations

BCG vaccinations to members of group X create a new system. This system is parallel to the one that described tuberculosis controlled only by prophylaxis and cure. A susceptible who receives BCG is transferred to class U, the group of vaccinated susceptibles. This individual's resistance to infection, however, is no different than that of any ordinary susceptible. Once he is infected, his risk of developing into an active case is markedly changed. The infection of a vaccinated susceptible moves him from class U to the nonactive class WB. The breakdown from WB to Y has been estimated to be as low as one fifth the risk of breakdown from WA to Y (British Medical Research Council, 1963). Furthermore, prophylaxis to an individual in WB would transfer him to a new group WE, where the risk of breakdown is still less. The number of individuals vaccinated with BCG and the number of nonactive cases in WB who receive prophylaxis are the last two control variables which will be considered (Figure 9-3).

EQUATIONS DESCRIBING TUBERCULOSIS EPIDEMIOLOGY

The system shown in Figure 9-3 can be described using nine differential equations similar in form to the ones proposed by Kermack and McKendrik (1932). The planning period is

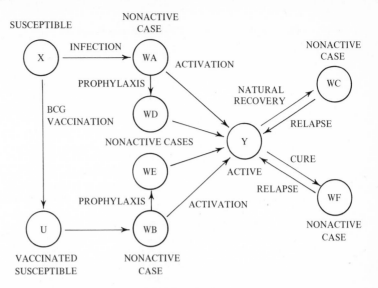

FIGURE 9-3. Tuberculosis controlled by prophylaxis, cure, and BCG vaccination. (Births and deaths are not shown.)

divided into intervals of one year, and equations are written for the rate of change of numbers in the various categories during the ith year.

The following equations can be derived by identifying (in Figure 9-3) the inflows and outflows into each labeled category or group. Because we have defined the system in terms of nine categories, we are required to generate nine equations to describe the dynamics of the system. Each equation is stated in differential form, i.e., the rate of change of the numbers of individuals in a category in a time interval is equal to the numbers of individuals entering from various categories less the numbers leaving the category.

Thus equation 1, asserts that the change in the number of susceptibles (category x) in time t (dx/dt), equals births in time t (μN_i) (see Figure 4), less the number infected ($\beta XY/N_1$) in time t, less the deaths of individuals in category x (λx), less those individuals who receive BCG vaccinations in time t (v_i), and finally, a special type of outflow that allows us to consider the efficacy of a mass vaccination campaign (v_x), or

$$\frac{dx}{dt} = \mu N_i - \beta \frac{xy}{N_i} - \lambda x - v_i - v_x. \tag{1}$$

The remaining equations are formed in a similar manner.

$$\frac{dx}{dt} = -\beta \frac{xy}{N_i} + \mu N_i - \lambda x - v_i - v_x. \tag{1}$$

$$\frac{du}{dt} = -\beta \frac{uy}{N_i} - \lambda u + v_i + v_x. \tag{2}$$

$$\frac{d(wa)}{dt} = \beta \frac{xy}{N_i} - m_A wa - \lambda wa - g_i. \tag{3}$$

$$\frac{d(wb)}{dt} = \beta \frac{uy}{N_i} - m_B w\dot{b} - \lambda wb - k_i. \tag{4}$$

$$\frac{d(wc)}{dt} = \gamma y - m_C wc - \lambda wc. \tag{5}$$

$$\frac{d(wd)}{dt} = g_i - m_D wd - \lambda wd. \tag{6}$$

$$\frac{d(we)}{dt} = k_i - m_E we - \lambda we. \tag{7}$$

$$\frac{d(wf)}{dt} = f_i - m_F wf - \lambda wf. \tag{8}$$

$$\frac{dy}{dt} = m_A wa + m_B wb + m_C wc + m_D wd + m_E we + m_F wf - \gamma y - \lambda_{TB} y - f_i. \tag{9}$$

189

The differential equation for total population over the entire planning horizon is

$$\frac{dN}{dt} = \mu N - \lambda(N - y) - \lambda_{TB} y, \tag{10}$$

where

X = the class of susceptibles.

x = number in class X at time t in interval i.

U = the class of vaccinated susceptibles.

u = number in class U at time t in interval i.

WA = the class of nonactive cases, members of which have not had lung damage, prophylaxis, or vaccination.

wa = number in class WA at time t in interval i.

WB = the class of nonactive cases, members of which have not had lung damage nor prophylaxis, but who were vaccinated while susceptible.

wb = number in class WB at time t in interval i.

WC = the class of nonactive cases, members of which have had lung damage and naturally recovered.

wc = number in class WC at time t in interval i.

WD = the class of nonactive cases, members of which have not had lung damage or vaccination, but who have had prophylaxis.

wd = numbers in class WD at time t in interval i.

WE = the class of nonactive cases, members of which have been vaccinated, have not had lung damage, but have had prophylaxis.

we = number in class WE at time t in interval i.

WF = the class of nonactive cases who have had lung damage and were cured via chemotherapy.

wf = number in class WF at time t in interval i.

Y = the class of active or infective cases.

y = number in class Y at time t in interval i.

v_i = number of vaccinations to newborn in interval i; v_i is an output from X and an input to U.

v_X = vaccinations in a mass campaign, zero in all intervals but the first; v_X is an output from X and an input to U.

g_i = number of prophylaxes to individuals in WA during interval i; g_i is an output from WA and an input to WD.

k_i = number of prophylaxes to individuals in WB during interval i; k_i is an output from WB and an input to WE.

f_i = number of cures provided to infectives during interval i; f_i is an output from Y and an input to WF.

The control variables, v_i, v_X, g_i, k_i, and f_i are the amounts of various strategies to be employed.

λ = death rate coefficient in all groups except Y.

λ_{TB} = death rate coefficient in group Y.

N_i = average population in the ith interval.

μ = birth rate coefficient in all groups.

μN_i = births in interval i, an input to X.

$\beta(xy/N_i)$ = rate of infection of susceptibles at time t in interval i; it is an output from X and an input to WA.

$\beta(uy/N_i)$ = rate of infection of vaccinated susceptibles at time t in interval i; it is an output from U and an input to WB.

γ = rate coefficient for natural recovery, the fraction of those in Y recovering per year.

m_A = rate coefficient for activation from category WA.

m_B = rate coefficient for activation from category WB.

m_C = rate coefficient for activation from category WB.
m_D = rate coefficient for activation from category WD.
m_E = rate coefficient for activation from category WE.
m_F = rate coefficient for activation from category WF.

The coefficients m_A, m_B, m_C, m_D, m_E, and m_F may be interpreted as the fractions of people moving from the appropriate nonactive classes to the active class each year. For instance, if $m_A = 0.01$, then one per cent of the individuals in WA enter Y each year.

The equations shown above are nonlinear because of the product terms $\beta(xy/N_i)$, and $\beta(uy/N_i)$ and their exact solution is exceedingly difficult, although equations (6), (7), and (8) have straightforward solutions.

These equations can be integrated numerically and thus used to predict the course of the disease under various predetermined forms of control.

This model attempts to describe the changes in the numbers of individuals in various categories of disease that we have identified. Although the model is only an approximation of the true epidemiology of TB we have introduced five *control variables* (v_i, xz, v_x, q_i, k_i and f_i) which allow us to evaluate the effectiveness of these modes of intervention.

Efficiency of BCG.   The rate coefficient for activation from class WB is less than that for class WA due to the effect of the BCG vaccination. Since m_B and m_A are composite rates for entire classes, the efficiency of BCG must be defined in terms of them. Mathematically stated, the BCG efficiency is

$$\frac{E_{BCG}}{E} = \frac{m_A - m_B}{m_A} \times 100.$$

As m_B decreases relative to m_A, the efficiency increases. If m_B equals m_A, the efficiency is zero. If m_B equals zero, the efficiency is 100 per cent. Since the efficiency of BCG is a controversial matter, several values of the parameter E_{BCG} (in particular, values of 70 per cent, 30 per cent, and 0 per cent) are used here; this is done in order to ascertain the utility of the vaccine under several conditions of efficiency. The rate of activation from class WB for different efficiencies of BCG is obtained by solving the above equation for m_B.

$$m_B = m_A \left(1 - \frac{E_{BCG}}{100}\right).$$

Numerical Example

Parameters, Initial Conditions, and Costs.   The estimates of parameters (Table 9-1), initial conditions (Table 9-2), and costs (Table 9-3) are not meant to be applicable to any specific tuberculosis situation. They are at best only representative of the values that might be found in some developing nations. The fact that in most situations such numbers are unknown points up the need for epidemiologic surveys. Where doubt clouds the use of some number, the use of several values may clarify how carefully that number must be estimated. The caveat can be summarized: *Application of the model to a particular epidemiological situation requires estimates of parameters for that situation.*

Natural Trend of the Disease.   In order to assess the impact of the control programs suggested in the next section, it is necessary to project the state of the tuberculosis system with no controls applied. This is done by integrating numerically the nonlinear differential equations (1) through (9); the "Improved Euler-Cauchy Method" is utilized. The parameters are those given in the preceding discussion.

The natural time trends are examined for two values of β. This is done on a trial basis because the United States estimates when used with the other parameters seem to indicate a rather excessive spread of the disease.

The adjusted estimate of Ferebee (1966) is $\beta = 3.45$ persons/person-year adequately contacted. The trend using this value is shown in Figure 9-4, where there is a "steep" increase in the number of inactive cases wa and thus in the number of active cases y and the number of recovered inactive cases wc. The number of susceptibles actually falls and then begins to recover. Such a projection would put perhaps two thirds of the population in the inactive category 30 years hence.

TABLE 9-1

Parameters of the Tuberculosis System

Parameter Values	Source of Comment
$\beta = 1.78$	Derived from data on Waaler, *et al.* (1962).
$\beta = 3.45$	Derived from Ferebee's (1966) estimate of $\beta'' = 3.0$.
$m_A = 0.0076$	Derived from data on Waaler, *et al.*
$m_B = 0.0076 \left(1.0 - \dfrac{E_{BCG}}{100}\right)$	E_{BCG} is subject to dispute and hence is varied to ascertain its utility at various levels of effectiveness.
$m_C = 0.017$	Ferebee.
$m_D = 0.0076 \, (1.0 = 0.52)$	52% efficiency for prophylaxis from PHS studies (Ferebee, 1966).
$m_E = m_B \, (1.0 - 0.52)$	No basis in data, an estimate only.
$m_F = 0.1$	Estimated from Ferebee.
$\lambda = 0.014$	Waaler, et al.
$\overset{\lambda}{\tau \beta} = 0.07$	Waaler, et al.
$\mu = 0.037$	Waaler, et al.

TABLE 9-2

Initial Conditions of a Hypothetical Population

$x_0 = 648{,}000$	Initial number of susceptibles.
$wa_0 = 297{,}000$	Initial number of inactive cases.
$wc_0 = 33{,}000$	Initial number of recovered inactive cases.
$y_0 = 22{,}000$	Initial number of active cases.
$N_0 = 1{,}000{,}000$	Total population at time zero.

TABLE 9-3

Costs

Cost/vaccination to newborn = \$0.30	Done twice in a lifetime (midrange of Piot's [1966]) estimate.
Cost/vaccination in a mass campaign = $0.20 \rightarrow \$0.40$	Cost increases as greater fractions of the population are covered (estimate from Piot).
Cost/prophylaxis = \$20	Estimate for one year (derived from Piot).
Cost/cure = \$200	Estimate for one year of chemotherapy (derived from Piot and from Fox [1964]).

This is contrasted (see Figure 9-5) to the trend using the estimate of $\beta = 1.78$ derived from the study of Waaler, *et al.* (1962) where both the susceptibles and the inactive cases grow at roughly the same rate. Clearly this number β affects not only the estimation of the tuberculosis problem but also the cost of the method chosen to solve it. The larger β foretells a much higher cost to control the disease. The smaller value would call for less costly control programs. Both values are considered in the numerical example in order to ascertain their effects on the controls chosen to accomplish given reductions of active cases. They are also considered so that their effects on the cost required to achieve those reductions can be determined.

Optimization

Once the model has been formulated it is desired to determine at what level these control variables should be applied. In order to find solutions that are optimal, i.e., the best solutions determined for a given set of assumptions, it is necessary to introduce optimization techniques. The area of mathematics dealing with maxima or

FIGURE 9-4. Natural trend of tuberculosis.

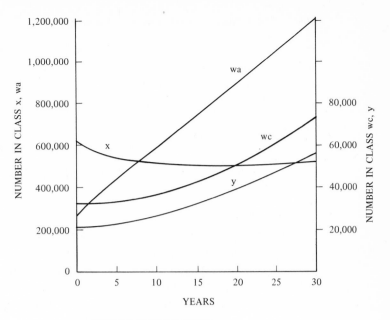

x = NUMBER IN SUSCEPTIBLE
    CLASS X
wa = NUMBER IN NONACTIVE
    CLASS WA
wc = NUMBER IN NONACTIVE
    CLASS WC
y = NUMBER IN ACTIVE CLASS
    Y
30 YEAR POPULATION = 1,910,000

FIGURE 9-4. Natural trend of tuberculosis.

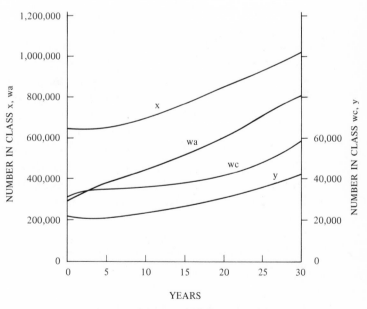

x   = NUMBER IN SUSCEPTIBLE CLASS X
wa   = NUMBER IN NON ACTIVE CLASS WA
wc   = NUMBER IN NONACTIVE CLASS WC
y   = NUMBER IN ACTIVE CLASS Y

30 YEAR POPULATION = 1,910,000

FIGURE 9-5. Natural trend of tuberculosis.

minima of functions subject to constraints is called *mathematical programing*. The objective function is the mathematical statement of the objective we wish to achieve, such as minimizing the cost of controls, and the constraints are the equations, which express the amount of resources available or the physical, biologic, or epidemiologic relationships to which any solution must conform. In general the statement of the mathematical programing problem is

$$\text{MAXIMIZE}$$
$$\text{or} \qquad U = F_j(x_j)$$
$$\text{MINIMIZE}$$
$$\text{Subject to} \qquad R_i = F_i(x_j).$$

If F_j and F_i are linear, the problem is called *linear programing;* and if F_j and F_i are nonlinear—*nonlinear programing*. Linear programing has undergone extensive development, and algorithms have been coded for practically all scientific computers.

In the TB model it is possible to obtain solutions for the set of differential equations (by numerical integration) that result in a set of nine simultaneous linear equations in the form of constraints

$$R_i = F_i(x_j) \qquad (i = 1, 2, \ldots, 9).$$

(For a detailed discussion of the development of the linear equations, see ReVelle [1967]. These are truly constraints in that any solution is required to conform to the predictive equations [1–9]. The use of the available controls is thus restricted to operate within the framework defined by the constraints.)

One additional set of assumptions is required for the optimization procedure. It is necessary to describe the criterion function (viz., $U = F_j(x_j)$) that is to be maximized or minimized. In our model we assert that our objective is to find the amount of each control to be used in each time period, such that the total cost of using the controls in all periods is minimized. (The trivial solution to this problem is to not apply any controls—with the result that the minimum cost is then zero. It will be apparent that other criteria are required and will be developed in the following sections.) We have assumed that the cost of using any control is a simple linear function of the amount that is used. For example, if the cost of administering a BCG vaccine to a newborn is 30 cents, then the cost of 100 vaccinations is $30 and 10,000 vaccinations is $3,000. This is not completely realistic because it is possible to obtain economies of scale in the administration of medical services and thus the cost in all likelihood is not strictly linear. The errors introduced by these assumptions must be carefully evaluated.

The formula problem can be stated as

Minimize the cost of achieving the specified active case reduction pattern by selection of the amounts of control variables to be applied to the system during various time intervals. The total cost is the sum of the costs of all controls. The constraints are the equations defining the states of the system.

Patterns for Active Case Reduction

For this model, it is incumbent on the decision-maker to specify the exact pattern of reduction of active cases that he desires. The justification of his specifications may be his expectation of the public's demand for adequate control. Because it is unlikely that he would have prior knowledge as to the relative expense of a number of patterns, it is useful to examine a sequence of reduction schedules.

Twenty-year Horizon. The initial condition is 22,000 active cases. From this starting value, four paths of reduction are chosen (see Figure 9-6).

 Schedule 1 allows for an initial gradual decrease in active cases to 14,400 at 12 years, followed by a sharp decrease to 2,000 actives at the end of 20 years. *Schedule 2* is a linear reduction of 1,000 active cases per year from 22,000 at the present to 2,000 at 20 years.

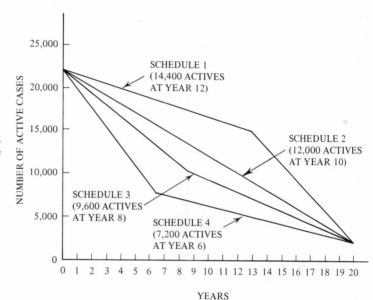

FIGURE 9-6. Four 20-year schedules for reduction of active cases of tuberculosis.

Schedule 3 considers a faster initial reduction to 9,600 actives at eight years, followed by a slower decrease to 2,000 by the twentieth year. *Schedule 4* represents the fastest initial decrease, to 7,200 at six years, and then a slow reduction to 2,000 by the end of year 20.

 These four schedules, although not exhaustive in terms of possible patterns, do reflect what might be considered feasible patterns of operation in that large oscillations in the state of the disease likely would be unacceptable to health authorities. Undoubtedly, the least costly way to achieve 2,000 actives in 20 years is not among the four schedules. Nevertheless, one hopes that by determining the lowest cost for each of these schedules, a glimmering of insight as to the least costly scheme may result. In addition, it may even be possible to ascertain whether or not the least costly scheme makes sense from a public health standpoint.

$$\text{Set I:} \quad \beta = 1.78, \; E_{BCG} = 70\%.$$

The costs and results of these four schedules are first compared in Table 9-4. The efficiency of BCG is 70 per cent and the value of β is 1.78 for these first calculations, designated as Set I. The programs are each optimal in the sense that no less expensive combinations of alternatives exist that will achieve the specified numbers of active cases.

 It should be noted that the conclusions drawn are from a particular set of parameters, initial conditions, and costs. Caution must be exercised in extrapolating to other situations.

 The fourth schedule is the most expensive of the four, the third next, the second still less expensive, and the first least expensive.

 The decision-maker presented with such costs must decide if the schedules with the more rapid initial reductions in active cases are worth the additional cost. Clearly, he must balance cost against the man-years of tuberculosis he allows (Table 9-4). From Schedule 1

TABLE 9-4

Optimal Schedules for Tuberculosis Control—Set I *for all Schedules*: No Prophylaxis

	Total Cost	Newborn Vaccinations*	Mass Campaign Vaccinations†	x_{20}	u_{20}	wa_{20}	wb_{20}	wc_{20}	wf_{20}	Thousands of Man-Years of Tuberculosis
Schedule	7,811,000	V1–V13	Full (648,000⁻)	349,000	697,000	209,000	241,000	33,000	32,000	284
Schedule	9,028,000	V1–V12	Full (648,000⁻)	393,000	692,000	209,000	202,000	31,000	36,000	240
Schedule	10,214,000	V1–V11	Full (648,000⁻)	435,000	690,000	209,000	164,000	28,000	40,000	196
Schedule	11,366,000	V1–V10	Full (648,000⁻)	478,000	689,000	209,000	125,000	26,000	44,000	162

E_{BCG} = 70 per cent
β = 1.78
Horizon = 20 Years

$wd_{20} = 0$
$we_{20} = 0$
$y_{20} = 2,000$

* V1–V13, for example, means that all newborn in years 1 to 13 are vaccinated in the least cost program.

† Full (648,000⁻) means that as many current susceptibles as possible were vaccinated in a mass campaign. On the order of 10,000 to 30,000, however, were missed because they were either infected or died before they could be reached.

to Schedule 4, the man-years of tuberculosis are reduced by 43 per cent, but the cost has increased by 45 per cent. The schedules are achieved by utilizing only two of the four possible types of control, drug treatment of active cases and vaccinations. In Table 9-5, the drug treatment recoveries required each year to meet the four schedules are compared. In Table 9-6, the yearly costs of Schedule 4 are listed. It is of interest that the maximum cost does not occur in the year when the mass BCG campaign is conducted. Rather, it occurs in the sixth year.

Schedules 1 through 4 all call for a mass campaign during the first year. In addition, vaccinations of the newborn are indicated each year for the first 13 years for Schedule 1, 12 years for Schedule 2, 11 for Schedule 3, and 10 for Schedule 4.

TABLE 9-5

Cures Required to Achieve Schedules 1, 2, 3 and 4 of Set I

Cures in Year 1	Schedule 1	Schedule 2	Schedule 3	Schedule 4
$i = 1$	256	652	1,246	2,236
2	391	845	1,525	2,660
3	504	1,014	1,780	3,057
4	614	1,181	2,030	3,447
5	722	1,344	2,277	3,831
6	829	1,505	2,520	4,210
7	934	1,664	2,759	2,317
8	1,037	1,820	2,994	2,354
9	1,139	1,974	2,234	2,390
10	1,239	2,126	2,319	2,426
11	1,338	2,276	2,402	2,462
12	1,436	2,423	2,485	2,499
13	2,524	2,569	2,568	2,537
14	2,764	2,716	2,652	2,576
15	3,004	2,863	2,736	2,615
16	3,243	3,009	2,820	2,654
17	3,481	3,154	2,902	2,693
18	3,714	3,296	2,984	2,731
19	3,945	3,436	3,064	2,769
20	4,170	3,573	3,142	2,805

$\beta = 1.78$, $E_{BCG} = 70$ per cent.

One must not construe this result on years of newborn vaccination as the answer to the tuberculosis problem in developing nations; it is not. The answer is limited by the horizon at which the decision-maker has chosen to look. As will be seen later, tuberculosis is not brought "under control" by these programs, and additional years of vaccinations may be required if the horizon for control is extended. The result is, however, testimony to the importance of BCG in a control program under the conditions of this example.

Also, vaccinations do not necessarily cease after some particular year. The cost for a vaccination to a newborn is given at 30 cents, implying a second vaccination often at school-leaving time (Piot, 1966). This second vaccination could be given to a newborn rather than to the individual already once vaccinated. If the individual does not receive a second vaccination, he may revert from class U to class X, but the newborn, instead of entering class X, will be put into U. Conceptually at least, the numbers in the classes will be unaffected if the vaccine is given to the newborn in years after those designated in the optimal program.

TABLE 9-6
Yearly Costs for Schedule 4 of Set I

Year	Total Cost of Cures	Total Cost of Newborn Vaccination	Cost of Mass Campaign	Total Cost for Year
1	$447,200	$11,222	$187,902	$646,324
2	532,000	11,471		543,471
3	611,400	11,727		623,127
4	689,400	11,990		701,390
5	766,200	12,262		778,462
6	842,000	12,541		854,541
7	463,400	12,828		476,228
8	470,800	13,122		483,922
9	478,000	13,424		491,424
10	485,200	13,732		498,932
11	492,400			492,400
12	499,800			499,800
13	507,400			507,400
14	515,200			515,200
15	523,000			523,000
16	530,800			530,800
17	538,600			538,600
18	546,200			546,200
19	553,800			553,800
20	561,000			561,000
			Grand Total	$11,366,021

$E_{BCG} = 70\%, \beta = 1.78.$

It is of interest that those schedules that initially accomplish the more rapid reduction in active cases require fewer years of newborn vaccination in the optimal program. This fact is presumably due to the greater degree of reduction of inactive cases accomplished by the higher numbered schedules.

This last observation is important in a comparison of the four schedules. Although the more rapid reduction schedules are more costly now, later they may result in a savings in cost due to the lower number of inactive cases in WB at 20 years. Essentially this means a lesser potential for new active cases.

The numbers in the various classes are plotted for Schedule 1 of Set I in Figure 9-7. This plot is typical of the trend in the various classes for the four schedules. The number in the susceptible class X falls to zero by the end of the first year owing to the mass campaign and the vaccination of all newborn in that year. For twelve subsequent years, because all newborn are vaccinated, the number in class X remains at zero. Then with the cessation of newborn vaccination in year 14, class X begins to expand. The expansion is not at an exponential rate, however, because individuals are still removed by death and transferred by infection to class WA.

The number in the vaccinated susceptible class U rises from zero to a value very near the initial number in class X. Class U thereafter expands each year, its inputs being the vaccinated newborns. Its expansion is slowed by deaths and by the infection process, which takes individuals out of U and into WB. After the thirteenth year, class U receives no further inputs and diminishes in size owing to deaths and infections.

The number of class WA rises during the first year, receiving inputs from class X,

FIGURE 9-7. Schedule 1 of
Set I. $\beta = 1.78$, $E_{BCG} = 70$ per
cent.

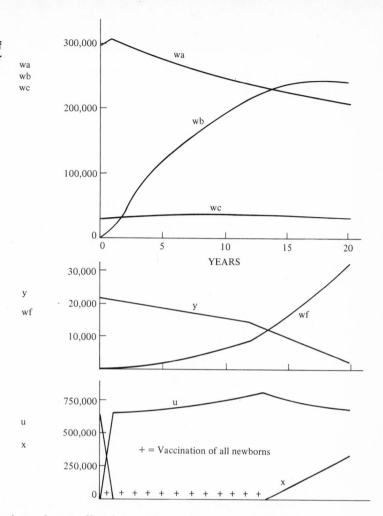

but in the following years, the input is cut off owing to the vaccination program; i.e., there are no individuals in X. Thus the size of WA decreases due to death and breakdowns to active cases. Even though class X begins to grow in year 14, class WA still does not expand because the sum of the death rate and breakdown rates exceeds the input rate from X.

Class WB, initially at zero, receives inputs injected from the growing class of vaccinated susceptibles. Thus the number of individuals in WB each year increases owing to the larger numbers in class U. However, eventually under the influence of a declining class U and a declining class Y, WB begins to fall. Class Y is controlled to fall slowly at first and then more rapidly. Therefore, class WF, containing the cured individuals from class Y, rises only gradually at the outset and then more quickly.

To summarize the results of Set I, the decision-maker finds that the higher numbered schedules, although representing substantially fewer man-years of tuberculosis, are considerably more costly. They provide, however, a lower potential for later spread owing to the presence of fewer inactive cases.

$$\text{Set II:} \quad \beta = 178, \ E_{BCG} = 30\%.$$

Because doubt exists over the exact effectiveness of BCG, the four schedules were repeated at an efficiency of 30 per cent for BCG, β remaining at 1.78 (Set II). The results

199

are presented in Table 9-7. The only additional conclusion that can be drawn from this set of schedules by itself is that fewer years of vaccinations to newborn are called for, but the mass vaccination campaign is still required in the optimal program. As before, the higher numbered schedules are more costly but result in fewer man-years of tuberculosis and fewer inactive cases in class WB at the end of 20 years. Of course, the cost to achieve the various schedules has increased from the previous set owing to the lower vaccine efficiency.

$$\text{Set III:} \quad \beta = 1.78, E_{BCG} = 0\%.$$

In order to assess the effect of allowing no BCG vaccinations, the efficiency of the vaccine was set at zero, and the same four schedules were rerun, β being still held at 1.78 (Set III, Table 9-8). This procedure constrains all vaccinations to be zero, because with zero efficiency obviously no advantage is gained by using the vaccine. Also, this method constitutes a verification of the model's properties. It is seen that the entire reduction is now accomplished by drug treatment of actives.

The results of these three sets of schedules, each set with a different efficiency for BCG, are compared in Tables 9-9 and 9-10.

As expected, the cost to achieve any one of the four schedules increases as the vaccine becomes less efficient (30 per cent) and is finally phased out (0 per cent) (Table 9-9).

If the vaccine is 70 per cent efficient, then a decision not to use it during the 20 years of control will require expenditures considerably above those necessary under the optimal plan (columns 4 and 6, Table 9-9). In meeting Schedule 1, use of the vaccine would save $3,096,000 or 28 per cent. In meeting Schedule 2, the saving would be $2,697,000 or 23 per cent. In meeting Schedule 3, a saving of $2,232,000 or 18 per cent is possible if the vaccine is utilized. In meeting Schedule 4, use of the vaccine would save $1,700,000 or 13 per cent. The savings are less but still substantial if the vaccine is only 30 per cent efficient (columns 5 and 7, Table 9-9).

However, this does not fully illustrate the cost advantage of the vaccine. In Table 9-10, the numbers in two of the inactive classes are compared for the three sets of schedules. Note that the sums of the numbers in classes WA and WB in Sets I and II are very close to the number of inactive cases in WA when no vaccine is used. For example, for Schedule 4, the sum is 334,000 if BCG is 70 per cent efficient and 329,000 if BCG is 30 per cent efficient. This compares to 326,000 in class WA when BCG is not used. Of the 334,000 inactive cases in Set I, there are 125,000 individuals who become active cases at a much lower rate (m_B) than individuals in class WA. This indicates that the potential for new active cases is much less at the end of 20 years if the vaccine is used. In consequence, including the vaccine in the program will lead to additional savings in the years beyond the 20-year horizon.

This last point is illustrated for Schedule 1 at a BCG efficiency of 70 per cent. If controls cease at the end of 20 years, the number of active cases trends back upward from 2,000. If the BCG were used in the amounts called for, this trend is considerably slower than if no BCG were used to achieve Schedule 1 (Figure 9-8).

$$\text{Sets IV, V, and VI:} \quad \beta = 3.45.$$

The combinations of control variables that achieve schedules 1 through 4 at minimum costs were determined for $\beta = 3.45$. The conclusions concerning vaccine use and savings in cost due to the vaccine are very similar to those for sets I, II, and III. The period of vaccinations of the newborn extends several additional years because of the larger value of β. Again, prophylaxis is ruled out of optimal programs.

TABLE 9-7

Optimal Schedules for Tuberculosis Control—Set II for All Schedules: No Prophylaxis

	Total Cost	Newborn Vacci-nations*	Mass Campaign Vacci-nations†	x_{20}	u_{20}	wa_{20}	wb_{20}	wc_{20}	wf_{20}	Thousands of Man-Years of Tubercu-losis
Schedule 1	9,800,000	V1–V10	Full	465,000	581,000	220,000	221,000	33,000	41,000	284
Schedule 2	10,777,000	V1–V9	Full $(648,000^-)$ Full	506,000	580,000	218,000	185,000	31,000	44,000	240
Schedule 3	11,684,000	V1–V8	Full	546,000	580,000	217,000	149,000	28,000	47,000	196
Schedule 4	12,517,000	V1–V6	Full $(648,000^-)$	618,000	549,000	218,000	111,000	26,000	49,000	162

$wd_{20} = 0$
$we_{20} = 0$
$y_{20} = 2,000$

$E_{BCG} = 30$ per cent
$\beta = 1.78$
Horizon $= 20$ Years
* and † same as Table 9-3

TABLE 9-8

Optimal Schedules for Tuberculosis Control—Set III for All Schedules: No Prophylaxis

	Total Cost	Newborn Vacci-nations	Mass Campaign Vacci-nations	x_{20}	u_{20}	wa_{20}	wb_{20}	wc_{20}	wf_{20}	Thousands of Man-Years of Tuberculosis
Schedule 1	10,907,000	0	0	1,045,000	0	435,000	0	33,000	47,000	284
Schedule 2	11,725,000	0	0	1,085,000	0	399,000	0	31,000	49,000	240
Schedule 3	12,446,000	0	0	1,126,000	0	362,000	0	28,000	51,000	196
Schedule 4	13,066,000	0	0	1,166,000	0	326,000	0	26,000	52,000	162

$wd_{20} = 0$
$we_{20} = 0$
$y_{20} = 2,000$

$E_{BCG} = 0$ per cent
$\beta = 1.78$
Horizon $= 20$ Years
* and † same as in Table 9-3

TABLE 9-9
Comparison of Costs of Sets I, II, and III

BCG Efficiency	Set I 70%	Cost Set II 30%	Set III 0%	Additional Cost if No BCG Is Used Even Though Its Efficiency Is: 70%	30%	Per Cent Savings Because BCG Was Used and It Had an Efficiency of: 70%	30%
Col. Number	(1)	(2)	(3)	(4)	(5)	(6)	(7)
How Obtained				(3)−(1)	(2)−(1)	(4)/(3)	(5)/(3)
Schedule 1	7,811,000	9,800,000	10,907,000	3,096,000	1,107,000	28%	10%
Schedule 2	9,028,000	10,777,000	11,725,000	2,697,000	948,000	23%	8%
Schedule 3	10,214,000	11,684,000	12,446,000	2,232,000	762,000	18%	6%
Schedule 4	11,366,000	12,517,000	13,066,000	1,700,000	549,000	13%	4%

$\beta = 1.78$
Horizon = 20 Years

TABLE 9-10
Comparison of Nonactive Classes of Sets I, II, and III

	Set I $E_{BCG} = 70$ per cent		Set II $E_{BCG} = 30$ per cent		Set III $E_{BCG} = 0$ per cent (No vaccine)	
	wa_{20}	wb_{20}	wa_{20}	wb_{20}	wa_{20}	wb_{20}
Schedule 1	209,000	241,000	220,000	221,000	435,000	0
2	209,000	202,000	218,000	185,000	399,000	0
3	209,000	164,000	217,000	149,000	362,000	0
4	209,000	125,000	218,000	111,000	326,000	0

$\beta = 1.78$
Horizon = 20 Years

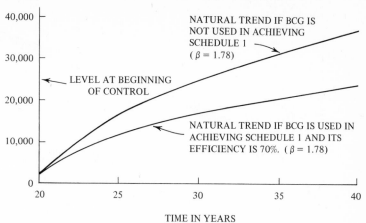

FIGURE 9-8. Trend after Schedule I is completed.

TIME IN YEARS

The significant feature that these calculations illustrate (Table 9-11) is the increase in the minimum cost to achieve these schedules. Set IV considers the BCG efficiency to be 70 per cent, and the costs of the four schedules are compared to those of Set I where the efficiency is also 70 per cent, but β is only 1.78. Set V is compared to Set II ($\beta = 1.78$), both sets having a BCG efficiency of 30 per cent. Set VI is contrasted to Set III ($\beta = 1.78$), these sets using a BCG efficiency of zero and thus excluding the vaccine from the program. All schedules show significant increases in cost, reflecting the necessity for both more vaccinations and more drug treatment recoveries to meet the planned pattern of active cases. A value of β equal to 3.45 is a high estimate of the parameter, and the resultant programs should provide the decision-maker with a conservative (high) estimate of the cost he will incur.

TABLE 9-11

Comparison of Costs for Two Values of β
Costs

	$E_{\mathrm{BCG}} = 70$ per cent		$E_{\mathrm{BCG}} = 30$ per cent		$E_{\mathrm{BCG}} = 0$ per cent	
	Set I	Set IV	Set II	Set V	Set III	Set VI
	$\beta = 1.78$	$\beta = 3.45$	$\beta = 1.78$	$\beta = 3.45$	$\beta = 1.78$	$\beta = 3.45$
Schedule 1	7,811,000	9,221,000	9,800,000	12,619,000	10,907,000	14,725,000
Schedule 2	9,028,000	10,344,000	10,777,000	13,382,000	11,725,000	15,238,000
Schedule 3	10,214,000	11,409,000	11,684,000	14,014,000	12,446,000	15,568,000
Schedule 4	11,366,000	12,406,000	12,517,000	14,497,000	13,066,000	15,694,000

The Natural Trend After 20 Years of Controls Are Complete. A logical query concerning the effect of these schedules is what measures, if any, must follow them in order to maintain the desired numbers of active cases. Clearly, some form of control is necessary. To ascertain initially what these 20-year programs have accomplished, the natural trend of the disease is projected for an additional 20 years. This device provides a preliminary picture of how effective the various schedules were.

Figure 9-9 shows the number of active cases of tuberculosis as a function of time, beginning at year 20 when controls ceased. The graphs are drawn for all four schedules of Set I where $\beta = 1.78$ and $E_{\mathrm{BCG}} = 70$ per cent.

The results are not encouraging; seemingly 20 years of control is not a long enough period to look at to make an appreciable change in the state of the disease. The large inactive classes and the large number of unvaccinated susceptibles cause the number of infectives to quickly rebound to undesired levels. A small difference between the schedules is seen in terms of the extent of the rebound, the higher numbered schedules producing the lesser rebound.

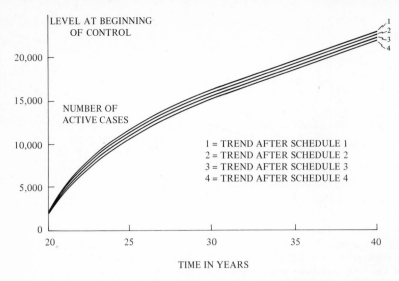

FIGURE 9-9. Natural trend after 20 years of control. $\beta = 1.78$, $E_{BCG} = 70$ per cent.

LEVEL AT BEGINNING OF CONTROL

NUMBER OF ACTIVE CASES

1 = TREND AFTER SCHEDULE 1
2 = TREND AFTER SCHEDULE 2
3 = TREND AFTER SCHEDULE 3
4 = TREND AFTER SCHEDULE 4

TIME IN YEARS

This fact leads to the necessity of considering even longer planning periods. This is needed even though the assumption of time stable parameters and unchanging medical technology becomes more difficult to justify.

Trend with Only BCG. The reduction schedules considered here have in all cases called for the use of BCG to achieve optimal programs. The only situation in which it was not called for was when its efficiency was set at zero. Invariably, substantial savings resulted from its use.

It is logical to question next the effect of BCG as the only form of control. Then the pattern that active cases follow cannot be specified. The only specifications are that a mass campaign of vaccinations be conducted in the first year and that all newborns be vaccinated each year. Thus, after the first year, class X disappears because all susceptible individuals are transferred to U.

The trend of active cases from 22,000 initially is again projected via numerical integration. Two efficiencies of BCG and two values of β are utilized in the examples.

In Figure 9-10, the trends are considered for $\beta = 1.78$. At a BCG efficiency of 30 per cent the number of actives rise slowly, reaching about 26,000 by the twentieth year. This is contrasted to the 31,000 active cases which the program with no controls produces by the twentieth year. That is, BCG holds the increase to 4,000 compared to 9,000 in the 20 years. At an efficiency of 70 per cent the results are more encouraging, BCG maintaining the number of active cases at almost exactly the initial value. A

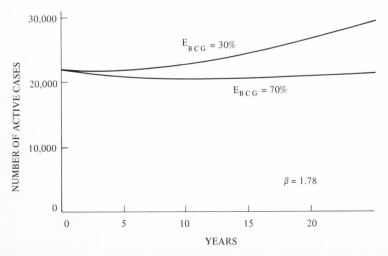

$E_{BCG} = 30\%$

$E_{BCG} = 70\%$

NUMBER OF ACTIVE CASES

$\beta = 1.78$

YEARS

FIGURE 9-10. Trend if BCG is only control.

slight rise near the end of 20 years is evident. Because the population is growing and the number of active cases nearly constant, the prevalence is actually falling.

The trends at a value of β of 3.45 are not so steady (Figure 9-11). A BCG efficiency of 30 per cent does hold the number of active cases to 34,000 by the twentieth year compared to 42,000 with no controls. Thus only 12,000 of a possible 20,000 new active cases actually occurred. When the BCG efficiency is 70 per cent, the active cases rise more slowly reaching only 24,000 by the twentieth year. Therefore, even at a β of 3.45, a 70 per cent efficient vaccine does assist the control effort considerably.

FIGURE 9-11. Trend if BCG is only control.

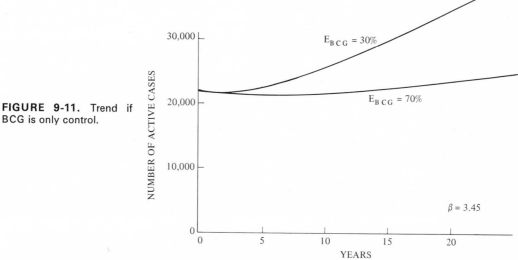

A Possible, Least Costly Pattern of Reduction.   It was noted earlier that the four schedules do not encompass all possible patterns of reduction, and that the least costly pattern is likely to make a prediction about the least costly pattern.

It is seen from the four 20-year schedules that the more slowly the reduction is carried out, the less costly the program is. For example, Schedule 1 allowed the greatest number of man-years of tuberculosis and cost the least, namely, $7,811,000 ($E_{BCG}$ = 70 per cent, β = 1.78). Having observed the pattern of active cases for 20 years when BCG is the only control used (Figure 8-1), one can immediately identify a pattern which provides the prescribed 2,000 active cases at 20 years at a cost far less than $7,811,000. The procedure is to use only BCG for 19 years and then undertake a drug treatment program at the beginning of the twentieth year to reduce the number of active cases from 22,000 to 2,000. This requires about 20,000 individual courses of treatment at $200 per individual, or a cost of about $4 million for the therapy portion of the program. The cost of the mass vaccination campaign and 19 years of newborn vaccination is about $460,000.

SUMMARY

The above illustration is indicative of a systems approach to problems in managerial medicine. The model is less than a *precise* reconstruction of the real situation, but in spite of its imperfections it assists in the development of additional insights that enable us to better evaluate alternative strategies and tactics.

This approach contains potential disadvantages if the user becomes transfixed by the quantitative information that the model produces. Decisions in public health require "good" quantitative information and "good" judgment. Without both ingredients the decision-maker is operating under a severe handicap. Systems analysis, by providing quantitative information, contributes to the first ingredient, *but it is not a panacea* that reduces decision-making to trivia.*

REFERENCES

ACKOFF, R. L., and SASIENI, M. W.: *Fundamentals of Operations Research*. John Wiley & Sons, New York, 1968.

BAILEY, N. T. J.: *The Mathematical Theory of Epidemics*. Charles Griffin & Co., London, 1957.

————: *The Mathematical Approach to Biology and Medicine*. John Wiley & Sons, London, 1967.

BARTLETT, M. S.: *Stochastic Population Models in Ecology and Epidemiology*. Methuen, London, 1960.

British Medical Research Council: BCG and vole bacillus vaccines in the prevention of tuberculosis in adolescence and early adult life; Third Report to the Medical Research Council by Their Tuberculosis Vaccines Clinical Trials Committee. *Brit Med J*, 1:973 1963.

BROGGER, S.: Systems/analysis in tuberculosis control. *Amer Rev Resp Dis*, **95**:419, 1967.

DUBOS, R. J.: *Man Adapting*. Yale University Press, New Haven, 1965.

FEREBEE, S.: Is eradication too much trouble? Paper presented at National Tuberculosis Association. Meeting, May 1966.

FOX, W.: Realistic chemotherapeutic policies for tuberculosis in developing countries. *Brit Med J*, 1:135, 1964.

KERMACK, W., and McKENDRICK, A.: A contribution to the mathematical theory of epidemics. *Proc Roy Soc Med (London)* **138A**:55, 1932.

PIOT, M.: Personal communication, August 1966.

ReVELLE, C. S.: *The Economic Allocation of Tuberculosis Control Activities in Developing Nations*. Doctoral dissertation. Cornell University, Ithaca, 1967.

————, LYNN, W. R., and FELDMANN, F.: Mathematical models for the economic allocation of tuberculosis control activities in developing nations. *Amer Rev Resp Dis*, **96**: 893, 1967.

WAALER, H., GESER, A., and ANDERSON, S.: The use of mathematical models in the study of the epidemiology of tuberculosis. *Amer J Public Health*, **52**:1002, 1962.

WEISBROD, B. A.: *Economics of Public Health*. University of Pennsylvania Press, Philadelphia, 1961.

World Health Organization: No truce for tuberculosis. *Amer Rev Resp Dis*, **89**:589, 1964.

---

* A Postscript: The discussions in the chapter have been restricted to what are called deterministic situations. Inasmuch as all managerial situations deal with actions for the future, we are confronted with the questions of how to deal with *risk* and *uncertainty*. Unfortunately, these stochastic approaches, albeit more realistic, are more difficult to implement because decision-makers are less able to incorporate these kinds of information into their decision processes.

Specific Problems
of
Public Health
and
Their Containment

10

Approaches to the Control of Human Infections

Edwin D. Kilbourne

INTRODUCTION

When man completes his first brief journey and emerges from the birth canal he is immediately beset with a host of microparasites with which he will live in a state of armed neutrality for the rest of his days. If he is unluckier than most, he may emerge already deafened, blinded, or crippled by the ravages of intrauterine infection, or he may quickly succumb to an ambush of pathogens within the canal itself. Toward the end of his life, as his strength ebbs and his defenses fail, his final illness, no matter how initiated, will be attended by recrudescence of earlier infections or fresh attacks from without.

The microorganisms that may invade the human host vary enormously in size and biologic activity and include metazoan (multicellular) organisms as well as protozoa, bacteria, rickettsia, and viruses. The inequities of circumstance dictate an unequal distribution of these parasites among the world's population, with the ironic result that economic "have-nots" have more than their share of parasites. Thus, the lives of whole populations are governed as much by the tertian tides of malarial plasmodia within them as by the diurnal tides of the ocean without. The incredible toll of such infestations cannot be measured in terms of mortality or even manifest morbidity in those who have never known true well-being. It is a basic problem of public health that the inverse ratio of man's economic and parasitic possessions is a self-perpetuating one. Much of the added burden of infectious disease in so-called "underdeveloped areas" is a corollary of a rural, crowded, impoverished existence in which the laws of economic survival require intimate contact among men in which they share one another's filth and the proximity of animals and their excreta. When man is thus forced to share the habitats of animals, he shares also their parasites and diseases. Or it may be that lesser beings will share their parasites with him—as does the malarial mosquito.

Chronically debilitated by these parasites, the impoverished population finds it difficult to develop the simple but expensive machinery of environmental sanitation to which the Western countries owe their relative freedom from all but the obligate parasites of man himself.

Yet in those countries with higher living standards, the problems of human parasitism are far from solved, and new problems have followed in the wake of sanitation, artificial immunization, and new antimicrobial drugs. Thus, the restriction in infantile fecal-oral contact resulting from modern sanitation has almost eliminated typhoid fever in some countries, but in those same countries "infantile" paralysis, now postponed from infancy, has become a disease of older children and adults (see Chapter 3).

It is the purpose of the discussions which follow to consider the parasitic or infectious diseases of man not as clinical entities but as complex natural phenomena influenced by both host and environment. It is the province of clinical medicine to define and study disease in the individual patient, and the province of medical microbiology to classify and study the microorganisms that cause disease. It is a major point and purpose of public health to study, and then influence, the interrelatedness of host, parasite, and environment. The discussions and classifications of disease in this chapter are unconventional by clinical and microbiologic standards, but they derive from the ecology and transmissibility of infectious diseases and provide a logical basis for public health practice. Infections such as malaria and typhus will not receive detailed consideration in these pages. Important as these infections are to large numbers of the world's population, they are, in a scientific sense, diseases of the past because their ultimate control awaits only the general application of well-established principles of sanitation. They are basically economic rather than medical problems.

A major emphasis of this chapter will be upon the control of communicable diseases directly transmissible from man to man. These are the diseases such as influenza that are relatively unaffected by the practice of environmental sanitation, and hence emerge as problems of the mid-twentieth century in industrialized societies. They are predictably the insipient problems of the near future for those areas that have not yet experienced industrial revolution.

The *relative* freedom of technologically advanced communities from the epidemic diseases of the past has not been realized by the complete elimination of microbial pathogens from the environment. In the great metropolitan area of New York City, salmonella in unhygienic delicatessens, rickettsialpox in multiple-family dwellings, psittacosis in pet stores, rabies virus in Connecticut foxes, and equine encephalitis virus in nearby New Jersey continually threaten this modern urban community. The costly machinery of environmental sanitation and public health are required for the continual maintenance of barriers between these microorganisms and the human population. There are other infections, such as tuberculosis and influenza, for which no physical barriers can be erected and for which different methods of control must be employed. In the hospitals of the city, patients are dying of self-derived "endogenous" infections with enteric bacteria for which there are no barriers except the preservation of the physiologic integrity of the individual. In this last half of the twentieth century, the great plagues of the past are rarely seen (see Chapter 3) but the problem of infection is still very much with us.

THE ORIGIN AND TRANSMISSION OF INFECTIONS

A rational approach to the control of infectious diseases obviously demands a knowledge of the distribution in nature of the causative microbes and an understanding of their modes of spread. All infections of man can be broadly grouped in two great categories including (1) those derived from the external environment and from other species and (2) those caused by primary or obligate human pathogens—the so-called contagious or communicable diseases. Control of infections of the first category can be achieved in most instances by environmental sanitation. This kind of control presents economic problems but few scientific ones. Most infections derived from the environment are sufficiently understood so that control measures can be designed to block the contact of parasite with man and thus ultimately to prevent infection.

Partly because of ignorance of the ecology of the contagious human pathogens, and partly because of their intimate relation to man, many of the communicable infections must be accepted as ubiquitous and perhaps "inevitable." In this latter case the goal is not necessarily prevention of *infection* but prevention or modification of *disease* by altering human resistance to these assaults from without that cannot be environmentally controlled.

INFECTIOUS HAZARDS OF THE EXTERNAL ENVIRONMENT

The infections with which environmental sanitation has been traditionally concerned are those in which the parasite either can or must exist for a time outside the human host. Such infections include:

1. The zoonoses, or infections primarily of animals.
2. Infections primarily human but with an arthropod vector (filariasis).
3. Human infections (typhoid) caused by agents that may survive without multiplication in soil or water.

To these may be added certain clostridia and staphylococci that induce the formation of toxins in food, thus contaminating the environment of man. Despite the diversity of these agents and the diseases they cause, it is useful to consider them together as threats of man's environment.

Infections Primarily of Animals That Are Transmissible to Man

In the case of certain infections, man is an accidental victim or "innocent bystander" who is attacked by a parasite that is a primary or usual pathogen in lower animals. In diseases of this sort the existence of man is not necessary for the continued survival of the parasite, and in most instances further transmission of the parasite directly from man to man does not occur. Infections that primarily involve animals are caused by a wide variety of microbial species and may be transmitted from animal to man in many ways. The more important infections of this type are considered in Table 10-1.

In general, human infections with the larger parasites (the helminths and bacteria) are derived from domestic animals or from animals such as the rat that live in close

TABLE 10-1

Animal Infections of Public Health Importance Transmissible to Man
Man an Accidental Host

Infection	Agent	Principal Hosts	Principal Methods of Transmission
Nemathelminthic			
Trichinosis	*Trichinella spiralis*	Swine, rat	Ingestion
Echinococcosis	*Echinococcus granulosus* (larva)	Dog (adult worm) Sheep, swine, cattle (larva)	Ingestion
Bacterial			
Anthrax	*Bacillus anthracis*	Herbivorous animals	Direct contact
Brucellosis	*Brucella abortus* *Brucella melitensis* *Brucella suis*	Cattle, swine, goats, horses Goats, sheep, cattle, swine Swine, cattle, horses	Contact, ingestion, inoculation, air-borne
Leptospirosis	*Leptospira icterohaemorrhagiae* (Many others)	Rodents, swine, cats, dogs, horses, poultry, calves	Direct contact(?)
Plague (bubonic)	*Pasteurella pestis*	Wild rodents	Insect (flea) bite
Salmonellosis (food poisoning)	*Salmonella typhimurium*, *S. cholerasuis*, *S. oranienburg*	Rodents, fowl, swine	Ingestion
Tetanus	*Clostridium tetani*	Horses, cattle	Inoculation or contact with animal feces
Tularemia	*Pasteurella tularensis*	Wild rodents	Contact, arthropod bites. ingestion
Tuberculosis (bovine)	*Mycobacterium tuberculosis*	Cattle	Ingestion, air-borne

Rickettsial			
Q fever	*Rickettsia burnetti*	Cattle, sheep, goats	Contact, air-borne ingestion
Spotted fevers			
Rocky Mountain spotted fever	*Rickettsia rickettsii*	?	Tick bite
Rickettsialpox	*Rickettsia akari*	Mouse	Mite bite
Typhus fever (murine)	*Rickettsia mooseri*	Mouse	Flea bite
Viral			
Psittacosis	Psittacosis (ornithosis) virus	Birds, including domestic fowl	Air-borne
Arbor viruses			
(group A)			
Western equine encephalitis	Western equine encephalitis virus	Birds	Mosquito bite
Eastern equine encephalitis	Eastern equine encephalitis virus		
(group B)			
St. Louis encephalitis	St. Louis encephalitis virus	Fowl, birds	Mosquito bite
Japanese B encephalitis	Japanese B encephalitis virus	Birds, heron (?)	Mosquito bite
Russian tick-borne encephalitis	Russian tick-borne encephalitis virus	Sheep, goats (?)	Tick bite, ingestion in milk
Yellow fever (jungle type)	Yellow fever virus	Monkey	Mosquito bite
Rabies	Rabies virus	Dog	Dog bite

TABLE 10-2
Infections Primarily of Man in Which the Infective Agent Has a Requisite Period of Extrahuman Residence Before Transmission

Infection	Agent	Extrahuman Phase	Intermediate Host or Vector	Transmission
Helminthic				
Schistosomiasis	*Schistosoma mansoni*	Water	Snail	Ingestion, skin penetration
	S. japonicum			
	S. haematobium			
Tapeworm	*Taenia saginata*	Cattle	—	Ingestion
	T. solium	Swine	—	Ingestion
	Diphyllobothrium latum	Fish	—	Ingestion
Whipworm	*Trichuris trichiura*	Soil	—	Ingestion
Ascariasis	*Ascaris lumbricoides*	Soil	—	Ingestion
Filariasis	*Wuchereria bancrofti*	Mosquito	Mosquito	Skin penetration
	W. malayi			Skin penetration
Hookworm	*Ancylostoma duodenale*	Soil	—	Skin penetration
	Necator americanus			
Protozoan				
Amebiasis	*Endamoeba histolytica*	Soil	(Fly)	Ingestion
Malaria *	*Plasmodium vivax*	Mosquito	Mosquito	Mosquito bite
	P. malariae			
	P. falciparum			
	P. ovale			
Trypanosomiasis	*Trypanosoma gambiense*	Fly	Glossina (fly)	Fly bite
	T. rhodesiense	Fly	Glossina	Fly bite
	T. cruzi	Triatoma	Triatoma	Insect bite
Leishmaniasis	*Leishmania donovani*	Phlebotomus (fly)	Phlebotomus	Fly bite
	L. tropica			
	L. braziliensis			
Mycotic				
Coccidioidomycosis	*Coccidioides immitis*	Soil	—	Air-borne
Histoplasmosis	*Histoplasma capsulatum*	Soil	—	Air-borne
Bacterial				
Relapsing fever	*Borrelia recurrentis*	Arthropod ? Wild rodents	Louse, tick	Skin penetration
Rickettsial				
Typhus (epidemic)		Louse	Louse	Skin penetration
Viral				
Yellow fever (urban)	Yellow fever virus	Mosquito	Mosquito	Mosquito bite

* Actually, an infection primarily of the mosquito.

proximity to human habitation. Human infection with these agents depends on close contact with the infected animals or upon ingestion of their tissues or secretions.

In the case of the rickettsia and viruses, transmission is usually effected through a variety of arthropod vectors and the source of infection may be the animal in the wild. The arthropod as a "flying hypodermic needle" greatly influences the possibilities for transmission to man. It is not necessary to live on a farm to be at risk from Eastern equine encephalitis. Communicability is predicated on the flight range of the mosquito and the proximity of certain wild birds as well as domestic horses.

Infections Primarily of Man in Which the Infective Agent Has a Requisite Period of Extrahuman Residence Before Transmission

Certain microorganisms, although they are primarily pathogenic for man, are not spread directly from man to man but have a requisite stage of existence in man's external environment. This can be a passing stage in water or soil, as with the agents of amebiasis or coccidioidomycosis, or it may be part of a complicated cycle involving intermediate animal hosts, as with schistosomiasis or tapeworm infestation. Infection from these environmental reservoirs may be initiated through direct transcutaneous inoculation of parasites by biting insects, overt invasion by free-swimming cercariae, or passive inhalation of mycotic spores (Table 10-2).

These infections, because most of them involve intermediate hosts or vectors of limited and circumscribed habitat, can be characterized as regional or geographically restricted infections. Therefore, they do not comprise universal and ubiquitous threats to the human population, although some—such as malaria—affect large areas of the globe and millions of people.

Infections Directly Transmissible from Man to Man in Which the Infective Agent May Persist in the Environment

The infective agents of certain diseases, although they may be transmitted directly from man to man, may be capable of survival for long periods in the external environment. From this location they threaten man through his water, his food—even through the air he breathes. This epidemiologically defined group of microorganisms is somewhat heterogeneous, but for the most part it includes bacteria and viruses that cause primarily enteric infections. The infections so classified are listed in Table 10-3. It should be emphasized that the infections of this group (with the exception of typhoid, dysentery, and cholera) are not usually or optimally transmitted from environmental sources.

Diseases Caused by Preformed Microbial Products without True Infection of the Diseased Host

Certain microorganisms while in the external environment may multiply and produce poisons or toxins. If eaten by man, these microbial products can induce severe symptoms and even death. These disease states are not true infections, as they can be induced experimentally by the exotoxin *in the absence of the bacteria*, and because

TABLE 10-3

Infections Directly Transmissible from Man to Man in Which the Infective Agent Persists or Multiplies in the External Environment

Infection	Infective Agent	Sites of Persistence	Trans- mission
Bacterial			
Cholera	*Vibrio comma*	Water, food	Ingestion
Dysentery (bacillary)	*Shigella*	Water, food	Ingestion
Typhoid fever	*Salmonella typhosa**	Water, food	Ingestion
Staphylococcal diseases	*Staphylococcus aureus** ⎫	Food, air, ⎫	
Streptococcal diseases	*Streptococcus pyogenes** ⎬	environment ⎬	Inhalation,
Tuberculosis	*Mycobacterium tubercu- losis* ⎭	in proximity to man ⎭	contact
Viral			
Smallpox	Smallpox virus	Air, dust, environment in proximity to patient	Inhalation
Infectious hepatitis	Hepatitis virus A	Water, food	Ingestion
Coxsackie virus disease	Coxsackieviruses	Water	Ingestion
ECHO virus disease	ECHO viruses	Water	Ingestion
Poliomyelitis	Polioviruses	Water, food	Ingestion

* May multiply in the environment.

the microorganisms are incapable of invading and multiplying in the tissue of the host. These toxic diseases are to be distinguished from such infections as diphtheria and tetanus in which disease results from exotoxin, following and coinciding with invasion of the host tissues by microorganisms. Because the diseases caused by preformed microbial toxins are food-borne, they are often confused with acute food-borne infectious gastroenteritis caused by the Salmonellae.

Botulism.   Botulism is a serious disease that fortunately is quite rare. It is reported more commonly in the United States in the Midwestern and Far Western states. The symptoms of the disease appear from 18 hours to four or five days after infected food has been eaten. Death results in one third to one half the cases.

The characteristics of the outbreaks are related to the ecology of the infecting organism. *Clostridium botulinum* is a spore-forming anaerobe. It is found in the intestines of many animals and is encountered freely in farm soils. It is not pathogenic to man or animals per se, but it grows freely in protein foods and produces a highly potent, soluble toxin. Even a few drops of fluid from a jar of infected home-cooked vegetables have caused death to man and to experimental animals.

The organism grows under anaerobic conditions, producing gas and a characteristic odor so that infected food has a "tainted" taste. The toxin has a special affinity for nerve tissues. Although six toxicogenic types are recognized, only two groups of organisms, A and B, are commonly encountered; type E as a contaminant of fish has become more common in the United States. Their toxins differ, so that type-specific antitoxin must be administered in order to save the patient's life. The toxin is killed by a temperature of 80 °C, maintained for 20 minutes. Boiling destroys it almost at once, The organism itself is quite heat resistant: a temperature of 120 °C maintained for 10 minutes is required to kill the spores.

Staphylococcal Food Poisoning. An unknown number of staphylococcal strains have the capacity to produce an enterotoxin (not to be confused with endotoxin) under appropriate culture conditions. Such conditions are provided by a wide variety of protein foods (notably those containing egg or milk products) and inadequate refrigeration. The widespread carriage of staphylococci in the nasal secretions and on the skin of healthy people makes contamination of food almost inevitable. If the protein food is not stored at refrigerator temperature, rapid multiplication of staphylococci can occur with concomitant production of enterotoxin (sometimes in less than six hours.) This preformed toxin is the agent of the acute and transiently devastating gastroenteritis that occurs in man within 3 to 12 hours of its ingestion.

The disease is obviously an intoxication and not a true infection. Symptoms are caused by the filtered toxin in the absence of the staphylococcus, and staphylococci capable of forming enterotoxin can be ingested without ill effect. These facts are reflected by the brevity of the incubation period, the course of the acute illness, and the absence of the fever and pyogenic sequelae that characterize staphylococcal invasion of tissues.

This form of food poisoning is by far the most frequent and contributes enormously to morbidity, if not to mortality. The difficulties in control of this disease, even in industrialized countries are related to—

1. The ubiquitous occurrence of *Staphylococcus aureus*.
2. The rapid rate of bacterial growth and toxin production in unrefrigerated foods.
3. The heat stability of the toxin, which can withstand boiling temperatures.
4. The absence of taint, odor, or other indication of food spoilage in toxin-containing foods.

THE CONTROL OF INFECTIOUS DISEASES ACQUIRED FROM THE EXTERNAL ENVIRONMENT
(the traditional mission of public health and environmental sanitation)

A number of infections of widely varying biological types have been categorized in relation to the problem of their transmissibility to man. These disparate infections have one common attribute: their agents threaten man from their residence in his general *biological* environment, which comprises the food he eats, the water he drinks, the air (and dust) he breathes, and the animals (vertebrate and invertebrate) with which he comes in contact. Literally, the environment also includes other people, but in terms of infectious disease "other people" constitute a very special environmental problem that will be discussed later as the contagious diseases.

It is obvious that control of infections emanating from the environment can be accomplished by appropriate manipulation of this environment. This fact was recognized long before the germ theory of disease was postulated. The ancients drained the marshes to control malaria because they recognized the association of filth and disease, and they also established empirical dietary laws against the eating of certain foods.

This manipulation of the environment of man is essentially the science of *sanitation* as it now exists in public health practice. It has been pointed out elsewhere in this text that public health legislation did not originate within the medical profession but was dictated more by esthetic and olfactory considerations (see Chapter 5).

The Changing Ecology of Infections

Details of public health practice with respect to sanitation will not be considered here, but the *rationale* of sanitation for infectious diseases is discussed in relation to the *ecology* and mode of transmission of infections. Before discussing the application of sanitation to the problems of environmentally linked infections, it should be emphasized that unplanned changes in the environment may change radically the relation of host and parasite to the advantage or detriment of either. Thus, floods are notoriously associated with epidemics of enteric infections because sewage and drinking water are mixed by rising water. An unusually rainy summer in New Jersey in 1959 increased the mosquito population and contributed thereby to a human epidemic caused by mosquito-borne eastern equine encephalitis virus.

The traditional human urge to "kill the vermin" resulted not only in the extermination of mice in a New York City apartment house but also in the appearance of a new disease, rickettsialpox, as parasitic mites left the cold bodies of their murine hosts to seek succor on the warm bodies of the human tenants of the buildings. This episode is, of course, no indictment of the killing of mice per se; if the mice had survived, they might have transmitted lymphocytic choriomeningitis virus instead. The lesson is the old one: the "balance of nature" even in a New York apartment house should be disturbed only with due appreciation of the consequences.

The Geographic Determination of Infections.   There is little evidence that the races of man differ in their susceptibility to the acquisition of infection. Therefore, differences in the geographic distribution of infectious disease may be assumed to result from factors determining local prevalence of the infectious agent. Such varying prevalences are in the large sense geographically determined, but they will depend definitively upon climate, the presence of an appropriate vector or intermediate host, or upon regional peculiarities of habit that permit man to come in contact with the parasite.

Thus, the "geographic" restriction of African sleeping sickness (trypanosomiasis) to Africa reflects the apparent restriction of the vector Glossina fly to that continent, although perpetuation of the infection is also dependent on the prevalence of infected mammals. On the other hand, the spotty global distribution of coccidioidomycosis and hookworm reflects primarily the occurrence of arid or damp climatic conditions, respectively. In the case of hookworm infection, however, the further requirements of poor sanitation (with respect to sewage disposal) and an unshod human foot are needed for the disease to occur.

Although it can be predicted that hookworm will never become a problem in Denver, Colorado, it cannot be said that yellow fever or malaria will never again threaten the continental United States. The insect vectors and susceptible population are present; only the introduction of human infection is required to complete the chain.

What factors, then, can be manipulated to prevent infections from the environment? The essential jobs of current public health sanitation are

1. Water purification.
2. Sewage disposal.
3. The control of food.

To a lesser extent public sanitation is concerned with insect and vermin control, housing, and other aspects of the socioeconomic environment. The newer and urgent tasks of control of air pollution and other twentieth-century environmental hazards are considered in Chapter 4.

The Control of Infections Carried by Water

Because the most common and important water-borne infections derive from the human intestine, the problems of sewage disposal and water purification are interlinked. Inadequate methods of sewage disposal can compromise the safety of water treated by optimal methods.

In cities of the United States the average daily consumption of water per capita is about 150 gal. Most of this water is used in industry. Only about 50 gal per capita are required for total household purposes. Because it is not feasible to have one water supply for domestic use and another for industrial use and fire protection, it becomes necessary for the entire water supply to be treated and purified as though every drop were to be used for drinking purposes.

Every community, from the small village to the largest city, has a primary obligation to provide a water supply that is adequate for all nutritional, household, industrial, and fire-protection requirements. Large cities may find it necessary to go great distances, to tap large watersheds, to tunnel mountains, to drain rivers, to inundate towns, and to depopulate large areas in order to provide storage facilities for their water supplies. Extensive and intricate systems of transportation of water, purification plants, and distribution systems must be supplied. These are all problems in sanitary engineering. It is sufficient for the physician to know that a water supply must be provided to each of the individual homes in the community that is adequate, potable (i.e., free from taste, odor, and color), and free from pollution, and that will not produce disease.

The development of community water supplies in the United States in the first half of this century was phenomenal. In 1900, only 3,200 cities and towns had community water systems. In 1950, nearly 15,000 cities had public water supplies that served well over 100,000,000 people. During this period the typhoid death rate dropped from 23 per 100,000 population to less than 0.5, and the death rate from diarrhea, enteritis, and dysentery was cut to one tenth of the former rate.

The physician is primarily interested in the water supply because it may be an important factor in the transmission of disease. Water-borne infection practically always results from pollution of the water supply with human wastes, particularly with the urine and feces of persons with active intestinal diseases, or perhaps by the carriers of disease agents.

There are exceptions to this rule—notably anthrax, which is a disease of animals that has been transmitted to human beings through water. Tulatemia also, another primary disease of animals, has been reported as being transmitted to human beings through infected water.

Water is used almost universally as a means of disposal of home and community wastes, especially the disposal of sewage. As areas become more densely inhabited, the problem of prevention of water-borne disease becomes more acute and difficult. During the developmental period of America, the great importance of water as a vehicle of infection was not fully recognized. Epidemic after epidemic of typhoid fever, cholera, and other intestinal infections occurred as a direct result of community-wide water pollution. The solution of these problems has been one of the great triumphs in sanitary engineering (Figure 10-1).

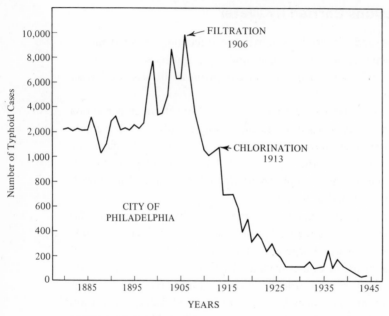

FIGURE 10-1. Reduction of typhoid fever in Philadelphia following treatment of the water supply. (Data supplied through the courtesy of Dr. Angelo M. Perri.)

Water-borne Epidemics. In former years, widespread epidemics of disease due to pollution of community water supplies were of annual occurrence. These outbreaks have almost entirely ceased in municipalities, and also in institutions having a common water supply. This result has been brought about through the vigilance of state and municipal divisions of sanitary engineering and by the development of proper methods of water purification, together with the establishment of suitable procedures for constant checking of possible pollution. From time to time, the methods that have been worked out so carefully fail to function, and disaster results.

In recent years, the constant vigilance of municipal and state health authorities has continued the decline in community-wide water-borne epidemics. Temporary labor camps, summer trailer parks, and other places where groups of people utilize primitive sanitation are now our chief source of water-borne outbreaks of disease.

Chlorination.   Long before the microbial nature of infectious diseases was appreciated, disinfectants were used empirically in the control of "putrefaction." Chloride of lime was so used as early as 1832, more than 50 years before the isolation of the typhoid bacillus. Chlorination of water has proved to be the most satisfactory method in the control of water-borne bacterial pathogens (see Table 10-4). Automatic devices are available that regulate the flow of the chlorine exactly in accordance with the need.

TABLE 10-4

Infections Transmissible Through Drinking Water

Infection	Susceptibility to Chlorination*
Metazoan	
Schistosomiasis	?
Ascariasis	?
Protozoan	
Amebiasis	0
Bacterial	
Cholera	+
Bacillary dysentery	+
Typhoid fever	+
Leptospirosis	+
Tularemia	+
Viral	
Infectious hepatitis	0
Coxsackievirus infection†	0
ECHOvirus infection†	0
Poliomyelitis†	0

* For amounts of chlorine currently used in standard sanitation practice.
† Theoretically transmissible, but not proved.

The method has the disadvantage that an excess of chlorine imparts an unpleasant taste to the water. Heavily polluted water, with a high degree of turbidity, will require such an excess of chlorine that the taste of the water becomes disagreeable.

The great value of chlorine is that it can be used as a supplementary procedure, to be added after other purification methods of storage and filtration have been employed. Thus the chlorine gives a further factor of safety.

Chlorination cannot be relied upon as an automatic and perfectly safe method of water purification. The method requires constant supervision, frequent testing of available chlorine by the use of the orthotoluidine test, together with daily bacteriologic checks of the efficiency of the procedures.

The Special Problem of Viruses and Water-borne Epidemics.   Recently the hypothetical threat presented by human enteroviruses and the virus of infectious hepatitis has proved to be more than theoretical. There is now little doubt that water-borne outbreaks of infectious hepatitis can occur. Twenty-eight water-borne epidemics in 13 countries have been reviewed (Mosely, 1959).

A particularly dramatic and well-studied epidemic occurred in Delhi, India, in 1955 (Melnick, 1957). Following a flood of the Jamuna River in October of that year, the water receded and the river changed its course (Figure 10-2), resulting in the

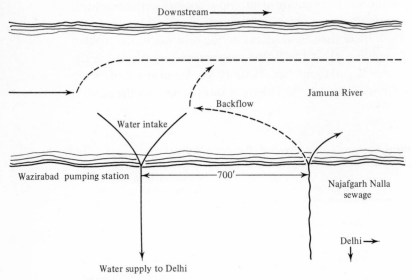

FIGURE 10-2.   Contamination of Delhi water supply with sewage doing backflow in the Jamuna River. (Reproduced from J. L. Melnick in F. W. Hartman *et al.* (eds.): *Hepatitis Frontiers: Henry Ford Hospital International Symposium*, No. 6. Little, Brown and Company, Boston, 1957.)

flow *upstream* of raw sewage that usually emptied below the water-purification plant. The raw sewage caused gross contamination of the city water supply as it entered the water pumping station. The situation was worsened by the absence of rain and storm water, so that the sewage entering the river from the *nalla*, or creek, was virtually undiluted. Study of the chloride concentration afforded a measure of the duration and degree of contamination of the city water and demonstrated that contamination occurred during one week in mid-November. It was calculated that during the peak of contamination about *50 per cent of the water entering the pumping station was made up of sewage*. This contamination was promptly recognized, and the alum and chloride concentrations were immediately increased—the chlorine from 0.5 to 2.1 parts per million. This treatment of the water was apparently sufficient to prevent any significant increase in typhoid or other enteric bacterial diseases, but it did not prevent the extensive epidemic of 35,000 cases of infectious hepatitis that became evident six weeks later. The well-defined period of water contamination provided a unique natural experiment for the definition of the incubation period of the disease. This proved to be 22 to 60 days with a mode of 40 days—longer than is usual with infectious hepatitis. Other epidemics of infectious hepatitis that were clearly spread by chlorinated water have been reported (Poskanzer and Beadenkopf, 1961).

Recent experimental studies have demonstrated not only the presence of poliomyelitis and other enteroviruses in raw sewage but also the resistance of certain enteroviruses to the concentrations of free and combined chlorine now recommended for sewage treatment. Although it is probable that water is a relatively unimportant vehicle for the spread of enterovirus infections, it is important to note that present-day sewage treatment does not truly "disinfect" or kill these pathogens.

The Control of Infections Transmitted by Milk and Other Foods

The important infections transmitted by milk are brucellosis, group A (beta hemolytic) streptococcal pharyngitis, and bovine tuberculosis. Less commonly, typhoid fever, bacillary dysentery, and staphylococcal "food poisoning" are traceable to contaminated milk. Of the rickettsial infections, Q fever can be milk-borne and, recently, milk has been implicated in transmission of the virus of the Russian tick-borne complex of infections (Table 10-5). Present methods of pasteurization are adequate for the destruction of any but the Russian tick-borne virus. The heat-stable enterotoxin of the staphylococcus also is not eliminated from milk by pasteurization if already present, although the staphylococci are destroyed.

If milk is not properly handled, it deteriorates rapidly as a food. It is an excellent cultural medium for bacteria and may act as a vehicle of pathogenic organisms. Thus, the procedures in the sanitation of milk are basically the application of simple bacteriologic principles to milk production. It has become a highly technical process, requiring the aid of veterinarians, bacteriologists, sanitary inspectors, and other specialists in dairy technology.

Bacteriologic Tests.   Normally, milk as it leaves the healthy udder of the cow contains few bacteria. Thus a high bacterial count in a milk sample may indicate that (a) the milk was not cooled promptly, (b) the milk is dirty, or (c) the udder of the cow was infected.

Before the advent of good dairy practice, milk frequently reached the consumer with a count of 500,000 bacteria per cubic centimeter, and 100,000 bacteria per cubic centimeter was considered as allowable in samples collected from the delivery wagon. The Certified Milk Commission set a standard of 10,000 bacteria per cubic

TABLE 10-5
Infections Transmitted by Milk or Milk Products

Infection	Eliminated by Pasteurization
Brucellosis	+
Salmonellosis (especially typhoid fever)	+
Tuberculosis, bovine	+
Q fever	+
Streptococcal infections (group A)	+
Staphylococcal enteritis	0
Russian tick-borne complex (encephalitis)	0

centimeter as allowable for certified milk. Gradually dairy practice has improved to such a degree that market milk now often comes to the pasteurizing plant with a bacterial count of only 10,000 to 20,000 bacteria per cubic centimeter.

The bacteriologic laboratory is the best means we have of measuring the cleanliness and sanitary quality of milk. Standard practice requires the determination of the total bacterial count of the sample.

Pasteurization of Milk.   The process of pasteurization is a final safeguard against milk-borne infection. It does not relieve the producer of the responsibility for employing cleanliness and all other proper dairy techniques: the milk must be clean and of good quality when it reaches the pasteurizer. Pasteurization, properly carried out, renders the milk *safe*.

Two common methods of pasteurization are used: the *holding* method and the *flash* method. The former method employs a temperature of 142 to 145 °F for 30 minutes, with rapid cooling of the milk to 50 °F and bottling by automatic machinery. Usually the milk is heated in large tanks with automatic temperature control and recording.

In the flash method there is a continuous flow of milk, with rapid heating to 160 °F for 15 seconds, followed by rapid cooling.

The purpose of pasteurization of milk is to destroy all pathogenic bacteria in the milk without injuring the quality of the product or changing its flavor. Pasteurization does destroy some of the vitamin C of milk, but milk is not an important source of this vitamin. It should, in any case, be obtained from other sources of food. Other theoretical objections have been raised, but the advantages so overwhelmingly outweigh the disadvantages that milk pasteurization has become almost universal in the United States.

PHOSPHATASE TEST.   The phosphatase test is used to determine whether or not milk has been suitably pasteurized. This enzyme is present in raw milk but is thermosensitive at pasteurization temperature. Thus a quantitative measurement of phosphatase in the milk is a good index of suitable pasteurization.

Boiling of milk is an unsatisfactory substitute for pasteurization. It renders the milk quite safe but changes the taste and even the quality of the milk. Boiling of milk is almost universal in the tropics; in many countries it is a household custom because it has been found empirically to be an important health safeguard.

Certified Milk.   Certified milk was developed by a Medical Milk Commission at a time when the quality of market milk was very poor and it was necessary to secure a safe supply of pure milk for infants. This milk is produced under the supervision of an official medical board, with very rigorous restrictions that give assurance of a high-quality product. All certified milk should be pasteurized in order to be safe as well as of good quality. The cost of certified milk is usually more than that of market milk.

Grades of Milk.   Formerly, milk was graded into different qualities in accordance with the fat content, the bacterial count, and other criteria. These grades included pasteurized and raw milk, grade A; and pasteurized and raw milk, grade B; together with other variable qualities of milk that brought confusion to the consumer and to the dairyman as well.

The general improvement in milk sanitation has almost nullified the necessity for the production of special grades of milk. The present tendency is to abandon the terms A, B, or C milk, and to produce one standard, high-quality, safe, pure milk that will be readily available to people in all walks of life at a reasonable cost. In promoting this standard of milk, primary insistence must be placed upon safety of the milk as an article of food.

Requirements for a Community Milk Supply.   The basic requirements for a satisfactory community milk supply are:

1. Intelligent dairymen who are familiar with all the details of modern dairy practice. They should seek the guidance of the state department of agriculture in all matters relating to dairy sanitation.
2. The cows should be healthy and well fed, free from bovine tuberculosis, brucellosis, and mastitis.
3. Provision should be made to chill the milk immediately after milking, and to keep it at 50 °F until delivered to the pasteurizer.
4. All milk should be pasteurized under carefully controlled conditions.
5. The milk should be placed directly after pasteurization into the container which will reach the consumer; it should be chilled at once and maintained at 50 °F until it is delivered.
6. A uniform state-wide sanitary milk code should be formulated, with provision for a proper system of inspection of dairies and of pasteurization plants.
7. Local laboratory service under health department auspices is essential, in order to act as a check on the purity, cleanliness, and safety of the milk.

Intestinal Infections.   Milk is seldom infected with human intestinal discharges, but when this does occur through careless dairy technique, the results can be very serious. Many widespread milk-borne epidemics of typhoid fever and bacillary dysentery have been reported from this source of infection. In practically every instance, the milk was unpasteurized. There are exceptions to this rule.

Typhoid fever epidemic due to pasteurized milk.   Typhoid fever began to appear sporadically in a large Western city. It occurred over a large area and lasted for a considerable period of time. The health authorities investigated all possible common sources of infection without success. They were sure it could not be a milk-borne outbreak, because these epidemics are characteristically explosive in onset, limited in time, and usually confined to a small area.

All the persons affected used milk from one large distributor, but this source was ruled out, because the milk was pasteurized. The distribution of milk by this company was very extensive, and the incidence of the disease was small and scattered. The milk came to the distributor from many sources, but all were under sanitary supervision. The pasteurization plant was well managed, all automatic temperature records were in perfect order, and the milk was bottled automatically and distributed in individual quart bottles. All employees of the pasteurization plant were examined, to be sure there were no typhoid carriers in the group.

The disease remained unchecked in the community, despite efforts to find a common source of infection. Fresh vegetables and fruits were studied, as well as butter and cheese, shellfish, and other possible modes of infection. Scattered cases of the disease continued to appear. The state epidemiologist was called into consultation, and on the basis of a statistical analysis of all the data, he made the following deductions.

1. The milk from one distributor was at fault.
2. The pasteurization process was working satisfactorily: otherwise the outbreaks would have been much more extensive, and would have occurred in spurts.
3. The delivery system was not at fault: else the cases would have occurred on a single or on individual delivery routes.

4. The infection must occur between the time the milk was pasteurized in bulk and the time it was placed on the wagons. This must be either in storage or in the operation of bottling.

The epidemiologist then studied the bottling operations, which were carried out automatically in a glass-enclosed room by two workers. He noted that the automatic capping machine failed, perhaps once in a hundred times; the two men at the bottling machines had a pile of caps nearby, so that they could cap the bottles by hand when the machine did not operate properly. Here was a possible source of contamination. One of these men was found, on repeated examinations, to be a typhoid carrier. He was an intermittent carrier—that is, only at times did he have large numbers of typhoid organisms in his stools. At other times they were difficult to find.

This outbreak had unusual characteristics because of the peculiar chain of circumstances that produced it, but it does illustrate the fact that milk may occasionally be infected even though it is properly pasteurized. The study also shows that a single negative stool examination is not sufficient proof that an individual is not a typhoid carrier.

Diseases Transmitted Through Milk Products: Cream, Ice Cream, Butter, and Cheese. Numerous outbreaks of disease are recorded that have been traced to cream and to ice cream. These foods are highly susceptible to infection and must be handled with the same scrupulous care as milk itself.

The procedures that are employed in the manufacture of butter and cheese tend to eliminate infection with the hemolytic streptococcus and with staphylococcus, but epidemics of typhoid fever, as well as paratyphoid and dysentry, have been traced both to infected butter and infected cheese. The bovine tubercle bacillus also may not be destroyed in the process of butter and cheese manufacture.

Thus, milk that is used in the manufacture of any milk products should be pasteurized; it should be of as good a quality and handled with the same sanitary precautions as is the bottled milk that goes directly to the consumer.

Cheese that is properly ripened is safe. Many health departments require that cheese be aged for not less than 60 days before it can be sold.

The Control of "Food Poisoning": Acute Diseases Caused by Toxic Microbial Products Formed in Foods Prior to Their Ingestion.   Although some acute illnesses derived from food are true infections (i.e., salmonellosis), much so-called food poisoning is caused not by microbial invasion of tissue, but by the effects of toxins elaborated in food before it is eaten. These entities have been described on preceding pages as botulism and staphylococcal enteritis. The prevention and control of these diseases are dependent to a large extent on public education concerning the handling and preparation of food.

Botulism has become a medical rarity in the United States because of the effective methods of sterilization introduced by the commerical canning industry. With home-canned products (especially beans) of dubious history, boiling of the food will destroy the heat-labile botulinus toxin. Specific antisera are available for the prophylaxis of infection in those exposed to toxin-containing food. These anti-toxins against the types A, B, and E toxins which affect man have also been used in therapy of the overt disease but their value is debated.

The prevention of the toxic enteritis caused by *Staphylococcus aureus* enterotoxin and the infective enteritis caused by *Salmonella*, and more rarely by other bacteria, may be considered together.

Prevention of *Staphylococcus aureus* and *Salmonella* Food Poisoning.   Although the epidemiologic investigation of an outbreak of food poisoning is always interesting and usually revealing, it invariably leaves the investigator with a sense of complete futility, for the outbreak is over when it is discovered, and no preventive measures can be instituted.

The prevention of these conditions is a long, slow process of education of food handlers and enforcement of regulations relating to the handling, processing, and storage of all types of food, together with special emphasis upon improvement in methods of preparation and storage of protein foods.

Effort should be concentrated in those places where outbreaks most frequently occur. Large banquets are the chief offenders. The banquet often overtaxes the resources of the hotel or the caterer: food is prepared in large quantities, well in advance of the dinner hour, and placed in individual serving dishes in order to avoid a last-minute rush. Salads, shrimp cocktails, creamed foods, and the like are prepared and allowed to stand for several hours before they are served. Food is carelessly handled and is not stored at sufficiently low temperatures. The result is that conventions of all types, church dinners, fraternity picnics—in fact, all large gatherings of people—are very frequently accompanied by outbreaks of food poisoning.

Prevention depends upon the simple facts that the bacteria and their products are readily destroyed by heat and cannot develop at low temperatures. Even though the salmonella actually enter the protein foods through careless handling, no harm results if the food is kept at proper refrigerator temperatures. However, a good general household rule is to reheat all protein food to boiling if the food has been kept in storage for any length of time, i.e., 24 hours in the refrigerator or 3 hours at room temperature.

Antemortem and postmortem abattoir inspection is of some value because animals with obvious diseases are condemned as unfit for food.

Scrupulous cleanliness in the preparation and handling of food, especially of meat and meat products, is an important safeguard. Pasteurization of milk and proper heating of milk products, such as ice-cream mix, custards, and all other such materials, are an essential part of the preventive program.

Constant supervision of restaurants, delicatessens, cold-storage plants, roadside eating stands, meat and fish markets, and all places that handle food in any way is a laborious and uninspiring but very important service that the health department gives to the people. It is never wholly successful because carelessness and negligence are almost universal human failings, and unintelligent food handlers cannot be expected to maintain strict standards of cleanliness at all times, even under most careful supervision.

New Problems in the Control of Food-borne Infections.   The increasing use of prepared foods and their processing in large quantities have increased the hazard of nontyphoidal salmonella infections. The major source of such infections is products made from raw or partially cooked dried eggs. The pooling of large numbers of eggs, including some contaminated with salmonella, inevitably increases the number of consumers at risk. The scattering of cases resulting from the wide distribution of such products may completely mask the relatedness of resulting cases of enteritis.

The prevalence of salmonella contamination of spray-dried egg powder is staggering. Almost 10 per cent of more than 7,000 samples of egg powder imported into England from the United States were contaminated with various salmonellae. The use of such powders by bakers and confectioners constitutes a special hazard, because cake and candy might not be sufficiently heated in their manufacture to kill the organisms. Perhaps related to the threat of raw-egg products and other processed foods, the incidence of salmonellosis has increased tenfold in Massachusetts between 1950 and 1956 and sevenfold throughout the United States at large in the period from 1946 to 1955 (Black *et al.*, 1960). Concurrently, typhoid fever has gradually declined. There is recent evidence that paratyphoid B in addition to the food-borne salmonella enteritides may also be carried by processed chicken eggs.

After several decades of virtual freedom from botulism derived from commercially processed food, the disease returned dramatically to prominence in 1963, probably as the result of a modern innovation in packaging. Smoked Great Lakes whitefish had been produced without mishap by a respected company for many years. A change to an attractive pliofilm package in which the fish were *vacuum packed* was made to extend the life of the product in retail markets (Figure 10-3). It is probable that this anaerobic environment contributed to the generation of spores of type E *Clostridium botulinum* and to an epidemic of botulism in Alabama and Tennessee (Rogers, 1964).

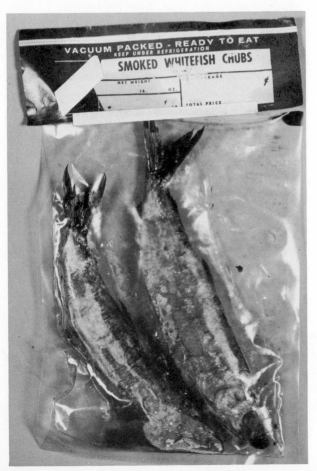

FIGURE 10-3. A package of vacuum-packed smoked whitefish in a pliofilm bag similar to those incriminated as the source of type E Botulinus toxin. (Reproduced from M. C. Koenig *et al. Medicine*, **43:** 520, 1964. © 1964, The Williams and Wilkins Company, Baltimore, Md. 21202, U.S.A.)

The Prevention of Food-borne Infections Related to Fecal Contamination. It is obvious that all infections that can be acquired via ingestion of water or milk (Tables 10-4 and 10-5) could be similarly acquired through food (Table 10-6). Therefore, the control of many of those infections classified literally as "food-borne" depends finally upon the elementary principles of sanitary sewage disposal and water purification. Thus the

TABLE 10-6

Common Infections Transmitted by Food

Infection	Usual Sources
Tapeworm infestations	
Taenia saginata	Beef
Taenia solium	Pork
Diphyllobothrium latum	Fish
Trichinosis	Pork
Amebiasis	Raw vegetables or fruit
Anthrax	Meat of sick animals (rare)
Brucellosis	Meat of sick animals (rare)
Bacillary dysentery	Meat products
Cholera	Raw vegetables or fruit
Streptococcal infections	Meat products
Salmonella enteritis	Meat and egg products
Typhoid	Shellfish
Tularemia	Rabbit meat
Tuberculosis, bovine	Meat of sick cattle
Staphylococcal enteritis*	Milk and egg products (custards, mayonnaise, etc.)
Botulism*	Sausage, fish, home canned legumes (beans)
Infectious hepatitis	Oysters,? clams

* Not true infections but intoxications.

hazard of food-borne amebiasis results from the grossest type of contamination of leafy vegetables with human feces (night soil) used for crop fertilization in the Orient. Other infections of the type in which uncooked vegetables are essentially a passive vector of human feces include schistosomiasis, ascariasis, and whip-worm infestation. In the absence of effective sanitation, infections of this type can be prevented by the cooking of contaminated vegetables.

The Control of Infections Carried by Meat and Fish. Unrefrigerated and improperly handled meat and fish provide, as milk does, a fertile culture medium for many bacteria. In the natural course of events, bacterial growth leads to the hydrolysis of proteins and to the "putrefaction" or "decay" of the animal flesh. Despite its stench and esthetically forbidding aspect, "rotten" meat is not intrinsically dangerous to the human organism unless the bacteria that have initiated decomposition include (a) enteric pathogens (salmonella or shigella) or (b) producers of toxins (staphylococci or clostridia). Putrefied seal meat is valued by the Eskimo as a delicacy and the hundred-year-old eggs of the Chinese are essentially a cheese produced by protein denaturation. In Western culture the hanging of beef or venison fosters protein and collagen breakdown through endogenous enzymatic action, which increases the meat's tenderness and palatability. For centuries man has devised many methods for delaying the decay of meat, all of them inadvertently directed at the suppression of bacterial growth.

There has been a tremendous improvement in the diet of man within a period of twenty-five years, owing to engineering advances in methods of preservation of foods. Formerly the diet of the average family was limited to certain staple foods—salted or dried meat and fish, potatoes, bread and other cereals, milk and milk products, with fresh meat at intervals, and vegetables and fruits only in their seasons.

The development of cold-storage facilities by the use of refrigerator railway cars on a large scale, the establishment of enormous community refrigerator plants, and the invention of simple family cold-storage units have revolutionized food habits and made most fresh foods, such as fruits and vegetables, fresh meat and fish, available to all people at all times of the year.

The principles of good food preservation are very simple. They depend upon the facts that—

1. Food spoilage is due largely to bacterial action. Thus, bacterial control results in food preservation.
2. Bacteria require certain favorable conditions for development. In general, they require: (a) a suitable—usually warm—temperature, (b) moisture, (c) protein food, and (d) a favorable medium for growth. For example, a high concentration of salt or sugar will check the growth of many bacteria.

Air is required for the growth of some organisms; others do not require it. Many bacteria require very special conditions for development, including a favorable hydrogen ion concentration and exact temperatures. Thus food preservation, developed for centuries on an empirical basis, has now become an exact science. It is, in great part, an application of simple bacteriologic principles to the processing of foods.

REFRIGERATION.   Most bacteria that destroy food, and most pathogenic bacteria as well, do not develop at low temperatures, though few organisms are killed by freezing. (Trichinae and cysts of the taenia are killed at—10 °F in a 20-day period.) Some foods, such as meat, fish, and fowl, are well preserved by being kept at temperatures below freezing, while other foods such as oranges, tomatoes, and potatoes are well preserved at low temperatures but injured by freezing.

The quick-freezing process, which is carried out at very low temperatures (-35 °F), with a holding temperature of -10 °F, has proved to be a very successful and safe method of preserving many fruits, vegetables, meats, and other farm products.

Cold storage foods lose little of their nutritive qualities, but they decompose rapidly when removed from storage and therefore should be consumed immediately.

CANNING.   The canning process applies the bacteriologic principles of the autoclave, or of fractional sterilization, and is a very safe and satisfactory method of food preservation. Commerical canning of food is done on a scientific basis and under health department supervision. This food may be stored for long periods at room temperature without spoilage. Gas formation, with bulging of the can, is a good index that this type of food is unfit for use.

Home-canned foods are often prepared under rough-and-ready conditions by unskilled hands. There is always a possibility of food contamination. Thus, home-canned foods—particularly meats and vegetables—should always be heated before use. (See the discussion on botulism.)

SALTING, DRYING, CORNING, AND PICKLING.   Salting, drying, corning, and pickling are methods of food preservation that utilize the principles that bacteria cannot develop without moisture and that they fail to grow in high concentrations of sugar, salt, or acids such as vinegar.

COOKING.   The cooking process is an invention of civilization that is, by far, the most important factor in the destruction of bacterial products and the preservation of food. Cooking frequently injures the flavor of food and destroys some of its nutritive value, but its advantage as a mode of health protection greatly outweighs its disadvantages. The use of heat in the preparation of food is one of the greatest methods of health conservation.

In areas or at times of economic duress, meat animals that are obviously sick are slaughtered and used for food. Under these conditions, certain unusual types of food-borne infection have occurred, including brucellosis, botulism, anthrax, and tuberculosis. Even this type of infection might be prevented by adequate cooking of the meat.

The principal hazard of meat that is obtained from manifestly healthy animals or fish and properly handled and refrigerated is from certain helminthic parasites, in which the larval form encysts in the skeletal muscle. These infections are the tapeworm infections and trichinosis. Intervention at any point in the life cycles of these parasites could control these diseases, but economic and political considerations make such attempts unrealistic. For example, if only cooked garbage were fed to hogs and if rats were excluded from their enclosures, trichinosis could be abolished by eliminating the sources of swine reinfection.

Inspection of meat is a virtually hopeless method of control because:

1. Even costly microscopic inspection cannot guarantee the safety of the entire carcass.
2. The consumer might be sold uninspected meat.

Therefore, the definitive and realistic control of these infections is based on accepting their probable occurrence and utilizing the principle of "terminal disinfection" by adequate cooking of the meat. In the case of trichinosis, recent studies have demonstrated that x-irradiation as well as freezing is also effective in killing encysted larvae in the meat. Interesting experiments with ionizing radiation for the preservation and microbial sterilization of food are now being conducted. At the present time, however, the final responsibility for avoiding meat-borne infection rests with the cook.

The Control of Animal Reservoirs and Arthropod Vectors of Infection

The Control of Infections of Domestic Animals as Related to Infections in Man. Infections of domestic animals that are transmitted to man (Tables 10-1, 10-5, and 10-6) could obviously be eliminated by the detection, then cure or elimination, of all infected animals. In the United States the virtual elimination of bovine tuberculosis has contributed less to the control of enteric tuberculosis (which is preventable by milk pasteurization) than to economic and nutritional welfare by insuring healthy herds of cattle. The problem of brucellosis is similar, and with trichinosis, too, prevention of animal (swine) infection is important. Therefore, it can be said, in brief, that regulation of disease in domestic food animals is critically important only in relation to the economic and nutritional importance of the animals. This is also true with respect to domestic animals that may serve as intermediate hosts for human parasites (e.g., African trypanosomiasis). Such infections are more readily controlled by attack upon the insect vector or by chemoprophylaxis in man himself.

An exception to the foregoing statement is the case of *psittacosis* in which careful supervision and control of the avian host are essential for the prevention of human infection. Such control is now aided by treatment of infected flocks with antimicrobial drugs (i.e., tetracycline).

Another exception is *rabies* in which there is now no substitute for strict supervision and control of domestic canines through licensure and rabies immunization. The hazards of currently available vaccines interdict routine immunization of any but certain high-risk groups of the human population.

In the case of wild animals and birds infected with viruses transmissible to man by arthropods (Table 10-1), prevention of such transmission is obviously best directed at the vector.

The Control of Arthropod Vectors of Infection.   Among the more dramatic accomplishments of modern medicine has been the control of certain arthropod-borne diseases by assaults upon the vector. The conquest of urban yellow fever in the West Indies by the elimination of the town-dwelling *Aëdes aegypti*, and the reduction of malaria in Europe and the United States by control of swampy anopheline breeding places were followed by the truly revolutionary discovery of DDT. This remarkable chlorinated hydrocarbon is relatively inexpensive, has low toxicity for man and other mammals, is effective against a wide variety of arthropods, and has residual killing activity long after it is applied to walls or other surfaces. Shortly after the discovery of its insecticidal potency in 1939, it was shown to be remarkably effective in controlling louse-borne epidemics of typhus in Italy during World War II by its direct application as dusting powder to the clothing and persons of those at risk.

In the winter of 1943 and 1944 the siege of Naples had driven people into large caves where they were crowded in indescribable filth and confusion. Typhus broke out in the city, and the danger of a serious widespread epidemic of the disease was apparent. The army in conjunction with the Typhus Commission organized a delousing campaign. Each person was deloused without removal of clothing. A simple technique was instituted of spraying the fine DDT powder into the hair and at the neckband. The hand-operated powder duster" also sprayed the dust up each sleeve and at the waistband, front and back. About one ounce of powder was used for each person. The DDT powder impregnated the clothing so thoroughly that the individual was rendered louse-free for about four weeks. In many thousands of persons treated there were no reports of dermatitis or other intoxication. The epidemic was promptly brought under control.

In recent times a serious effort is being made by the World Health Organization to eradicate malaria by intensive, carefully planned nationwide cycles of DDT spraying.

Typical examples of such programs have been cited in the *WHO Chronicle*, **14** (8) 297, 1960.

The delegate of Afghanistan stated that malaria was the greatest public health problem in his country. The eradication campaign there had started 18 months earlier, and more than 4 million persons were now protected in areas where malaria prevalence had been almost 75 per cent.

The malaria eradication programme in Colombia is considered to be the most successful of the country's health activities. An agreement on the programme of the campaign was concluded with WHO in 1956, and spraying started in 1958. The fourth spraying cycle has just ended, and it is hoped to finish the fifth cycle, thus completing the first stage of eradication, in March 1961. Eradication is expected to be achieved by 1962. Insecticide resistance has developed in some localities among certain *Anopheles*, but the question has been studied thoroughly by experts and it is hoped to overcome this difficulty. Evaluation of the campaign started with the end of the first spraying cycle and every care is being taken to ensure that it is as complete as possible. Technical staff for the Colombian campaign has been trained with WHO assistance, and 25 per cent of the national health budget is being devoted to the campaign. Agreements have been concluded with neighbouring countries—Venezuela, Peru, Ecuador and Panama—for joint eradication efforts, aimed in particular at freeing the Pan American Highway from malaria hazards.

In India, practically the whole population of 400 million is being protected by spraying, and complete eradication of malaria is one of the aims of the country's third five-year plan which starts next year. "The plan for (malaria) eradication," said the chief of the Indian delegation, "will go down in history as one of the most fascinating endeavours on a global scale for the welfare of mankind."

Such bold campaigns for the reduction or elimination of biological species require not only the international political cooperation reflected in the foregoing citation, but also detailed knowledge of geography, topography, and climate, as well as of the biology of the mosquito and its habits. This indeed is true of any type of vector or vermin control. As pointed out in "Insecticide Resistance and Vector Control," *WHO Technical Report series*, no. 191, p. 98, 1960:

Application of pesticides by routine methods and on a nonselective basis often leads to unsatisfactory and costly results. Frequently, the period of activity of an insect is restricted, so that effective use of a chemical measure is limited to that period. For example, the application of insecticidal fogs before dusk is unsuccessful in controlling infestations of certain species of mosquitoes, whereas, the same treatment at dusk, or shortly thereafter gives excellent results. Some species of anophelines (e.g., *Anopheles sergenti* in Israel and Jordan) are semi-domestic in their habits, and residual treatments are only partially effective in reducing or interrupting malaria transmission. In contrast, in the same countries a domestic species (*A. sacharovi*) has been almost completely eradicated by similar applications.

But the greatest deterrent to eradication campaigns is the selection, by widescale use of a chemical insecticide, of genetically resistant insects within a species. This problem has become of great practical importance recently, and it is reported that at least 50 arthropod species of public health importance (including flies, mosquitoes, lice, and ticks) are resistant to one or more of the commonly employed insecticides, including DDT. This problem, which is similar to microbial resistance to antibiotics, has been partially circumvented by the development of other chlorinated hydrocarbon insecticides (dieldrin, Chlordane, and lindane), which may be effective against DDT-resistant flies or mosquitoes. The inevitable development of resistance to these newer

compounds has already occurred and emphasizes the need for "saturation" eradication programs to forestall the gradual genetic development of resistance in arthropod
populations.

A SUMMARY OF METHODS FOR THE CONTROL OF ARTHROPOD DISEASE VECTORS.   The
important human infections borne by arthropods are listed in Table 10-7 together
with chemical methods for their control. This highly simplified summary emphasizes
the diversity of approach to the chemical (insecticidal) control of arthropod disease
vectors. Although this chemical approach is of major importance in disease eradication programs, it must be supplemented by the older methods of arthropod control,
which include:

1. Elimination of breeding sites.
2. Control of infected animals which may carry fleas, mites, or ticks.
3. Use of insect repellants for personnel exposed in the field.

Control of ticks, mites, and culicine mosquitoes, which inhabit rural, forest, or
jungle areas, is obviously difficult or impossible at times. In such areas, special ecologic
problems are encountered because the use of toxic residual insecticides could kill
birds, fish, and game animals. In these circumstances it is more reasonable to protect
man by immunization or chemoprophylactic procedures. Such prophylaxis is indeed
used and includes vaccines against yellow fever, as well as quinacrine (Atabrine) and
chloroquine for malaria, and broad-spectrum antibiotics for scrub typhus.

The complexity and interdependence of changes in man, environment, mosquito,
and parasite with respect to the control of malaria are summarized in Figure 10-4.

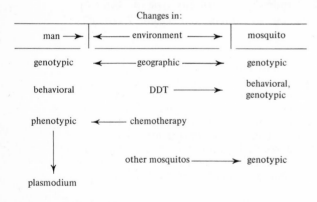

FIGURE 10-4.   Complexity and interdependence of changes in man, environment, and
mosquito in relation to control of malaria.

The physical environment selects and influences both men and mosquitoes, and man
is able to (and does) modify the environment. Geographical location in association
with malaria prevalence has induced genetic selection of man (see Chapters 2 and 3)
and also determines the species of mosquito in residence. The behavioral patterns of
man (sleeping and working habits) determine the probability of his contact with
malarial mosquitoes, and man's manipulations of the environment with DDT
influence mosquito behavior as well as genetic selection of resistant variants. The
transient change in human phenotype by malaria chemotherapy or chemoprophylaxis
has resulted in the emergence of drug-resistant plasmodia. Environmental changes

TABLE 10-7

Important Diseases Transmitted by Arthropods: Chemical Control of Vectors

Arthropod	Disease Transmitted	Chemical Control*	How Applied
Lice	Epidemic typhus, relapsing fever, plague (rare)	DDT, lindane	To person
Fleas	Plague, murine typhus	DDT	To rat runs and harborages
Ticks	The spotted fevers, plague, tularemia, Russian tick-borne encephalitis, relapsing fever	DDT, chlordane, dieldrin, parathion	Area control by sprays and dusting
Mites or chiggers	Scrub typhus, rickettsialpox	Dieldrin	Area treatment
House flies	Enteric infections, especially typhoid and bacillary dysentery	DDT, dieldrin, lindane (organophosphorus compounds)†	Residual spray (dwellings)
Biting flies			
Tsetse fly	Trypanosomiasis	DDT	Area control
Black fly	Onchocerciasis	DDT	To watercourses for larva control
Sand fly	Leishmaniasis	DDT	Residual spray (dwellings)
Cone nose bugs (triatoma)	American trypanosomiasis	Dieldrin	Residual spray (dwellings)
Mosquito			
Anophelines	Malaria	DDT, dieldrin, BHC‡	Residual spray (dwellings), larva control
Culicines	Yellow fever, filariasis, dengue, encephalitis	DDT	Dwellings (yellow fever)
		DDT, dieldrin, BHC‡	Area and larva control (filariasis encephalitis)

* For complete information on chemical names and other data see WHO Technical Report Series, **191**.
† Other DDT-like compounds are chlorinated hydrocarbons.
‡ The insecticide benzene hexachloride (hexachlorocyclohexane).

235

that have resulted from human intervention have led to changed infection cycles with different mosquito variants or species "taking over" transmission of the malarial parasite.

The Control of Disease-carrying Rodents. The basis of rodent control is proper environmental sanitation with respect to food handling, garbage disposal, and adequate human dwelling places. In addition, relatively specific and powerful poisons have been developed that, when ingested, kill rats or mice rapidly. These poisons include

1. Warfarin, a dicoumarin derivative.
2. Pival (2-pivaloyl-1-3-indandione).
3. ANTU α-naphthyl thiourea).
4. 1080 (Sodium monofluoroacetate)—the most potent compound, but also extremely toxic for man and other animals.

As with the insecticides, knowledge of the biology and habits of the species is needed so that baits will be taken. Actual eradication of rodents is almost impossible. Anti-rat campaigns that are only partially effective may cause an actual increase in the number of rats because of the adaptable birth rate of the animals, which may have been previously suppressed by stress and crowding. Rats have also shown genetic adaptation and resistance to poisons.

A new approach to rat control is the use in rat baits of the steroid mestranol as an oral contraceptive. This compound acts to sterilize fetal and newborn animals.

MAN AS AN INFECTIOUS HAZARD TO MAN (the "contagious" or "communicable" infections transmitted directly from man to man)

There is a large group of infections whose perpetuation depends on the direct transmission of their infective agents from man to man *without the necessary intercession of intermediate hosts, arthropod vectors, or prolonged survival in the environment.* These are truly human infections and are caused only by the smaller parasites—bacteria and viruses—which are obligate and specific parasites of man. Intimate human association and contact are required for the spread of these infections, and certain of them (smallpox, measles) have been recognized as contagious for centuries on the basis of circumstantial evidence and high clinical attack rates. Others of these infections such as poliomyelitis have only recently been recognized to be equally contagious because the clinical attack rate or incidence of manifest *disease* is low, although the incidence of inapparent *infection* is high in susceptibles.

It is appropriate to consider together in this section infections as manifestly dissimilar as cholera, syphilis, and influenza because the problems concerning their spread and, conversely, their containment are basically similar.

Infections That Are Primarily Enteric

The so-called enteric infections are those in which the parasite primarily invades and multiplies in the gut, usually the small intestine. Such infections are almost invariably acquired by ingestion; therefore it is predictable (and a matter of fact) that the infective agents are hardy enough to pass the acid barrier of the stomach and that they possess the ability to survive for a time outside the host. It is also apparent that all those agents potentially could be borne and spread by food and water in the absence of direct human-human contact (Table 10-6).

Bacterial Infection.   The evidence that the bacterial enteric infections (Table 10-8) are spread directly by fecal-oral contact is for the most part epidemiologic. In the case of bacillary dysentery, outbreaks of the so-called asylum type have occurred in the absence of food or water contamination and have been correlated with the grossly poor sanitation of inmates in institutions and with bacteriologic evidence of fecal contamination of doorknobs, and so on. The epidemiology of cholera and shigellosis is influenced by the fact of subclinical or inapparent infection; in the case of typhoid the epidemiology is affected by the occurrence of a protracted carrier state in almost 3 per cent of cases. These factors result in the shedding of organisms into the environment in the absence of diarrheal disease. In areas of poor sanitation and high population density, a relative immunity develops in survivors of infection, thus complicating further the accurate assessment of endemic infection. Furthermore, typhoid in infants and young children can be so mild as to be unsuspected and thus constitutes an unrecognized infection focus. The more prolonged course of typhoid coincides with protracted (one to eight weeks) excretion of bacilli in the feces, so that the recognized case is a constant hazard.

The Enteroviruses.   In a little more than a decade the development of revolutionary approaches in virology has resulted in the recognition of more than 50 "new" viruses and a completely altered concept of the previously recognized diseases that they have since been found to cause. Among these viruses, the 30 Coxsackie viruses and 28 antigenic types of ECHO viruses comprise (together with the 3 polioviruses) the biologically related enteroviruses, which cause varying disease states in man but primarily infect his intestinal tract. The neurotropic potential of these viruses, especially the polioviruses, initially obscured their relationship to non-neurotropic disease and complicated the understanding of their epidemiology. It is now clear that the viruses of this group are epidemiologically not unlike typhoid in their primary invasion of the enteric tract, their subsequent spread to other organs, the mildness of their disease if engendered in childhood, and their protracted persistence in the gut.

The formulation of new laboratory methods (tissue culture, use of infant mice) for virus isolation and antibody studies has led to recognition of the importance of clinically inapparent infections and to the concept that the enterovirus infections are among the most contagious of diseases.

Twenty-four distinct types of group A and 6 of group B Coxsackie virus have been categorized. The Coxsackie viruses of both groups A and B have pathogenicity for the infant mouse in common but differ in their pathologic effects. The group A and B viruses differ also in the diseases that they induce in man. Although viruses of both groups can cause lymphocytic (aseptic) meningitis, the group A strains cause herpangina and also an exanthematous fever, whereas the group B strains cause epidemic myalgia or pleurodynia, pericarditis in adults, and fatal myocarditis in infants.

The Coxsackie viruses are isolable from the pharynx but are present in highest

TABLE 10-8

Infections Directly Transmitted from Man to Man: The "Communicable" or "Contagious" Diseases

I. Infections that are Primarily Enteric

Infection	Infective Agent	Nonenteric Sites of Infection	Persistence of Agent in Stool
Bacterial			
Cholera*	*Vibrio comma*	—	One or 2 days, or duration of illness (carried 30 days)
Bacillary dysentery*	*Shigella* species		Duration of illness (occasional carrier state)
Infantile diarrhea	*E. coli* (certain species, e.g., 0111, 055), possibly viruses		?
Typhoid*	*Salmonella typhosa*		Thirty days or more; carrier state in 3 per cent for 1 year
Viral			
Enteroviruses			
Coxsackie group A	Coxsackie A, types 1-24	Pharynx, vagina	Up to 30 days
Herpangina, summer grippe, meningitis, exanthem			
Coxsackie group B	Coxsackie B types 1-6	Pharynx	Variable
Pleurodynia, summer grippe, meningitis, pericarditis			
ECHO virus infections	ECHO virus, types 1-28	Pharynx	Variable
Pharyngitis, meningitis, exanthem, diarrhea, colds			
Poliomyelitis	Poliovirus, types 1-3	Pharynx	Pharynx: 10 to 14 days; stool: 7 to 123 days
Reovirus infections	Reoviruses	Pharynx	?
Infectious hepatitis	Hepatitis, virus A	?	Unknown but occasionally 5 months
"Viral" or nonbacterial gastroenteritis	Two or more filter-passing agents	?	?

* Rarely transmitted directly man to man. Controllable by environmental sanitation.

concentration in the gut. Virus can be carried for as long as 30 days after acute infection.

Whereas the Coxsackie viruses are separable from other enteroviruses by their pathogenicity for infant mice, the ECHO viruses (with few exceptions) are pathogenic only in primate tissue culture. Indeed, their recognition is a direct outgrowth of the use of tissue cultures in poliomyelitis research. When tissue culture became widely used for the isolation of poliovirus from suspected cases of poliomyelitis, pathogenic agents that were not polioviruses were found in increasing number. Because some of these agents were initially recovered from patients without apparent disease, they were originally known as orphan viruses or "viruses in search of disease," then, more definitively as enteric cytopathogenic human orphan (ECHO) viruses.

The 28 types of ECHO virus have been implicated as have the Coxsackie agents in lymphocytic meningitis, but more frequently than the other enteroviruses in illnesses associated with rash (ECHO types 4, 9, 16). The indication that certain types cause diarrhea is the first evidence that a virus propagable in the laboratory can cause that syndrome. It is remarkable, in fact, that the *entero*viruses do not usually cause *enteric* symptoms.

Only twenty years ago poliomyelitis loomed as a virtually unassailable fortress on the medical horizon. At that time research was tremendously handicapped by the lack of convenient and reliable methods of cultivating the virus and measuring antibody against it. The inadequacy of earlier methods had led to the erroneous concept that poliomyelitis was a unique type of viral disease, a disease of low contagiousness (as indicated by paralytic cases), a disease that defied the usual laws of immunology, an infection predominantly of "civilized" society that produced "infantile paralysis." Because the virus was neurotropic in the chimpanzee and monkey, it seemed unlikely that it could ever be propagated in tissue cultures of nonneural cells. The enormous progress within the past twenty years in the understanding of the true nature of poliomyelitis is specifically related to the acquisition of evidence that

1. Poliovirus is excreted in human feces.
2. There are three separate types of poliovirus, which induce little or no immunity to one another.
3. Most infections with poliovirus are nonparalytic.
4. Most so-called nonparalytic poliomyelitis is caused by other enteroviruses.
5. Certain other enteroviruses cause paralytic poliomyelitis.
6. Poliovirus can be cultivated in cultures other than neural tissues.
7. Virus so cultivated can produce effective immunity to paralysis in man.

The cornerstone of much of this evidence is the Nobel prize-winning discovery by Enders, Weller, and Robbins (1949) that the polioviruses could be cultivated in non-neural tissue culture. There is no stronger argument for the "practical" importance of basic research than the poliomyelitis story. Epidemiologic research, no matter how brilliantly conceived or logically executed, is finally dependent upon the specificity and precision of its methods.

Renewed investigation of poliomyelitis soon confirmed earlier suspicions that poliomyelitis was not an infection principally of civilized countries. On the contrary, infection with poliovirus—as with other enteric pathogens—is more common in areas of poor sanitation where it occurs at an earlier age. Because infection in infancy is less often associated with manifest disease or paralysis, the paralytic *disease* is less common in poor areas, although, paradoxically, *infection* is more widespread. The emergence of the apparently "new" disease of infantile paralysis in this century has occurred initially in nations with the highest level of sanitation (the Scandinavian countries, the United Kingdom, and the United States) and closely parallels the decline of other enteric infections such as typhoid. The postponement of poliovirus infection until later childhood or even adulthood resulted more frequently in the paralytic effects of the infection (poliomyelitis) in the older host, which is *more vulnerable to the effects of the infection* than the very young infant (see Chapter 3).

Reovirus Infections.   A newly recognized group of viruses that apparently cause disease of both the respiratory and enteric tracts has recently been separated from the ECHO viruses and termed the "reoviruses."

It is too early to assess the importance of these viruses as agents of human disease, but it is interesting that at least one such virus has been associated with a steatorrheic enteritis in adults and diarrhea in children. These or related viruses apparently infect many animal species as shown by serologic methods.

"Viral" or Nonbacterial Gastroenteritis.   Often called "intestinal flu" but having no relation to true influenza, "viral" enteritis causes an immense morbidity in the winter months of the year. The acute onset and brief but prostrating course can be mistaken for the vomiting and diarrhea of food poisoning. However, the sequential onset of cases within family groups aids in the differential diagnosis.

Two clinical patterns of illness are recognized:

1. An afebrile diarrheal disease attended by nausea and vomiting.
2. A febrile disease with abdominal pain but usually without diarrhea.

The two diseases appear to be immunologically distinct. The etiologic agents of "viral" enteritis have not been cultivated in the laboratory so that evidence for its viral etiology comes from studies in human volunteers.

Infectious Hepatitis.   Infectious hepatitis is an infection of widespread prevalence with a peak incidence in childhood. On the basis of human volunteer studies, the infective agent appears to be a filter-passing virus (termed hepatitis virus A), which is remarkably resistant to thermal and chemical inactivation, withstanding exposure to one residual part per million of chlorine for 30 minutes or more.

Study of this disease has been badly handicapped by the lack of laboratory methods for isolating and cultivating the causative virus. Nevertheless, clinical and epidemiologic studies have drawn a tentative picture of the natural history of hepatitis. It is probable that infection by the fecal-oral route is prevalent in childhood, particularly in areas of poor sanitation. Such infection is often without jaundice and is sometimes completely inapparent in infants and young children. Certain geographic areas such as the Middle East and Mediterranean Coast seem to have an unduly high endemic prevalence. In Denmark, a country of good sanitation where accurate disease reporting has been carried out, seasonal trends of incidence have been noted with increases beginning in late summer and peaks in midwinter; yearly variation in "epidemic waves" was also observed.

The presence of antibody against the virus in gamma globulin from pooled human blood suggests that most adults have had infection and have developed immunity. However, as with poliomyelitis, the overt, severe *disease* is more common in older children and adults and is *less* common in areas of poor sanitation where the incidence of inapparent childhood infection (and consequent adult immunity) is high. Here again is the misleading clinical suggestion that in underdeveloped areas there is "no polio" and "no hepatitis." It is probable that the asymptomatic infant (who carries virus for months in his stools) could be an important source of infection in all areas.

The epidemiology of infectious hepatitis is further confused by the existence of the virus of serum hepatitis (virus B). That virus produces a similar clinical picture but may be immunologically different and it is probably not spread by the fecal-oral route.

Infections Primarily of the Respiratory Tract

The most common and troublesome of human infections are those in which the infective agents multiply primarily in the respiratory tract. These agents, which almost invariably are spread by intimate human contact, are specific and demanding in their requirements, and thus cannot exist for long in the external environment, in contrast to the enteric pathogens. They are thus unaffected by environmental sanitation, so that by exclusion they become relatively more important in contemporary "civilized" societies. The causes of many of these infections have only recently been identified, and the causes of many minor infections of the respiratory tract are still unknown (Table 10-9).

Diphtheria. In almost all countries diphtheria remains an important medical problem despite the fact that it is one of the best studied of microbial diseases. In underdeveloped areas in which immunization is not practiced, *Corynebacterium diphtheriae* is a killer of infants and children; in countries such as the United States in which childhood immunization is widespread, the disease is a constant threat to the increasing number of adults who lose their artificially induced childhood immunity. The continuing immunity of adults in impoverished areas is related to endemic prevalence of *C. diphtheriae* among carriers in the population, so that immunity is continually reinforced by re-exposure and latent reinfection.

Diphtheria is primarily a local infection of the upper respiratory tract by one of three types of *C. diphtheriae: gravis, mitis,* and *intermedius,* which apparently cause disease of the varying severity indicated by their names. The exotoxin liberated by bacilli growing superficially in the mucous and dead epithelial cells of the upper respiratory tract destroys adjacent living cells, which in turn become the sites of further bacterial multiplication and local "membrane" formation. Unless the infected individual possesses appropriate blood concentrations of specific antitoxin, systematic absorption of toxin may result in toxic damage to peripheral nerves and heart muscle— much of which is reversible with time.

TABLE 10-9

Infections Directly Transmitted from Man to Man: The "Contagious" Diseases

II. Infections Primarily of the Respiratory Tract

Infection	Infective Agent	Nonrespiratory Sites of Infection	Persistence of Infective Agent in Respiratory Tract
Bacterial			
Diphtheria	*Corynebacterium diphtheriae*	Skin, myocardium, nervous system	2 to 4 weeks
Hemophilus influenzae infections	*Hemophilus influenzae*	Meninges	6 to 8 weeks
Pertussis	*Hemophilus pertussis*		
Meningitis (epidemic)	*Neisseria intracellularis*	Meninges, skin, joints	
Pneumonia	*Diplococcus pneumoniae, Klebsiella pneumoniae*	Meninges, urinary tract	Variable
Staphylococcal infections	*Staphylococcus aureus*	Skin, endocardium	2 to 4 weeks
Streptococcal pharyngitis and scarlet fever	*Streptococcus pyogenes*	Skin	
Tuberculosis	*Mycobacterium tuberculosis* (var. *hominis*)	Multiple	Variable
Leprosy	*Mycobacterium leprae*	Multiple	?
Viral			
Adenovirus infections ("ARD," pharyngitis)	Adenoviruses (types 1–18)	Eye, gut	4 days or less
Common cold cough, rhinitis, and fever	Rhinoviruses (types 1–55)	?	5 days or more
	Respiratory syncytial virus (CCA)	?	?
Parainfluenza (croup, colds)	Parainfluenza viruses 1–4	?	?
Influenza	Influenza viruses A,B,C	?	1 to 7 days
Mumps	Mumps virus	Meninges, central nervous system, salivary glands, gonads, pancreas	Up to 9 days
Smallpox	Variola virus	Skin, viscera	? 14 to 21 days
Chickenpox and herpes zoster	Varicella virus	Skin, posterior roots	7 to 14 days, lifelong*
Herpes simplex	Herpes simplex virus	Skin, eye	Lifelong*
Measles	Measles virus	Skin, C.N.S.† (?)	Up to 9 days?
Rubella	Rubella virus	Skin, C.N.S.† (?)	Up to one year‡
Primary atypical pneumonia	PPLO	?	?
Infectious mononucleosis	Virus ?	Liver, spleen	?

* In latent, noninfective form.   † Central nervous system.   ‡ In congenitally acquired infection.

Because of the immunity of artificial immunization is specifically antitoxic and not antibacterial, it is interesting that nevertheless *Corynebacterium diphtheriae* has almost disappeared in communities in which childhood immunization is prevalent. It seems probable that perpetuation of the bacterium in the population depends in part on its capacity to injure the host with its toxin sufficiently to permit its further local multiplication and subsequent dissemination.

Hemophilus Influenzae Infections.   The importance of *H. Influenzae* in human disease remains controversial. In the sense that the bacillus is not etiologically related to influenza, it is misnamed. Although studies during the pandemic of 1918 suggested an association of *H. influenzae* (Pfeiffer's bacillus) and influenza, other studies indicated the equal or greater importance of pneumococci, streptococci, and staphylococci in secondary bacterial invasion. It has since been learned that many (up to 50 per cent) normal people carry *H. influenzae* in the respiratory tract in the winter months. However, most of these organisms are "untypable," nonencapsulated, and nonpathogenic.

Nevertheless, there is no question that *H. influenzae*, especially type B, causes primary pyogenic respiratory tract infections, which are often complicated by otitis media, pneumonia, septicemia, and meningitis—especially in young children.

Pertussis (Whooping Cough).   Pertussis is a highly contagious and potentially fatal air-borne infection of childhood caused by *Hemophilus pertussis*. A related bacterium, *H. parapertussis*, causes a similar but milder clinical syndrome, which includes the classical symptom of "whooping cough" and evidence of peribronchitis.

Pertussis is endemic throughout the world and occurs at any season. In the United States, peak incidences occur in early winter in the North and in the spring in the South. The spread of the infection seems to be related to cases of clinical disease; healthy carriers are not considered important in this regard. However, the prevalence of partial immunity from vaccination may so modify the disease that it is misdiagnosed; such undiagnosed cases could become unrecognized sources of infection.

Mortality from pertussis occurs principally in patients less than one year of age. The mortality has progressively declined in the United States since 1920.

Meningococcal Infections and Meningitis.   As in the case of poliovirus infections, meningococcal infections are frequent, but they are only rarely associated with manifest disease or central nervous system involvement. During epidemics the carrier rate can reach 95 per cent. Although the interepidemic carrier rate is 5 to 15 per cent, examination of a given population over a winter period has disclosed that most of the population have carried meningococci at some time during the observation period. In temperate climates, minor epidemics occur yearly with fluctuations to major epidemics at five- to twelve-year intervals.

In most individuals, meningococcal infection of the nasopharynx is either wholly asymptomatic or attended by mild rhinitis or pharyngitis. The next most common manifestation is a subacute septicemia with recurrent fever, rash, and polyarthritis. Least common are the severe and potentially fatal manifestations of fulminating septicemia or meningitis. Acute septicemia and meningitis with their fatal sequelae are most common in infants and children. In contrast to *H. Influenzae* meningitis, which is more common in girls, meningococcal disease appears to be more common in boys.

Crowded living conditions seem to foster the dissemination of organisms, for the incidence is higher in crowded urban areas and in army barracks and institutions. Undiseased carriers are important in the spread of infection, and one clinically apparent case is rarely traced to another.

Pneumococcal Pneumonia.   It is estimated that in adults 95 per cent of primary bacterial pneumonia is caused by the pneumococcus (*Diplococcus pneumoniae*). Even in the so-called secondary or bronchopneumonias, which may complicate chronic lung diseases or surgery, the pneumococcus is the most common etiologic agent. In view of the fact that 40 to 70 per cent of the healthy population may carry pneumococci, many of them virulent types, it has long been evident that factors other than the presence of pneumococci in the nose and throat are important in the pathogenesis of pneumococcal pneumonia. Epidemiologic studies of man and experimental observations in animals suggest that damage to the respiratory mucosa by noxious agents (especially viruses) and factors that depress the defenses of the lower respiratory tract (alcohol, pulmonary edema, and so on) lead to aspiration of pneumococci so that they reach the alveoli.

Although pneumococcal pneumonia is so sporadic in occurrence that it is not considered to be a "contagious" disease, it may become epidemic if: (a) the pneumococcal carrier rate of a population becomes high and (b) the concomitant incidence of viral respiratory disease is high. Such conditions are sometimes seen in institutional groups or military populations.

Although more than 75 antigenic types cause human disease, most cases of pneumonia are caused by the "lower-numbered" types of pneumococcus, types 1, 2, and 3. Of these types, 1 and 2 are not commonly carried by normal subjects. The type-specific immunity associated with recovery from pneumonia appears to reduce the chance of a subsequent carrier state in the convalescent.

Primary pneumococcal pneumonia is most common in young adults, in males (perhaps because of occupational exposure), and in workers in steel mills and coal mines.

Primary pneumonia caused by *Klebsiella pneumoniae* (Friedländer's pneumonia) may be confused diagnostically with pneumococcal pneumonia. The ecology of this infection is very different, however. *Klebsiella* is found both in the throat and in the normal intestinal tract, and can be naturally carried by species other than man. It rarely causes pneumonia in the absence of obvious general debility, previous infection, or alcoholism. It is a rare cause of pneumonia.

Staphylococcal Infection.   Among bacteria that cause respiratory tract infection, the staphylococci are unique in their capacity to resist environmental stress and in their apparent capacity for mutation to withstand such stresses. Thus while meningococci, group A streptococci, and pneumococci remain susceptible to most antibiotics, increasing numbers of antibiotic-resistant staphylococci have appeared. Basic knowledge of the pathogenesis and immunity of staphylococcal disease is less advanced than with most other bacterial infections; this fact also contributes to emergence of staphylococcal infection as a current problem of modern society.

It is *Staphylococcus aureus* strains of certain types (coagulase positive) that are of principal importance in human disease. Such strains can be carried nasally and cutaneously by 30 to 50 per cent of the general population. Yet overt disease as evidenced by furuncles, osteomyelitis, or pneumonia is relatively uncommon. In recent years it has become apparent that *epidemic* staphylococcal disease (as in hospitals and nurseries) seems to be engendered by relatively few types of staphylococci. Most such strains are of bacteriophage group III; coincidentally they are antibiotic resistant. Of group III, the phage subtype 80–81 has caused most hospital infections in the United States in the last decade; in the United Kingdom and Australia, phage types 80 and 52A have been responsible. Because typing staphylococci has not been done routinely until recently, it is not clear whether the ostensibly "virulent" strains of today differ from those of the past. Another question is whether or not staphylococcal infections are becoming more numerous and more serious as the proportion of antibiotic-resistant strains increases.

Staphylococcal infections are most common in infancy and childhood. However, they are a constant threat to the debilitated or organically damaged host of any age, e.g., the diabetic or the patient with influenza.

Although the epidemiology of staphylococcal infections has not been definitively established, it appears that nasopharyngeal carriage of the organisms is of major importance in spreading infection. The staphylococcal type carried cutaneously is usually the same as that in the nose of the carrier.

Streptococcal Pharyngitis and Scarlet Fever.   Only hemolytic streptococci categorized serologically as group A are important in the causation of respiratory disease in man. The usual manifestation of such infection is acute pharyngitis. If a rash occurs concomitantly, the disease is termed "scarlet fever," although epidemiologically it does not differ from pharyngitis without rash. Erysipelas was once thought to be a different disease, but now it is recognized as a cutaneous manifestation of streptococcal infection.

Group A streptococcal infections represent a special problem among infectious diseases because of the serious and sometimes permanent damage that may occur as late sequelae in some patients. These sequelae of infection include acute rheumatic fever and the permanent cardiac damage that may occur during its course. Another sequela is a form of acute glomerulonephritis, which is initiated only by specific group A streptococcal types, particularly type 12; this rarely leads to permanent renal damage.

Although immunity following streptococcal infections is type-specific, there are indications that general nonspecific immunity to streptococcal disease may develop with age. Infections in infants and young children may be mild and protracted and difficult to diagnose clinically. Apparently healthy individuals, as well as convalescents, may harbor pathogenic streptococci during epidemic seasons in the winter and spring. A rise in this carrier rate may herald an epidemic. Streptococcal infections are world-wide in distribution, but the incidence of disease is higher in cold climates. Infection is spread by intimate association of a susceptible person with one carrying streptococci in his upper respiratory tract. Although the clothing and adjacent environment of such a carrier may contain organisms, spread probably occurs directly from one respiratory tract to another.

Tuberculosis.   Most human tuberculosis is caused by the human type of *Mycobacterium tuberculosis*. Ten per cent or less may be caused by bovine or avian variants of this bacterium. In the United States, tuberculosis caused by the bovine strain has been essentially eliminated through pasteurization of milk and careful supervision of dairy herds.

The spread of tuberculosis from man to man is dependent upon close human contact and presumably occurs as an air-borne infection. The genesis of most tuberculosis is within the family, and the incidence of tuberculosis within family groups in which an adult has an open or cavitary lesion is extremely high. Indeed, the demonstration of a positive tuberculin test in an infant or a young child may serve as a casefinding method for "open" disease in an adult with whom the child has been in close contact.

Tuberculosis differs from most infections of the respiratory tract in its chronicity and in the limited efficacy of both the healing process and the immunity engendered by the infection. These circumstances influence the epidemiology of the disease. Thus, supposedly cured or arrested tuberculosis may be endogenously reactivated in the absence of external reinfection, and the patient may become a threat to society years after the primary infection.

Because primary (or childhood) tuberculosis and reinfection (or adult) tuberculosis behave like two different diseases, they are often considered separately with respect to their pathogenesis and epidemiologic significance. Man is intrinsically quite resistant to infection with *Mycobacterium tuberculosis*, and most such infection does not result in disease. However, the initial invasion by tubercle bacilli, whether in the child or in the adult, may be followed by an acute illness associated with caseation of the lymph nodes and by rapid progression of healing within a brief period of time. If hematogenous spread of the organism occurs, generalized or miliary tuberculosis or tuberculous meningitis may result. Paradoxically, this more acute form of the disease is rarely contagious because of the absence of necrotic lesions, which permit the egress of myobacteria into the bronchi.

In the postprimary or reinfection type of disease, the prior development of significant but incomplete immunity causes the disease to be localized to the lungs and bronchi and to their lymphatics, and the disease has a less acute and more protracted course. Disease of this sort is of paramount importance in the spread of pulmonary tuberculosis.

THE INFLUENCE OF AGE, RACE, SEX, AND ENVIRONMENTAL FACTORS ON THE EPIDEMIOLOGY OF TUBERCULOSIS. No infection is more influenced by the environmental conditions of the host and his physiologic state than is tuberculosis (See also Chapter 3). It is notable that significant decline in the incidence and the death rate of tuberculosis occurred long before the advent of chemotherapy. Nevertheless, in the world at large, tuberculosis still causes 3 million deaths a year. It is significant that in the United States a declining *mortality rate* from tuberculosis has not been paralleled by an equal decrease in *morbidity and prevalence* of infection. Outside of Western Europe, North America, and Australia, both moribidty and mortality rates are still very high.

In the United States, the characteristic peak mortality previously observed in the third decade of life has changed; now the highest mortality rate from tuberculosis is in elderly males. In underdeveloped countries, however, the peak mortality is still observed in the third decade.

The occurrence of severe disease and death is generally higher in very young infants, in males, in nonwhite races, in poorer economic groups, and in the malnourished. It is obvious that there is a considerable overlap of these various variables. For this reason it is not clear whether the apparent racial differences in susceptibility to serious tuberculous disease are on a genetic basis or are coincidentally related to environmental factors. Physiologic and psychologic stresses, such as pregnancy and mental illness as well as intercurrent disease or infection, appear to predispose to postprimary tuberculosis.

Epidemiologic Implications of Disease Caused by Chromogenic or Atypical Mycobacteria.   Within the past decade there has been increasing recognition of the pathogenic potential of so-called atypical or chromogenic mycobacteria. Because some of these organisms appear to be geographically restricted in their distribution and may come more from the environment than from human beings, they can confuse considerably the picture of tuberculosis unless their existence is recognized. These mycobacteria confound epidemiologic surveys because some are of low pathogenicity and cause virtually no disease; yet they may induce hypersensitivity to tuberculin in a majority of the population. The role of most of these organisms in human disease is only now being explored.

Viral Infections of the Respiratory Tract.   In recent years, tremendous progress has been made in the study of acute infections of the upper respiratory tract. Many new viruses have been isolated, categorized, and related to specific disease processes. Many viruses have now been isolated from patients with the common cold syndrome—usually defined as an acute, brief, benign illness, which is afebrile and predominantly manifested by rhinitis.

The importance of minor respiratory tract infections lies in the enormous incidence of illness they occasion rather than in their threat to life. Nevertheless, it is probable that even the most minor of these infections may pave the way for secondary bacterial infections and their sequela of chronic pulmonary disease. It is also true that such "minor" infections in the aged or those with underlying cardiopulmonary disease occasionally result in severe and even fatal illness. In addition, it is apparent that respiratory symptoms of presumed viral etiology comprise a surprising burden to ostensibly healthy people even when the symptoms are not severe enough to cause absenteeism from work.

Adenovirus Infections.   Twenty-eight types of adenovirus have been identified since the discovery of this group in 1953. However, the importance of these viruses in human disease is still being established. It is apparent that certain specific types (types 3, 4, and 7) are important causes of illness under certain restricted conditions. For reason that are not clear, these viruses cause a very high incidence of infection and disease in military recruits in training camps. These viruses, with the exception of type 3, seem to be of little importance in causing disease in the civilian population at large.

In civilian populations, other virus types (including types 2 and 5) may cause outbreaks or sporadic cases of acute pharyngitis or pharyngoconjunctival fever and "pink eye" or swimming pool conjunctivitis. Type 8 adenovirus has been clearly related to *epidemic keratoconjunctivitis*.

The adenoviruses of greatest biologic interest are those that appear to be truly latent in the adenoidal and tonsillar tissue of man. The adenoviruses may persist for years within those tissues without inducing disease, as is true of herpes simplex and herpes zoster viruses in other sites. Such adenoviruses are detected only when the tissue is removed and cultivated *in vitro*. The oncogenic (tumor-inducing) potential of certain adenoviruses has been discussed in Chapter 3.

The Common Cold and the Rhinoviruses.   Because of its mild and poorly defined characteristics, as well as its obvious association with changing climates and temperatures, there has been question in the past whether the common cold was indeed a contagious and infectious disease.

Until recently, the best data have been provided by studies of isolated communities in which the common cold occurred as an epidemic disease after its apparent introduction by people from outside the community. For many years there has also been evidence that the common cold could be induced in human volunteers by inoculation of nasopharyngeal washings from patients with the syndrome. Within the past ten years there has been adduced conclusive evidence for a virus etiology. It has been shown that agents capable of causing the common cold syndrome can be propagated in tissue culture and that they are, in fact, viruses. Although many unrelated viruses including the adenoviruses and influenza viruses can induce mild illness indistinguishable from the common cold, a group of small RNA viruses (picornaviruses) termed *rhinoviruses* can be isolated from about one quarter of acute respiratory infections (Hamre, 1968). Fifty-five antigenically different rhinoviruses have now been classified. Studies in volunteers have established that infection with a rhinovirus is followed by durable immunity. This fact coupled with the evidence for multiple common cold viruses suggests that the individual who has "one cold after another" has no deficiency in immune response to colds but simply is encountering a series of pathogens with which he has had no prior experience. Colds occur with greatest frequency in childhood (in the immunologically inexperienced) and progressively less frequently with advancing age.

Rhinovirus infections are probably spread as contact infections—perhaps by droplets. There is little direct evidence on their degree of communicability. Volunteer studies have shown that experimental colds are more readily induced by nasal drops than by aerosol sprays of small particles, suggesting that contact spread may be more important in nature than true airborne spread through small droplet nuclei. In natural infections, virus is shed for at least one week after the onset of symptoms. In the case of experimental colds it has been learned that virus shedding may occur in the early asymptomatic phase. Thus individuals may be contagious before they develop symptoms.

Parainfluenza Viruses.   The parainfluenza viruses are so named because they fit biologically into the myxovirus group, of which influenza viruses are the original prototypes. Again, as with the adenoviruses and the common cold viruses, the importance of these agents in human disease is only now being defined. However, it is clear that the four types of parainfluenza virus thus far identified in man are associated with acute upper respiratory infection in infants and children, which may be attended by laryngotracheitis or croup; it is also probable that a milder "common cold" type of disease may occur in adult infection. The limited data now available suggest that a considerable percentage of croup and acute respiratory infections in young children may be accounted for by these viruses (at least in certain years).

The identification of similar viruses in nonhuman species, including the monkey and the bovine, has suggested a possible animal reservoir of infection, but this possibility remains unproved.

Respiratory Syncytial Virus.   The respiratory syncytial virus was first isolated in 1956 from chimpanzees, and originally termed the *chimpanzee coryza agent* (CCA). Its current name reflects the cytopathic effect it induces in tissue culture. It has been demonstrated that the virus is important in causing febrile illness in children. The disease may be related to involvement of either upper or lower respiratory tracts. The highest incidence of infection appears to be in children one year of age. Confusion with influenza is possible because fever and cough are the principal presenting signs.

Influenza.   The virus of influenza appears to be unique among the infectious agents of man in its capacity for undergoing mutation so extreme that it can circumvent immunity produced by its pre-existing forms. This fact, together with the relative brevity of even its specific immunity, has allowed it to persist in modern times as the last great unconquered plague.

It is unlikely that bubonic plague or smallpox will ever recur as pandemics because of (a) the advances of environmental sanitation and chemotherapy for the containment of plague, and (b) the triumph of smallpox vaccination. The "white plague" of tuberculosis is also yielding to improved environmental conditions and newer chemotherapeutic measures. Yet even with our ability to produce a specific vaccine rapidly, influenza occurred again in pandemic form in 1957 and 1968. Specific immunization did prevent the disease in a minority of the world's population, and the fatal effects of secondary bacterial pneumonia were appreciably curtailed by modern antibiotics. Nevertheless, the impact of this brief but prostrating infection was felt throughout the world.

Although there are three distinct types of influenza virus (A, B, and C), only influenza A virus is an important cause of epidemic disease in the general population. Since the original isolation of influenza A virus in 1933, three major antigenic changes have occurred—the first in 1947, the second in 1957, when the first pandemic in the era of

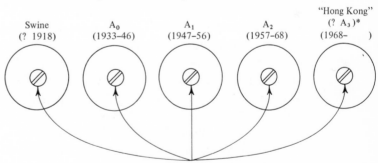

Swine (? 1918) A_0 (1933–46) A_1 (1947–56) A_2 (1957–68)   "Hong Kong" (? A_3)* (1968–   )

All share in common a "CORE" nucleoprotein antigen (not involved in immunity) that identifies these variants as influenza A viruses

*Note: A minor (neuraminidase) antigen of the Hong Kong virus is similar to the neuraminidase of recent A_2 strains. Therefore some cross immunity may be expected.

Influenza A & B are complete distinct from (i.e. share no antigens with) influenza C viruses.

FIGURE 10-5. Shifting antigenic nature of influenza A viruses.

modern virology occurred, and the third with the recent "Hong Kong" variation (Figure 10-5). Although the virus was still recognizable in the laboratory as influenza A, its mutations were so great that members of the population who had been vaccinated with pre-existing strains of virus had no immunity to the new variants. (The problem that such mutation poses with respect to control of the disease is discussed fully in Chapter 3.)

In light of the evidence that an influenza virus can demonstrably cause pandemic as well as sporadic epidemic disease, the inference that the great 1918 pandemic was caused by a similar virus seems more and more justifiable. Although no virus was isolated from human beings in 1918, a virus causing influenza in swine at that time was subsequently isolated from those animals and shown to be closely related to the human influenza A viruses that were later discovered. The relation of these viruses is schematically shown in Figure 10-5.

When influenza appears in the community, the two major public health problems are

1. A sometimes explosive onset of morbidity that involves large numbers of the population with a brief, usually benign, but prostrating disease.
2. Increased mortality in certain members of the population principally in the aged or those with underlying cardiopulmonary disease.

The rapid spreading of what was then a "new" virus, to which everyone was susceptible, is illustrated in Figure 10-6 showing the extremely rapid dissemination of A2 (Asian) influenza within a hospital ward. The protective effect of vaccination of attending personnel is shown in the lower part of Figure 10-6. It must be emphasized, however, that the spread of influenza is sometimes puzzlingly slow; within family groups it may not have a uniformly high attack rate, and secondary cases may appear only after six or seven days. Factors of virus dose, environment, and differences in age may influence markedly the incidence of influenza even in populations without any specific immunity to the virus.

Influenza virus alone may induce a fatal pneumonia in elderly or cardiac patients, but it more frequently increases mortality indirectly by preparing the way for secondary bacterial pneumonia. Indeed, so constant is this relationship that an excess mortality related to pneumonia is widely used by public health officers as a subtle indication of the presence of influenza in the population. This mortality occurs chiefly in those over 45 years of age. Because older, less active people may escape the first wave of infection in the community, their infections may occur later, when evidence of influenza morbidity in the population at large has disappeared. Thus, a puzzling increase in mortality may be observed in the older age groups in the apparent absence of clinical influenza in the community.

It is possible that influenza not only predisposes to secondary bacterial infections in the individual patient but that it also increases the carrier rate and prevalence of pathogenic bacteria in the community.

Pandemic, Epidemic, and Endemic Influenza.   Influenza may exist in the community in pandemic, epidemic, or endemic form. Pandemics of the disease are rare and occur at roughly 30- to 40-year intervals. (Identification of "Hong Kong flu" as pandemic

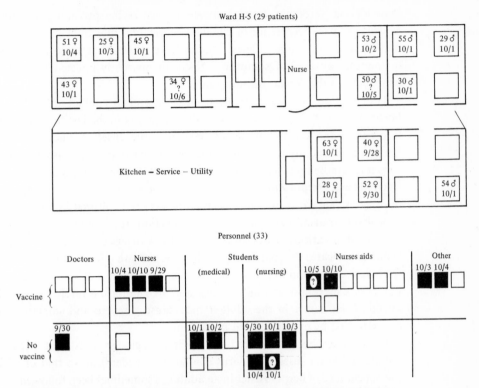

FIGURE 10-6. An influenza epidemic on a hospital ward (A2 [Asian] influenza in 1957). Topography of ward H5 and make-up of ward personnel. Shaded blocks represent individual patients and personnel who develped influenza symptoms. The date of appearance of symptoms is indicated within or above the blocks. (Reproduced from H. L. Blumenfeld *et al.: J Clin Invest,* **38**:199, 1959.)

is still conjectural.) During interpandemic periods, the virus continues to cause sharp localized epidemics in closed or isolated communities and sporadic disease (sometimes fatal in the elderly) in larger open population groups. The question of "what happens to the virus between epidemics" has not been completely answered. It seems reasonable to surmise, however, that as population immunity rises, *continuing infection is less frequently evidenced by disease* (see Figure 3-4). Therefore, the disappearance of epidemics of disease does not necessarily reflect the absence of virus in the community. There is evidence of such "endemic" persistence of influenza virus following the 1957 pandemic.

Mumps.   Mumps or epidemic parotitis is caused by a virus biologically similar to the influenza and parainfluenza viruses. It is a myxovirus that apparently does not vary in its antigenic constitution. For this reason, one attack of infection appears to confer lasting immunity, although second or even third attacks have been reported.

The disease is acute and incapacitating; however, in children (the usual victims), it is almost always benign. In adults a painful and feared complication is orchitis, which occurs in 20 per cent of male cases. However, sterility or sexual abnormality after such a complication is rare.

Although case histories indicate that only 60 per cent of adults have had mumps in childhood, serologic studies indicate a much higher percentage of infections. This evidence of past occurrence of clinically inapparent infections has been confirmed by human volunteer studies. These studies have shown that subjects may excrete virus in the total absence of symptoms. Such unapparently infected people undoubtedly contribute to the spread of infection.

Transmission of disease results from close human contact and is presumably airborne. Virus is detectable in the saliva and pharynx in the last few days of the incubation period and for as long as six days after the onset of illness. Probably because mumps is essentially a systemic infection, which does not cause necrosis of respiratory tract epithelium, secondary bacterial complications are notably infrequent.

Varicella and Herpes Zoster.   Varicella, or chickenpox, is one of the most contagious of diseases. The virus, which only recently has been cultured in human tissue culture, is probably transmitted as an air-borne infection. It is notoriously difficult to prevent the spread of varicella virus within a hospital with susceptible children. Epidemiologic evidence indicates that patients with the infection are infectious for the duration of the fresh vesicular eruption or, on the average, for a period of seven days after the onset of illness. Chickenpox is a mild disease and, like mumps, is rarely followed by bacterial infection. However, in the adult it may cause a severe and sometimes fatal illness characterized by extensive viral pneumonia.

It has long been suspected on epidemiologic grounds that herpes zoster, or "shingles," was caused by a virus similar, if not identical, to that of varicella. Thus the appearance of herpes zoster in an adult has sometimes been followed by chickenpox in his children. Culture of both viruses has proved their biologic and immunologic identity. There seems to be little doubt that herpes zoster represents the reactivation of pre-existing latent varicella virus in posterior nerve roots or their dermatomes.

Herpes Simplex.   Herpes simplex is a perfect illustration of the differing pathogenic potentials in a given infectious agent under varying circumstances. In premature infants, the virus may cause a fatal generalized infection characterized by visceral necrosis. In some infants it assumes its more usual manifestation of acute stomatitis with fever; in other infants, it causes clinically inapparent infection. In older children or adults, it may be present as an acute pharyngitis or aseptic meningitis; in younger children, it may cause fatal encephalitis. Its recurrent manifestations may be asymptomatic or may be evidenced as the common fever blisters or cold sores, that attend other acute infections.

Herpes simplex per se is not an important infection; however, it is a fascinating prototype of the latent viral infection (see Chapter 3) that can be reactivated in later years in spite of demonstrable and persisting serologic immunity.

Smallpox.   One of the plagues of ancient times, smallpox is endemic throughout most of the world with the exception of North America and Australia, but remains a constant threat to all people. The virus of smallpox is unique among respiratory-borne viruses in its hardihood and, may exist in the environment for significant periods of time. However, such extrahuman residence is of little importance in the epidemiology of the disease because most cases originate from an actively infected patient with a discernible skin rash.

Sustained immunity to the disease seems to depend on its endemic prevalence in the community. In endemic areas, mild or inapparent infections in partially immune persons may contribute to the spread of the disease.

Two types of smallpox have been described, (a) variola major, the classical severe type attended by a high mortality, and (b) variola minor, or alastrim, a relatively benign disease, which has appeared in Africa, Western Europe, and America during the last 60 years. The high mortality of approximately 30 per cent that can result from variola major is not due to secondary bacterial pneumonia per se, although this may occur as a complication.

Measles.   This ubiquitous and highly contagious virus disease is worldwide in distribution. It is chiefly a childhood disease except in populations that remain isolated for long periods of time. When isolated communities such as the Faroe Islands or Greenland are infrequently attacked by measles, the attack rate of clinical disease is close to 100 per cent, and the disease involves all age groups. In this situation, mortality from pneumonia occurs in the very young and the very old, as is the case with influenza.

Measles occurs at any time of year, but most outbreaks take place in the late winter and early spring. The disease occurs in epidemic cycles of two- to three-year intervals. This epidemic periodicity has been explained as the result of introduction of new susceptibles into the population by birth or immigration.

Unlike most other viral infections, infection with measles virus appears to provoke manifest disease in almost all patients; i.e., the clinical attack rate is extremely high, and inapparent infection is virtually unknown. Therefore, new epidemics must result from the exogenous introduction of virus in the communities into which new susceptibles have also been introduced.

Secondary to viral multiplication and damage in the respiratory tract, bacterial invasion may occur so that as many as 15 per cent of patients could suffer otitis media or pneumonia related to pneumococcal or streptococcal infection. As with influenza, most mortality (particularly in primitive populations) is the result of secondary bacterial pneumonia. Encephalitis is a dangerous but relatively infrequent complication, occurring in fewer than 1 per cent of cases.

Rubella.   This mild exanthematous viral infection (also known as German measles) is almost always benign in children but can produce a more serious illness in young adults who have escaped childhood infection. It has the potential for causing serious congenital malformation if contracted during pregnancy. Because the clinical syndrome is essentially that of a low-grade febrile disease with transient erythematous rash, it is probable that many other infections have been confused with it, including the recently recognized enteroviruses, which may produce rash.

It may be inferred that rubella is not as widespread nor as contagious as measles because many adults escape childhood infection only to suffer the disease in later life. Transmission of the infection is presumably via the respiratory tract.

Infants infected *in utero* continue to shed the virus in respiratory tract secretions for months after birth and during this period are capable of transmitting infection. Secondary bacterial infection is rarely encountered. The major importance of this disease is as a cause of congenital malformation.

Primary Atypical (Mycoplasma) Pneumonia.   During World War II, an atypical type of pneumonia emerged to prominence. This pneumonia differed from the acute bacterial pneumonias in (a) its relative indolence of course, (b) its lesser severity, and (c) its failure to respond dramatically to sulfonamides and penicillin. This disease was only sporadically encountered in civilian practice, but it often became epidemic in military camps or in institutions such as boarding schools. Bacterial pneumonic pathogens such as pneumococci or group A streptococci were rarely isolated from patients with this disease. The disease is now known to be caused by *Mycoplasma pneumoniae*—an organism that produces a spectrum of illness including mild upper respiratory disease and otitis. It is contagious via the respiratory route. Broad-spectrum antimicrobial agents such as the tetracyclines are effective in treatment of the infection.

Venereal and Other Infections Acquired by Direct Contact

The human infections that are spread by direct contact of untraumatized skin or mucous membranes include the venereal diseases:

Syphilis (*Treponema pallidum*).
Gonorrhea (*Neisseria gonorrhoeae*).
Chancroid ("soft chancre") (*Hemophilus ducreyi*).
Lymphogranuloma venereum (LGV virus).
Granuloma inguinale (*Donovania granulomatis*).

Treponemal diseases other than syphilis that are transmitted by nonvenereal contact are:

Yaws (*Treponema pertenue*).
Pinta (*T. carateum*).
Bejel (nonvenereal syphilis: *T. pallidum*).

The viral ocular infections, trachoma and epidemic keratoconjunctivitis, are possibly transmitted by direct contact.

The primarily cutaneous infections of ringworm of the scalp *Microsporum audouni* and impetigo (staphylococcal or streptococcal) are also considered to arise from contact infection.

Syphilis and Gonorrhea.   Syphilis is a disease in which the social and moral implications are so closely interwoven with its medical and public health aspects that it is difficult to discuss this infection without becoming involved in matters that have little bearing upon the epidemiology and the control of the infection.

Syphilis is caused by *Treponema pallidum* and is transmitted, in practically every instance, by direct venereal contact with an active superficial lesion of the skin or mucous membrane. Although the disease is restricted to no one special class or ethnic group, the majority of cases are to be found in the sexually promiscuous and the economically deprived. The incidence of infection is significantly higher in Negroes.

Gonorrhea is an acute infectious venereal disease attributable to *Neisseria gonorrhoeae*. The incubation period of the disease is short—three to six days—and the period of communicability continues as long as the organisms are present in the discharge. Relapses are not uncommon, and female patients may be infectious for a long period. Communicability of the disease may be determined very satisfactorily by cultural methods, and to a less satisfactory degree by direct microscopic examination of the discharges.

Gonorrhea is transmitted by intimate personal contact, usually sexual, with the infected person. Newborn babies may acquire a very serious conjunctival infection, ophthalmia neonatorum, from the mother at the time of birth. Children, particularly little girls, may acquire the infection occasionally from contact with materials that have been freshly soiled with the discharges of the patient. The organism survives for only a short time in an unfavorable environment; thus practically all infection occurs by direct contact. All individuals are susceptible to infection, and a single attack does not confer immunity.

It is a discouraging fact that syphilis and gonorrhea are far from being under control, despite the susceptibility of both infections to penicillin therapy. Indeed, after a dramatic decline in the incidence of acute cases after the general introduction of penicillin in 1946, a recent recrudescence of both diseases has been noted throughout the world. This increase in syphilis has occurred in both developed and developing countries. A new danger is the possibility that in Africa syphilis might now move into areas in which yaws (with its accompanying antisyphilitic immunity) has been extirpated.

In the United States, reported infectious syphilis reached a nadir in 1958 (6,661 cases) but has since tripled within the last decade (23,250 cases in 1965). In New York City the increase was even more precipitous and dramatic being over 400 per cent between 1957 and 1961. A concerted program of patient and physician education with an emphasis upon improved reporting of cases has recently reversed this increase in New York.

An important epidemiologic fact has been a shift in the age incidence of both gonorrhea and syphilis since 1950 so that they have been facetiously termed "childhood diseases," because a significant proportion of cases now occurs in 15- to 19-year-old age groups.

The decline in gonorrhea has not paralleled that for syphilis, being less precipitous and less sustained.

Factors thought to contribute to the persistence of gonorrhea and syphilis are

1. More cases are being treated by private physicians; hence they are less adequately reported and followed up by finding and sustained treatment of contacts.
2. Increase in moral laxity and sexual promiscuity in the post-World War II era.
3. Paradoxically, the availability of antibiotics and contraceptives and the efficiency of health education campaigns in their use may foster promiscuity.

The development of penicillin-resistant gonococci has been greatly feared and watched for, but has not yet become a problem.

Chancroid. Chancroid is due to *Hemophilus ducreyi* and produces a deep, painful, ulcerated pustule, often with enlargement of the inguinal glands. The incubation period is from three to twelve days after exposure, and the disease is almost always acquired by sexual contact. It remains infectious as long as the open lesions contain the organisms. The disease is highly communicable, but is not so prevalent as the other venereal infections. In the U.S. Army, for example, it constitutes only about 5 per cent of all the venereal infections. One reason for this is that the lesions are so obvious that exposure to infection does not often take place.

The diagnosis is easily made by direct microscopic examination of smears, but multiple dark-field examinations of the lesions should be made to rule out concomitant syphilis.

Preventive measures are the same as for other veneral infections. Direct prophylaxis does not protect as well against chancroid as it does in gonorrhea and syphilis.

Sulfonamides, streptomycin, and the broad-spectrum antibiotics are effective in syphilis and might confound interpretation of response.

Granuloma Inguinale.   The etiologic agent of this disease is *Donovania granulomatis*. It is a venereal disease with a long incubation period of three to six weeks after exposure. It is rarely encountered in the United States. The chronic indolent ulcerative lesions is spread by direct contact, and the prevention is that of the other venereal diseases. Treatment is similar to that used in chancroid.

Lymphogranuloma Venereum.   Lymphogranuloma venereum is carried by an agent now classified with the chlamydia. This infection is almost always acquired by sexual contact, though laboratory workers have contracted the disease in the handling of heavy concentrations of the virus under cultivation. It is very widespread. Lymphogranuloma has been described more frequently in Negroes, but all races and all ages are susceptible. It is more common in men than in women. Those groups having a high prevalence of lymphogranuloma venereum.

The incubation period of the disease is from 14 to 21 days. The infection is communicable as long as the open lesion contains the virus. Because the disease is a chronic suppurative lesion, the period of communicability may be rather long. Virus has been isolated from asymptomatic individuals.

The infection responds rather indolently to the prolonged administration of sulfonamides or tetracyclines.

The preventive measures in lymphogranuloma venereum are exactly the same as those employed in the prevention of other venereal diseases. Because the condition is so difficult to recognize clinically and so frequently confused with syphilis, and because persons with syphilis so frequently have this disease also, it has been suggested that each person with recently acquired syphilis should also have a Frei test (for cutaneous hyperactivity to the antigen) or a complement-fixation test with the Frei antigen.

The Nonvenereal Treponematoses

A number of clinically distinct nonvenereal contact infections are caused by spirochetes very similar if not identical with *Treponema pallidum*. These infections appear to be geographically restricted to certain tropical or subtropical areas and to involve family groups or communities of low socioeconomic level. In contrast to venereal syphilis, childhood infection is most common.

Transmission is by direct or indirect contact from man to man. Congenital transmission is rare. The incubation period approximates six weeks. The period of communicability is highly variable but depends upon the presence of moist dermal lesions.
YAWS. Yaws occurs in Equatorial Africa, the Philippines, Burma, Thailand, throughout the South Pacific, and in scattered areas in the West Indies and Central and South America.
BEJEL. Bejel, or nonvenereal syphilis, involves arid regions in Africa, Turkey, and the Balkans.
PINTA. Pinta, which differs from the other infections in its vitiligoid lesions, occurs among dark-skinned people of Mexico, Columbia, Venezuela, and Ecuador. It is also sporadically observed in Africa and Asia. The incubation period is from one to three weeks.

With all these infections, some cross immunity and cross serologic reactions with syphilis exist.

Trachoma. Trachoma is a progressive, destructive infection of the conjunctiva, which is estimated to involve 400 millions of the world's population. Some 10 millions of these victims will eventually become blind if untreated. The disease is caused by an agent of the lymphogranuloma—psittacosis group of "virus-like" agents now classified as the Chlamydia. The trachoma agent can be cultivated in the chick embryo and in human amnion cells in tissue culture and is susceptible to the action of sulfonamides and most antibiotics.

Trachoma is associated with filth, poverty, poor personal sanitation, and usually, but not invariably, with hot, arid, dusty environments. The incidence is notably high in North Africa and India. It is present among the Indians of the American Southwest but appears to be rapidly declining in that area.

Control of the disease is theoretically feasible with mass campaigns of antibiotics or sulfonamide administration, but education in personal sanitation together with economic improvements among the involved population may be equally important.

Infections That Can Be Artificially Transmitted by Inoculation

A derivative of the modern practice of medicine is the growing problem of infections transmitted inadvertently from man to man by man (see also Chapter 3). These infections are transmitted by hypodermic injection and are of two principal types.

1. Those transmitted by inadequately sterilized needles or syringes or other skin-piercing instruments that are contaminated with human blood.
2. Those transmitted by the injection of human blood or blood products that contain the infectious agent.

Infections in the first category include serum hepatitis, infectious hepatitis, malaria, and syphilis. Certain of these infections may be transmitted outside of medical practice through the badly contaminated needles of narcotic addicts. Outbreaks of hepatitis have also been traced to tattooing parlors.

In addition to the obligate human parasites that may be transmitted by needle, tetanus bacilli and other bacteria resident in the environment may be inoculated by grossly contaminated instruments. Such gross contamination usually involves the hastily cleaned equipment of drug addicts.

Serum Hepatitis.   Serum hepatitis may be truly a disease of modern times. It appears to be unique among infections in that it is not known to be transmitted by any other means than by artificial parenteral inoculation. However, study of this disease has been curtailed by the lack of laboratory techniques to identify and propagate the infective agent. Limited studies in human volunteers have established that the causative agent is a virus of small size (hepatitis virus B) that is demonstrable in the blood of certain subjects at intervals as long as five years apart. Presumably, blood from such individuals contains virus continually and represents a constant threat to others if used for transfusion or in the preparation of plasma, albumin, or other blood products. Such carriers of virus—who are discovered after they have donated blood and transmitted the disease—are usually asymptomatic and often give no history of jaundice or liver disease. Even chemical tests of liver function may not disclose abnormalities at the time of demonstrable viremia. It is therefore almost impossible to screen out carriers in blood donor centers. The problem is complicated by the fact that the virus of infectious hepatitis (virus A) may also be transmitted by blood or blood-contaminated instruments. In this case, history taking or liver function tests may be of value in excluding potential transmitters of infection. The virus of infectious hepatitis has been demonstrated in the feces of those infected, and the disease is clearly "infectious" by personal contact or through food or water.

The two forms of hepatitis are distinguished not only by their epidemiology but by differences in incubation period and immunity. Indeed, it is on the basis of these differences that the two viruses A and B have been provisionally identified. The 60- to 160-day incubation period of serum hepatitis contrasts with the shorter 15-to 40-day period of infectious hepatitis. However, intermediate periods up to 60 days have been recognized in epidemics of infectious hepatitis.

The increasing use of blood products and of subcutaneous injections in general has increased the relative importance of serum hepatitis as a cause of both morbidity and mortality. In the civilian population, infection rates as high as 11.9 per cent have resulted from the use of large pools of plasma. During military campaigns rates have been much higher. Basic research on the disease and search for effective methods of inactivating the virus in blood are confounded by the present lack of methods for cultivating the virus, which can only be detected by inoculation of human volunteers.

In addition to the major problem of serum hepatitis, a number of other infections have been inadvertently transmitted from man to man by needle; these include syphilis, malaria, measles and cutomegalovirus infection (see Chapter 3). It is evident that any infection with a stage of blood stream invasion could in theory be so transmitted.

The Intrauterine Transmission of Infection (Congenital Infections).   Another way in which man-to-man transmission of infection occurs is *in utero* by transplacental transmission. In general, most infections severe enough to induce bacterial septicemia in the mother result in spontaneous abortion, with or without actual infection of the fetus. However, a variety of infectious agents (from protozoa to viruses) are able to traverse the placental barrier and to infect the fetus yet allow its survival into the post-partum period. Most infections that permit survival of the infant are acquired late in pregnancy (toxoplasmosis, syphilis, tuberculosis, poliomyelitis), but the viruses of rubella and cytomegalic inclusion disease may induce nonfatal but teratogenic infection of the fetus in the first trimester. It is not yet clear whether other viruses may cause congenital defects.

The prevention of this sort of disease transmission must obviously be directed at prevention of the specific infections in the mother prior to or early in pregnancy. There is some evidence that vaccinia may compromise the outcome of pregnancy if inoculated in the first trimester. If live virus vaccines of other types are developed in the future, their use in pregnant women must be undertaken with caution.

THE CONTROL OF INFECTIONS DIRECTLY TRANSMISSIBLE FROM MAN TO MAN

There is surprisingly little direct evidence concerning the mechanisms by which most infectious agents are transmitted from man to man. Certain widely held assumptions have been made about mechanisms of transmission, which are based on

1. Epidemiologic (circumstantial) evidence.
2. Knowledge of the site of multiplication of the parasite in the host.
3. Studies in experimental animals.
4. Limited experiments in human volunteers.

On the basis of these methods of study, it has generally been concluded that the enteric infections (Table 10-8) are transmitted by ingestion of fecally contaminated material and that the infections resulting from primary invasion of the respiratory tract (Table 10-9) are "air-borne," i.e., are caused by inhalation of microorganisms suspended in the air. It is possible—even probable—that such assumptions are correct, but it should be remembered that the only established *sine qua non* for the transmission of both enteric and respiratory infections seems to be close contact, proximity, and association between the donor and recipient of the infection. Earlier impressions that measles and other respiratory viruses were more communicable than, for example, poliomyelitis have been changed following recent recognition of the high communicability of poliomyelitis when suitable methods for the detection of cases *and the recognition of subclinical instances of infection* are utilized.

Also, the relative inefficacy of attempts at air sterilization or decontamination stress indirectly the need for close physical proximity in transmission of many alleged "airborne" infections. On the other hand, with such enteric infections as poliomyelitis, virus is detectable and apparently multiplies in the pharynx, where it is at least potentially a source of contagion. Adenoviruses multiply in both the upper respiratory tract and the small bowel. The shedding of virus from the pharynx is best correlated with the contagious period of the infection. The spread of streptococcal infections may require direct contact with nasopharyngeal discharges rather than aerosol dissemination of streptococci. This point and the others mentioned above have obvious importance with respect to control measures.

With the few exceptions listed in Table 10-3, it is unlikely that the environment is an important source of infective agents transmissible from man to man. These exceptions include bacteria, which may actually multiply in the environment, such as staphylococci, streptococci, and *Salmonella typhosa*, as well as the stable enteroviruses and the virus of infectious hepatitis. In general, the pathogens of the respiratory tract are extremely unstable and cannot survive long in the external environment.

Even more unstable in the environment are the microorganisms responsible for direct contact infections, especially those involved in venereal diseases. It is therefore understandable that transmission of such infections occurs largely across membranes or at mucocutaneous junctions and rarely through the intact skin, because a moist, warm, nutritionally favorable milieu must be found quickly by such organisms. Even so, the acquisition of venereal infection can be prevented by prompt washing of even these highly susceptible sites.

The Inevitability of Certain Infections.   In those special situations in which infections are transmitted from man to man by artificial means (e.g., through the hypodermic needle by physicians or drug addicts), there is an obvious opportunity for destruction of the parasite during its trip from one man to another. With the vast majority of infections transmitted from man to man, however, other methods of control are needed. It will be seen in the subsequent discussion that the most effective of these methods of control accept the inevitability of transmission, or indeed, sometimes, of infection, and it is their purpose to create a last line of defense within man himself, by the administration of specific drugs or the mobilization of specific immune mechanisms in the potential victim.

Even if it were possible by ultraviolet irradiation or other means to insulate the child from contact with the causative agents of the "diseases of childhood," *such a procedure would put the child in undue jeopardy if infection were postponed until his adult years.* Almost without exception, primary infections result in more severe disease in the adult than in the child. Therefore, methods of disease control that merely postpone the infection without inducing specific resistance are not only unrealistic, but dangerous.

Some General Considerations in the Control of Infections Transmissible from Man to Man.   It is obvious that realistic methods of disease control depend on definition of the source of the infectious agent and identification of the susceptible host. These problems should be considered:

1. Is the chief source of infection the clinically diagnosed case?
2. Do subclinically infected carriers contribute to the spread of infection?
3. If subclinically infected carriers do not spread the infection, which groups are most susceptible: young, old, male, female?

The answers to these questions will vary with each individual disease, and the natural history of each disease must be defined before the appropriate methods of control, based on knowledge of transmission, can be implemented. If the clinical case (as in tuberculosis) is a major source of infection, then case-finding methods will be of value in control. On the other hand, case finding will offer little in the control of poliomyelitis, in which most infections are subclinical or inapparent and where specific methods of therapy for the identified case are nonexistent.

Not too long ago, it was the general assumption of public health practice that the clinical case was the important source of contagion in almost all childhood infections. This attitude led to the formulation of legislation (much of it now scientifically obsolete) that required the isolation of patients with "communicable" diseases at home or in "pest houses," the placarding of homes, and often the quarantine of contacts. Increasing awareness of the equal or greater importance of the nondiseased carrier, as well as the development of antimicrobial drugs that rapidly suppress pathogenic bacteria in the patient, have led to revision of much of this legislation.

Case Detection, Antimicrobial Therapy, and Chemoprophylaxis in the Control of Contagious Diseases*

Infections Controllable by Case Finding of Clinically Apparent Infections (Disease). Certain infections can be controlled by the case finding of clinically apparent infections (that is, disease). Infections in this category include those with high clinical attack rates (in which inapparent infections are therefore not important) and certain chronic infections in which contagiousness and exposure may be protracted. Infections in which case finding is useful include

Pulmonary tuberculosis (adult or nonprimary type).
Leprosy.
Infantile diarrhea.
Typhoid.
Serum hepatitis (by screening of blood donors by history).
Measles (high clinical attack rate).
Venereal infections (in the male, and indirectly, in the female named as his contact).
Smallpox.

Tuberculosis is the prototype of infections in which case finding is of great importance in the control of the disease, despite the fact that most tuberculous infections are not manifest by disease. Such infections, which are of the primary type and noncavitary, do not contribute to the dissemination of *Mycobacterium tuberculosis*. In recent years, case finding has become even more important as specific antituberculous drugs have been developed; now the result of case finding is not only the isolation and public health education of the patient, as carried out in the past, but also the administration of specific therapy simultaneously to aid the patient and serve as prophylaxis for the dissemination of infection in the community.

In the case of venereal infections, case finding is peculiarly efficient in the control of

* There are a number of points of attack in the control of contagious diseases. It is obvious that in the classification of diseases in accord with their vulnerability to one or another method of control, the same disease could be considered in several categories. Thus, in the several categories in this chapter, tuberculosis appears in each, although the best method of control depends on specific circumstances.

the disease. Knowledge of the epidemiology of these diseases permits certain predictions about the patterns of spread in the community. Because venereal infections are transmitted almost exclusively during the sexual act, only sexual contacts of the index case are at risk and need be sought. Promiscuity has its social patterns and often involves groups of individuals of both sexes who perhaps frequent a single bar and grill. Within such groups venereal infection may be traded back and forth so frequently that therapy of less than the entire group becomes meaningless. Recently developed techniques of personal interviewing have been surprisingly effective in tracking down contacts of reported cases of clinical disease. This type of "cluster epidemiology" is exponentially effective as it (1) uncovers multiple cases from a single one and (2) permits a more sensible (namely community) chemotherapeutic attack among the potentially infected and reinfectable.

Infections Controllable by Specific Treatment of Clinical Cases. The availability of highly effective chemotherapy in the form of such orally administered drugs as isoniazid has partially resolved the need for legal restraint and hospital confinement of "open" or infectious cases of pulmonary tuberculosis. Not only may the period of hospitalization be reduced, but the contagiousness of patients who "sign out" or refuse hospitalization may be demonstrably lessened. This has been shown by a study of the occurrence of secondary cases among contacts of treated and untreated cases.

There are other infections that are not considered in the foregoing section in which the clinical case is *not* the most important method of transmission, yet certain of these infections are amenable to specific antimicrobial treatment, and such treatment will contribute to the curtailment of transmission in the community. These infections are listed here in addition to tuberculosis, in which treatment of the case is a major method of prevention of spread.

Tuberculosis.
Leprosy.
Streptococcal infections.
Staphylococcal infections.
Typhoid fever.
Bacillary dysentery.
Venereal infections (chiefly male).
Malaria (not transferable man to man but reduction in parasitemia may interfere
    with mosquito transmission).
Ringworm of the scalp (treatable with griseofulvin).

Infections Controllable by Case Finding of Clinically Inapparent Infections by Laboratory Procedures. Certain infections can be controlled in part by the detection of nondiseased carriers. Infections in this category are few in number because (a) the detection of such infections is dependent upon the availability of easily implemented laboratory procedures, and (b) this method of control is only important in certain limited epidemic situations. Appreciable numbers of the population may carry pathogenic organisms in the absence of epidemics. However, the presence of this reservoir of undiseased carriers is usually suspected on the basis that sporadic manifest disease has occurred. This group of infections includes

Typhoid fever (detection of carrier by stool culture).
Meningococcal infections (nasopharyngeal culture).
Staphylococcal infections (nasopharyngeal or lesion culture).
Streptococcal infections (nasopharyngeal or lesion culture).
Tuberculosis (chest x-ray revealing cavitary but asymptomatic infection).
Gonorrhea in the female (by culture or fluorescent antibody techniques).

The prospects for terminating the typhoid carrier state are not good even if the carrier is subjected to cholecystectomy. Penicillin in large dosage may occasionally be effective; otherwise prevention of infection depends upon the education of the carrier and his supervision with respect to food handling. In the case of the other infections, potentially effective antimicrobial therapy is available; with staphylococcal infections in particular, carriers among hospital personnel can be restricted to prevent their contact with the unduly susceptible, such as the newborn infant or the surgical patient.

The amount and duration of antimicrobial therapy used for significant reduction in secondary disease transmission may be much less than that needed for therapy of active disease. Such chemoprophylaxis will not usually eliminate the organism carried except in the case of the exquisitely sensitive meningococci and gonococci. However, the number of bacteria can be so reduced that transmission of infection is similarly diminished. It should be noted that this type of infectious disease control is useful only in certain epidemic situations and sometimes only at particular times of the year. The epidemic prevalence of meningococcal meningitis is associated with an increase in carriers of type I meningococci. This increase may last for several years. *However, the seasonal fluctuation in the occurrence of meningitis during this period cannot be related to the carrier rate per se.* Still another determinant of meningitis in the military is its predilection for the young recruit. However, the carriage of meningococci (and hence the risk of meningitis in future contacts) can be dramatically reduced by the administration of relatively small doses of sulfadiazine quite inadequate for the treatment of the established disease. As indicated in Figure 10-7 the effect of a single dose of 8 gm is sufficient to eliminate the detectable carriage of type I meningococci for as long as 16 weeks after its administration. Recently, in accord with principles of microbial genetics, emphasized in Chapter 3, sulfonamide resistant meningococci have emerged to practical importance in the genesis of epidemics.

The development of immunofluorescent techniques for the detection of bacterial antigens offers promise for better detection of the female carrier of gonococci who is (usually) asymptomatic. Penicillin treatment of sexually promiscuous individuals so detected will materially reduce the spread of the disease and might eventually lead to its elimination. Therapy of the male in whom sexual activity is restricted by his acute and painful symptoms contributes to the reduction of gonorrhea only insofar as such therapy prevents evolution of the infection to a chronic state that results in protracted carriage of gonococci.

However, the prophylactic use of antigonococcal drugs is so effective as to be actually conducive to promiscuity. This fact together with evidence that the acquisition of syphilis may not be prevented by penicillin doses that are adequate to prevent

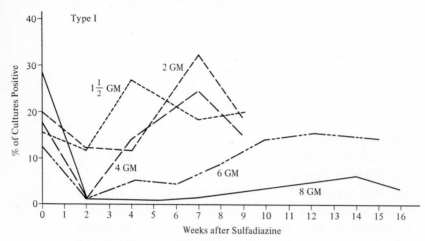

FIGURE 10-7. Type I meningococcus carriers before and after graded doses of sulfadiazine. (Reproduced from Aycock W. L. and J. H. Mueller. *Bact Rev*, **14**: 155, 1950.)

gonorrhea is already posing new public health problems. A special danger is the fact that penicillin may prevent the primary chancre from appearing, as well as other manifestations of the infectious state, yet the individual may later develop the more serious sequelae of syphilitic infection.

Prophylaxis with Specific Antimicrobial Drugs (Chemoprophylaxis) to Prevent or Postpone Infection in Susceptible Contacts. It would seem to be a reasonable and obvious procedure to reduce the spread of infections treatable with drugs by administration of the appropriate antimicrobial drugs to contacts exposed to such infections. As a matter of fact, this measure contributes very little to the control of infectious diseases and is employed only in certain limited circumstances. These circumstances are related to

1. The biology of the etiological parasite.
2. The nature of the infection that it causes.
3. The mechanism of its transmission.
4. The availability of a specific antimicrobial drug.

Thus, antimicrobial prophylaxis is most effective in infections in which

1. The parasite is highly drug susceptible (to low, briefly maintained concentrations of drug). Such parasites are usually incapable of establishing persistent or latent infection after antimicrobial treatment.
2. Infection is manifested by easily recognizable disease in the primary case.
3. The time of contact can be sharply defined.
4. Antimicrobial drugs of low toxicity are available that may be conveniently administered.

Of all the infectious diseases only gonorrhea meets these "ideal" requirements for contact chemoprophylaxis, and then only with the reservation that the male contact must anticipate the probability of infection in his partner, because her symptoms may not be evident.

Infections caused by the biologically similar meningococcus are similarly amenable to prophylaxis with antimicrobial drugs, but the recognized case of meningococcal disease is not an important factor in spread of infections.

In World War II, the incidence of bacillary dysentry was reportedly reduced by mass sulfonamide prophylaxis. However, the rapid evolution of sulfonamide-resistant shigella limited the value of this approach to controlling the disease. As in the control of other enteric infections, environmental sanitation remains the most important factor in dysentry control.

The administration of the antituberculosis drug, isoniazid, to children who are family contacts of sputum-positive adults is an effective method of tuberculosis prevention. The Expert Committee on Tuberculosis of the World Health Organization has recognized the use of two types of chemoprophylaxis, each directed at a different stage in the infectious process. In the terminology of the Committee,

Primary chemoprophylaxis—the use of anti-tuberculosis drugs in those not infected, i.e., non-reactors to tuberculin; *secondary chemoprophylaxis*—the use of anti-tuberculosis drugs in those who are infected as demonstrated by a significant reaction to the tuberculin test, but who have no pathognomonic signs or symptoms of tuberculous disease.

Primary chemoprophylaxis has not been widely endorsed because of the greater usefulness of BCG vaccination in the tuberculin-negative person who is heavily exposed to infection. On the other hand, secondary chemoprophylaxis, which is essentially the prevention of disease in those recently and already infected, offers great promise in controlling childhood tuberculosis in areas of high tuberculosis prevalence.

It should be pointed out that it is not clear with respect to other infections whether chemoprophylaxis actually prevents the acquisition of infection or merely its sequel of disease, even if drug is given prior to contact with the parasite. It is probable that for any given disease either primary or secondary chemoprophylaxis may be operative, depending upon whether or not circumstances of host-parasite contact permit the establishment of the parasite in the tissues of the host. The effectiveness of anti-gonococcal and antimeningococcal prophylaxis may reflect the inability of these organisms to "get started" and initiate infection in the presence of antimicrobial drugs. It is clear, however, with the arthropod-borne diseases, malaria and scrub typhus, that administration of specific drugs such as quinacrine (Atabrine) or tetracycline, even for long periods of time, does not prevent infection but only postpones the eventual advent of disease.

Chemoprophylaxis in Persons Peculiarly Vulnerable to Infections or Their Sequelae. Probably the greatest value of chemoprophylaxis at present is in the control of the late sequelae of Group A streptococcal infections, rheumatic fever, and nephritis, and definitively, the chronic residual of rheumatic heart disease. During World War II, and in military and civilian studies since, it has clearly been shown that the mass administration of penicillin can reduce the streptococcal carrier rate, lower the incidence of streptococcal pharyngitis and scarlet fever and, most importantly, reduce the incidence of rheumatic fever and other late manifestations of streptococcal infection.

It is also true that antistreptococcal therapy for developed streptococcal pharyngitis may still reduce the expected rate of subsequent rheumatic fever.

Only a minority of hypersensitive individuals are vulnerable to rheumatic fever following a streptococcal infection. Once this vulnerability is recognized by the occurrence of the initial attack, the protracted administration of penicillin may prevent both future streptococcal infections and their threatening sequelae in the vulnerable (rheumatic) subject. This type of chemoprophylaxis has received wide acceptance and is a good example of preventive medicine and public health directly administered by the individual medical practitioner.

The prophylactic use of antibiotics to prevent bacterial infection in other potentially vulnerable patients is less clear-cut and generalizations cannot be made. It is popular in academic circles to view with horror the "promiscuous" use of antibiotics in the absence of a specific therapeutic indication. This commendable caution can be carried too far sometimes, because of unwarranted extrapolations among basically differing problems. For example, the prophylactic use of penicillin to prevent the pneumococcal pneumonia that may follow influenza in an elderly or cardiac patient, is quite different from the administration of a tetracycline drug to prevent recurrent urinary tract infections in a patient with a congenital anomaly of the urinary tract.

In the first case, it is reasonable to anticipate that pneumonia may occur within a certain brief period of time; and that if pneumonia does occur, it will probably be pneumococcal and the pneumococcus will be susceptible to the action of penicillin.

In the second case, eventual infection is almost inevitable, but the time of infection and the nature of the bacterial pathogen are unpredictable. Chemoprophylaxis in this case may indeed tend to select a bacterial invader that is resistant to the drug being employed chemoprophylactically.

Another type of chemoprophylaxis that appears to hold promise is the protracted daily use of broad-spectrum antibiotics in chronic pulmonary disease to prevent the recurrent acute infections accompanying such disease, infections which may be life threatening.

The whole concept of antimicrobial prophylaxis or chemoprophylaxis deserves continuing re-evaluation.

Specific Artificial Immunization and the Control of Infectious Diseases

The Prevention, Modification, and Treatment of Infectious Diseases with Preformed Antibody or Gamma Globulin (Passive Immunization).   It would seem that the use of specific antibody would be a logical method for the prevention and therapy of infectious diseases. Yet this approach has limited applicability.

1. Antibody, whether in the form of specific immune serum or the purified serum fraction, gamma globulin (immunoglobulin), is costly to produce and limited in supply.
2. Antibody must be administered parenterally and in relatively large amounts.
3. Whether the antibody is of human or animal origin, it is rapidly eliminated from the

recipient who is "passively immunized" with it, so that effective immunity rarely persists beyond two to three months.

4. If nonhuman in origin (heterospecific), the antibody, with accompanying or contaminating serum proteins, will induce the formation of other antibodies, which 7 to 14 days after injection may be associated with "serum sickness" in the recipient. Repeated or booster injections of antibodies may cause immediate and occasionally fatal anaphylactic reactions.

The immunoglobulins, even if derived from man, are sufficiently antigenic in the homologous species (man) so that recipients of multiple transfusions may develop agglutinating antibody against foreign human gamma globulin so introduced (Allen and Kunkel, 1963). The clinical significance of these observations is unknown, but the recognition of this potential is important in assessing the use of repeated injections of isologous (i.e., nonheterologous) antigens. In at least one instance severe reaction has been associated with the presence of antibody to aggregated human gamma globulin (Henney and Ellis, 1968).

In the decade prior to the introduction of antibacterial chemotherapy, antibody was used with fair success in the treatment of several acute pyogenic infections including pneumococcal pneumonia and meningococcal and *Hemophilus influenzae* meningitis. Specific antibody has not been of any importance in the prevention of bacterial infections except in rare individuals with abnormally small amounts of serum gamma globulin (agammaglobulinemia or hypogammaglobulinemia). (See Chapter 3.)

In the case of diphtheria and tetanus in which disease is dependent on *in vivo* production and absorption of microbial toxins produced during infection, the administration of antitoxin antibody in large amounts may be therapeutically useful in binding unabsorbed toxins. The injection of smaller amounts of antitoxin provides effective immunity for two to three weeks after exposure. The increasing use of active immunization with toxoid and the use of human immune globulin have largely superceded heterologous antitoxin (which is usually of horse serum origin) in the prevention of diphtheria and tetanus.

The most important use of preformed antibody is with human gamma globulin for the prevention of those diseases in which (1) the pathogenesis of the disease is dependent upon a stage of blood stream invasion (viremia), during which time the parasite is accessible to humoral antibody; (2) the contact period may be precisely defined; (3) the infection is sufficiently common so that high titer antibody may be found in the gamma globulin fraction of serum pools derived from the general population.

Among the diseases that may be prevented or modified by the injection of gamma globulin during the early incubation period are measles, rubella, mumps, poliomyelitis, and infectious hepatitis (see Table 10-10). Of these diseases, only measles consistently meets the criterion of a readily definable contact period, because clinically mild or inapparent infection may characterize the other diseases. There are circumstances, however, as in institutional or household epidemics of hepatitis, when the period of contact is similarly definable.

Gamma globulin is of little use in poliomyelitis because of rapid spread of infection (often inapparent) within households, so that by the time the paralytic "index" case is recognized, all members of the household are infected. In any event, the problem is academic because of the success of active immunization with polio vaccines.

The relative mildness of rubella and varicella and the apparent variability of protection of different lots of gamma globulin have not led to widespread use of gamma globulin prophylaxis in these infections. Indeed, human immunoglobulins have proved ineffective in preventing fetal infection when administered as a prophylactic for maternal rubella. Furthermore, disease (but not infection) may be suppressed in the mother, thus eliminating an important guide in the management of the case.

The control of those viral diseases listed in Table 10-10 will ultimately depend on active immunization with vaccines not yet available (except for poliomyelitis and measles). Passive immunization with preformed antibody (gamma globulin) is an extravagant and cumbersome stopgap procedure, but nevertheless it is of real value in special circumstances—especially in the prevention of disease in children with pre-existing disability.

The Principles of Active Immunization.   A brief review here of the principles of immunization is relevant to an understanding of the limitations and potential of this method for the control of human infections.

The introduction into the host, either through infection or artificial inoculation, of living or dead microbes results in an irrevocable change in that host associated with the production by lymphoid cells of specific antibodies (immunoglobulins). Although the exact role of antibodies in recovery from infection is uncertain and highly controversial, there is no doubt of their value in the prevention of bacterial, rickettsial, and viral diseases. Altered tissue or cellular immunity sometimes associated with dermal hypersensitivity (as exemplified by the tuberculin reaction) may be induced by artificial immunization, but here again, the exact relation of this state to resistance to infection is still under investigation.

It is important to point out that immunity—whether naturally or artificially induced—is never absolute and may be overridden to a degree with a sufficiently large quantity of challenge antigen (infection). In most instances specific immunity prevents the evolution of *disease* or lessens its severity but probably does not actually prevent *infection*.

The parenteral injection of protein or small molecular weight antigens is followed initially by the appearance in regional lymph nodes and in the serum of IgM or 19S high-molecular-weight antibody. This antibody is very efficient in binding antigen. Soon thereafter another molecular species of antibody of identical specificity but smaller size (IgG or 7S antibody) makes its appearance. The avidity of IgG antibodies for antigen—initially low—increases with time. If a second injection of antigen is given, IgM is formed only to new or previously unrecognized antigens in the preparation; the principle response is a rapid outpouring of high avidity IgG antibody to the antigen administered earlier. This is the anamnestic, or "booster," response. Most antibacterial and antiviral antibody measured in conventional serologic tests is IgG.

The recognition of these different molecular species of antibody and their different kinetics of appearance (and disappearance) has proved of value in the diagnostic study of infections and in predicting the immunity of vaccinated individuals. IgM, because it appears early and declines soon after infection, is indicative of *recent* infection or vaccination. The production of IgG but not IgM suggests previous immunologic experience (secondary response) to the agent in question. When children previously given inactivated measles vaccine were challenged, children who produced IgG antibodies were immune to challenge with live virus vaccine, but children who produced IgM (and hence had not responded to the earlier vaccine) were not immune to infection. (Schluederberg and Karelitz, 1965).

The timing of the second injection is important in the attainment of a true accelerated secondary, or "booster," response. The interval between initial and second injections should be at least 40 days.

Live Versus Dead Vaccines.   As mentioned earlier, immunity may be induced with either living (multiplying) or dead (inactivated) agents. However, the duration of immunity—particularly with the viral vaccines—is greater when induced with living organisms. This effect is probably explained by (1) the greater antigenic mass presented by a replicating agent, (2) the greater antigenic heterogeneity revealed as the agent multiplies, i.e., "minor" antigen attains sufficient concentration to provide an antigenic stimulus as well as the major antigen identifiable in inactivated preparations, and (3) priming of cells adjacent to the site that is vulnerable to subsequent challenge infection (if the vaccine virus has been administered by the natural route, as with polio vaccine).

The *route of vaccine administration* may prove to be of critical importance in engendering local secretory IgA antibody. Recent studies suggest that such antibody may be induced with inactivated antigens.

The dangers and problems inherent in the use of both types of vaccine are considered in detail in Chapter 3.

How Many Antigens Can Be Given?   As more vaccines are developed, the exceedingly practical question arises as to whether an increase in the number of antigens can "overwhelm" the antibody-forming machinery so that production of immunity to the individual components of the vaccine is compromised. In the case of living virus vaccines, interference is already recognized as a practical problem—hence the spacing of administration of polio vaccine viruses. On the other hand, when unrelated virus vaccines such as measles and smallpox are injected at different sites, no reduction in the number of sero-conversions (individuals forming antibody) is detectable (Budd et al., 1967). However, when multiple inert protein antigens are administered parenterally a reduction in antibody response has been observed. This question deserves much more study.

The Optimal Time for Immunization.   Each vaccine must be evaluated separately with respect to the question of the optimal time for its administration. Basic immunologic studies in the past few years have demonstrated, first, that the young infant—indeed even the fetus *in utero*—is capable of immunologic response. Secondly no generalization can be made about the timetable of development of immunologic competence. Rather this has to be determined for each antigen. Another limitation to the early administration of antigen is the presence in the infant during the first few months of life of passively transferred maternal antibody that may bind or neutralize the immunizing antigen.

Active Immunization by Vaccination. The Prevention of Disease by the Artificial Induction of Specific Immunity.   The induction of disease-specific immunity by artificial active immunization (vaccination) is a major triumph of preventive medicine (specific recommendations are given in Chapter 15). Ideally, the effective vaccine induces protracted immunity by presenting the recipient with antigen identical with the disease-producing agent, yet so modified that it is not injurious to the subject or his associates. Although no such perfect vaccine exists, several, such as live polio vaccine, are virtually free of toxicity yet highly effective in producing lasting immunity.

TABLE 10-10

The Prevention or Modification of Disease with Specific Preformed Antibody

"Passive" Immunization

Antitoxic Antibody	Usual Antibody Source
Tetanus*	Equine
Diphtheria	Equine
Antiviral Antibody	
Measles	Human (gamma globulin)
Infectious hepatitis	Human (gamma globulin)
Poliomyelitis†	Human (gamma globulin)
Mumps†	Human (gamma globulin)
Rubella†	Human (gamma globulin)
Rabies*	Equine

* Not acquired by human-to-human contact.
† Rarely of practical value.

Because the ultimate producer of vaccine-induced immunity is the host himself, the reagents used in the activation of this immunity may be (and often are) relatively crude preparations. The final reagent (antibody) that is manufactured in the host is pure and specific. Furthermore, the initial or primary immunization of the subject induces a state of altered reactivity to the antigen so that its reinjection subsequently as a "booster" is followed by a secondary immune response, which is more rapid and of greater degree than before (Figure 10-8).

Because all infective agents of human disease (as a result of containing protein or polysaccharide) are potentially antigenic, vaccines could, in theory, be developed to stimulate antibody production against any of them. In fact, effective vaccines have been produced using living bacteria (BCG)*, nonviable bacterial cells (typhoid), modified exotoxins (diphtheria), type-specific polysaccharides (pneumococcal pneumonia), and infective and inactivated viral particles. Even so, the universal application of artificial immunization to the control of infectious diseases would be completely unwarranted.

For example, there would be little point in injecting the population at large with the undeniably potent vaccines that have been used experimentally for pneumococcal pneumonia. Even if only the more important lower-numbered types were included in such a vaccine, the incidence of primary pneumococcal or lobar pneumonia is small and unpredictable in its distribution. When the disease does occur, it can be contained readily in most cases by the use of powerful chemotherapeutic agents such as penicillin.

* Vaccine prepared from Bacillus Calmette-Guérin.

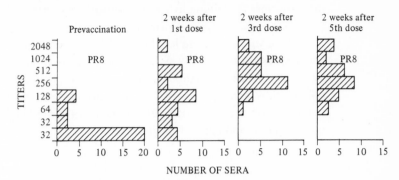

FIGURE 10-8. Booster response to immunization with influenza A (PR8) vaccine. (Reproduced from J. J. Quilligan et al.: *J Clin Invest*, **27**:576, 1948.)

Somewhat different examples are the vaccines for typhoid and tuberculosis. In the United States, these vaccines contribute relatively little to the control of their respective diseases, but they are of value in certain populations at high risk of infection.

The special importance of vaccination in the general population is in the control of the intrinsically human contagious diseases that are perpetuated by human-human contact (Tables 10-8 and 10-9). These infections are as world-wide in their distribution as man himself. They know neither geographic nor absolute seasonal limitation because they are not dependent upon the nuances of the environment or the life cycles of vectors but only upon the vagaries of human-to-human contact and human susceptibility. Thus, contact of man with these agents is almost certain and is not subject to environmental control.

Because many of these contagious agents may infect and be transmitted without producing manifest disease in all cases, the time at which contact occurs is unpredictable and cannot be defined for any given human being. Therefore, the inevitability of recurrent contact with the obligate human parasites must be accepted as a fact of life, for the finest of sanitary engineering cannot block the measles virus in its brief journey between two wrestling four-year-olds. Instead, the four-year-old must himself be so modified that contact, or even infection, with the virus does not result in disease.

It is particularly important at the present time, with new viruses identified every year, to consider carefully not only the indications for vaccination against these agents in the individual patient, but also the contraindications, i.e., whether the contribution of the virus to human morbidity warrants the production of a vaccine. With the great plagues eradicated, we are now entering a period with the leisure and the methods to examine the public health aspects of morbidity from minor diseases as well as those with directly fatal issue. Thus, whereas there was no real cause for debate about the need for vaccination against smallpox and its devastating mortality, the place of adenovirus vaccine in the medical scheme of things still awaits definition. **The Nature of the Vaccines Currently in Common Use.** Although many vaccines can be commercially produced, only those with the characteristics summarized in Table 10-11 are currently in common use. These vaccines include two bacterial toxoids, three vaccines containing living or inactivated bacterial cells, and living and inactivated vaccines made from six viruses.

Of these vaccines, those for diphtheria, pertussis, tetanus, smallpox, poliomyelitis, and measles are used widely in the general population. The first three (DPT) are usually administered in combination in infancy and early childhood. Immunization against poliomyelitis and measles is also recommended for preschool children. Smallpox immunization is also carried out routinely in the United States before admission to public schools and before foreign travel.

TABLE 10-11
Vaccines in Common Use

Vaccine	Source	Constituents
Toxoid		
Diphtheria	Culture	Formalin-modified toxin (filtrate of broth culture)
Tetanus	Culture	Formalin-modified toxin (filtrate of broth culture)
Bacterial (noninfective)		
Pertussis*	Culture	Formalin-modified toxin (filtrate of bacterial cells)
Typhoid, paratyphoid	Culture	Heat-killed bacterial cells
Bacterial (infective)		
BCG†	Culture	Viable tubercle bacilli (Calmette-Guérin) of reduced virulence
Viral (noninfective)		
Influenza	Chick embryo	Formalin- or ultraviolet inactivated A and B strains
Poliomyelitis (Salk)	Monkey kidney tissue culture	Formalin- or ultraviolet inactivated virus types 1, 2, 3
Rabies (Semple)	Rabbit brain	Phenol- or ultraviolet inactivated
(Lilly)	Duck embryo	"virus fixe"
Adenovirus (3, 4, 7)	Monkey kidney tissue culture	Formalin-inactivated types 3, 4, 7
Viral (infective)		
Smallpox	Calf lymph	Vaccinia virus
Yellow fever (17D)	Chick embryo	Tissue culture-adapted yellow fever virus
(Dakar)	Mouse brain	Mouse brain-passaged yellow fever virus
Poliomyelitis	Monkey kidney tissue culture	Polioviruses 1, 2, and 3 (reduced neurovirulence)
Rabies (Flury LEP‡)	Chick embryo brain	Flury strain chick embryo passaged rabies virus
(Flury HEP§)	Chick embryo	
Measles (Enders)	Chick embryo tissue culture	Measles virus of reduced virulence

* Bacterial cell suspension; usually included with diphtheria and tetanus toxoids as DPT.
† Vaccine prepared from Bacillus Calmette-Guérin.
‡ Low egg passage (less attenuated).
§ High egg passage (more attenuated; less antigenic potency).

The other vaccines listed in Table 10-11 as being in common use are not utilized in mass immunization; however, they are valuable in certain special circumstances. **Vaccines Less Commonly Used.** Other vaccines in less common use or of less established efficacy include

1. Vaccines now largely superseded by the availability of antimicrobial drugs (the rickettsial vaccines for spotted fever, typhus, scrub typhus, and Q fever). These vaccines are still useful for the prevention of disease in special groups at high risk, such as laboratory or field workers.
2. Vaccines that may be only temporarily effective but that may postpone infection to a time more dangerous for the host. This is the case with the inactivated mumps virus vaccine. This vaccine has not yet received sufficient study to determine the duration of induced immunity. Because such complications of the disease as orchitis are more common and more severe after puberty, it would be unwise to postpone the disease to that time. A newly licensed live virus mumps vaccine is promising, but because the duration of its effectiveness is still being studied, it is currently recommended only for older children who have no definite history of mumps.
3. Vaccines still in the experimental stage and of limited effectiveness (vaccines for arbovirus infections, especially Japanese B encephalitis).
4. Vaccines of questionable effectiveness for which it seems unreasonable to anticipate success. (The vaccines for cholera and bacillary dysentry—essentially focal diseases of the bowel without systemic invasion.)

The Evaluation of Response to Vaccination. Vaccines are designed to induce specific immunity to disease. The ultimate measure of their effectiveness is their capacity to reduce the incidence of disease (morbidity) or mortality in human beings exposed to infection under natural conditions. A "protection ratio" may be derived from controlled studies by comparing the attack rates in vaccinated and unvaccinated members of the exposed populations:

$$\text{Protection ratio} = \frac{\text{(incidence in vaccinated)}}{\text{(incidence in unvaccinated)}}.$$

For most vaccines the arithmetic value of this ratio is less than 0.6.

Because many factors influence response to vaccination, it is desirable to have some ready indication other than challenge by the natural infection (which may never occur). Such indications of response may not necessarily be analogous to immunity, but they may serve as a guide to the antigenic potency or viability of the vaccine or the ability of the subject to respond. The same tests used in determining past or present natural infection may be used in the evaluation of vaccines directed against them. Thus, delayed cutaneous hypersensitivity to tuberculin or diphtheria toxin (Schick test) may be used as a test of successful vaccination with BCG or diphtheria toxoid.

Similar convenient skin tests are not available for other commonly employed vaccines. However, the cutaneous site of smallpox vaccination is easily observed, and the characteristic course of the dermal infection is an obvious indication of successful inoculation with vaccinia virus. The local lesion produced with BCG is a less exact indication of inoculation, but it is of some value in indicating vaccine viability.

The presence of humoral neutralizing antibody has been frequently and consistently correlated with specific immunity, especially in studies of influenza and poliomyelitis vaccines. However, except in experimental studies, it is hardly practicable to assess the adequacy of immunization by serologic studies. Furthermore, recent studies of immunization against infection with parainfluenza type 1 virus have shown a lack of concordance of serum neutralizing antibody and resistance to experimental infection However, there was a good correlation between resistance (as measured by failure to shed virus) and the presence of antibody in nasal secretions (Figure 10-9) (Smith *et al.*, 1966).

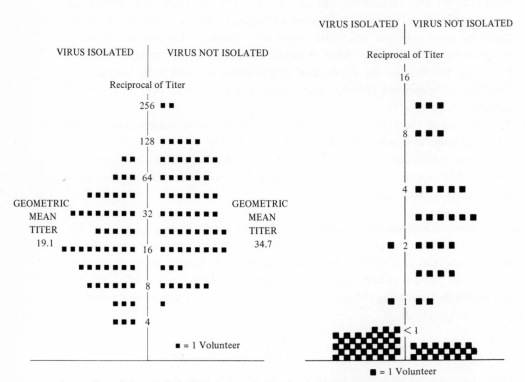

A *Serum Neutralizing Antibody Titer before Challenge with Parainfluenza Type 1 Virus.*

B *Neutralizing Activity of Nasal Secretions before Challenge with Parainfluenza Type 1 Virus.*

FIGURE 10-9. The lack of correlation of serum neutralizing antibody and immunity to challenge with parainfluenza Type 1 virus and the correlation of immunity with antibody in nasal secretions. (Reproduced from C. B. Smith *et al: New Eng J Med*, **275**:1145, 1966.)

For the most part, the potency of most vaccines is inferred from
1. Past experience in field trials with comparable antigen doses and immunization schedules.
2. Tests of vaccine viability (measurement of infective virus) when live virus vaccines are used.
3. Antigenic potency in experimental animals. (Much work needs to be done in this direction, particularly with respect to correlating the results of animal and human immunization with identical lots of vaccine.)

Neither natural nor vaccine-induced immunity is absolute, and either may be overridden by large challenge doses of infecting organisms or by environmental or endogenous factors that impair the nonspecific resistance of the host. The relative inefficacy of typhoid vaccine may reflect the large numbers of bacilli that may be ingested in contaminated water or food in this enteric infection. In contrast, the challenge dose of respiratory-borne pathogens (which cannot multiply in the environment) is not susceptible to such wide variation.

The Duration of Artificially-induced (Vaccine) Immunity: Relation to Mechanisms of Vaccine Immunity. It cannot be stated categorically that vaccine-induced immunity will be more or less "solid" or enduring than the immunity that results from a natural infection. Neither can it be said that "live" vaccines in general induce more lasting immunity than "dead" ones. For example, immunity from tetanus toxoid (a nonviable antigen) persists for at least as long as that following inoculation with living vaccinia virus. Furthermore, the immunity from tetanus toxoid far exceeds that of the natural infection, following which reinfection and disease may occur, whereas the immunity following smallpox far outlasts that from vaccinia.

The foregoing comparisons are somewhat spurious, but they serve to emphasize the imprecision involved in speaking of vaccination in general rather than in terms of the particular disease.

In the first place, the route by which tetanus toxoid is given permits better dissemination of antigen to antibody-forming lymph nodes than occurs during natural tetanus infection in which toxin migrates along peripheral nerves from the local lesion. Also, the immunity from tetanus vaccine is specifically antitoxic. Infection and invasion by tetanus bacilli are not, and need not be, prevented to prevent the disease. Furthermore, the amount of toxin formed during infection is small, and may itself serve as an effective booster of pre-existing toxoid-induced immunity.

On the other hand, the cutaneous route by which smallpox vaccine (vaccinia) is given is presumably less effective in disseminating antigen than the extensive viremia of smallpox. Furthermore, the respiratory route by which the challenge virus enters is remote from the site of cutaneous vaccination so that factors of local immunity are less operative in containing infection. That local or regional immunity occurs is illustrated by the need for rotation of vaccination sites in certain repeatedly vaccinated persons in order to effect a "take." It is clear that certain inactivated vaccines (mumps and poliomyelitis) do not prevent infection, yet the sequel of infection of the gut with either wild or vaccine strains of live polioviruses is a relative immunity to enteric reinfection.

The immunity of inactivated influenza vaccine is said to be equal to the relatively brief immunity that follows the natural disease. Yet the assumption that naturally acquired immunity to influenza is brief has been derived from a few studies in military or institutional situations. In these cases, attack rates (and presumably challenge doses) were high and probably unrepresentative of exposure within the general population. Certainly, population immunity to influenza does rise and remains high following the introduction of new viral strains, but the role of continuing reinfection in such population immunity is probably important (Kilbourne, 1961).

It is only reasonable to suppose that vaccination procedures most closely simulating natural infection will induce immunity comparable to that of the disease. It is suspected (but unproved) that those infectious agents that induce enduring immunity may (1) persist within the host for his lifetime, acting continually or recurrently as antigenic stimuli; or (2) recurrently reinfect the host from exogenous sources without producing disease.

Yellow fever vaccine, a live, parenterally introduced vaccine against a parenterally introduced infection, appears thus far to have induced persisting immunity for as long as ten years as judged by persistence of neutralizing antibody.

Immunization with "killed" or inactivated vaccines would appear to be less promising in inducing persisting immunity without frequent "recall," or booster, injections. However, it is entirely possible that natural challenge with the infection itself may "boost" primary vaccine immunity in time to forestall its late effects, or disease (Salk, 1959). This postulate remains to be proved, however. In the case of diphtheria, childhood immunization with toxoid clearly does not produce enduring immunity. It is now a cause of grave concern that diphtheria may occur during epidemics among previously immunized adults who have not had recent booster injections. The problem is compounded by the hypersensitivity to toxoid that exists in immunized adults, so that low doses of toxoid must be cautiously administered.

With inactivated viral vaccines a new and potentially serious problem is the danger of hypersensitization to the viral protein. Individuals previously given inactivated measles vaccine may suffer an unusual type of illness characterized by rash and pulmonary symptoms when they are subsequently injected with live virus measles vaccine or are naturally infected with measles.

The Anamnestic or Secondary Response to Booster Injections. The declining immunity that follows primary injection of nonliving antigens may in most instances be quickly "recalled" by later "booster" injections (Figure 10-8). Even in the absence of residual detectable antibody, the latent immunity from the initial priming with antigen may be evidenced by an accelerated production of antibody in the subject. If the incubation period of the disease to be prevented is sufficiently long, or if contact has not yet occurred, booster injections in previously immunized subjects may be used effectively to supplement the less desirable passive transfer of preformed antibody. The situations in which booster injections are most frequently used are in the prophylaxis of tetanus, diphtheria, and typhoid. It has long been recognized that the incidence and severity of unfavorable "reactions" are greater in subjects who have been previously injected with, and hence sensitized to, diphtheria toxoid. For this reason, prior skin testing with *toxin* (Schick test) to determine immunity status, or with *toxoid* (Moloney test), to determine sensitivity to toxoid has been carried out before reimmunization of adults. Simple reduction of toxoid dose may obviate such tedious pretesting and yet provide an effective antigenic stimulus for both diphtheria and tetanus (Levine, 1961).

The waning immunity following smallpox vaccination must be periodically "boosted" by revaccination. In this case, the secondary immune response is visibly accelerated ("vaccinoid") as evidenced by the more rapid progression of the vaccinia lesion, which reaches its peak in less than a week in contrast to 8 to 10 days in the case of the primary reaction. Immunity to smallpox is concomitantly accelerated.

The Use of Adjuvants with Inactivated Vaccines. Another method for prolonging the immunity induced by nonliving vaccines is to use adjuvant materials with the antigen. Such "adjuvants" are chemically diverse, and include aluminium phosphate and mineral oils. Their mechanism of action is not fully understood, but they seem to enhance and prolong the response to primary immunization. The use of adjuvants is still experimental, and the possibility of chronic toxicity has deterred their general acceptance. This important problem deserves further study, however.

The Route of Administration.   It is well established that immunizing antigen must be injected into or beneath the skin to evoke immunity. Such parenteral administration is necessary to deliver intact protein antigen to the antibody-forming cells of the reticuloendothelial system. An obvious exception to this rule is live poliovirus vaccine, which must be delivered by oral (enteral) ingestion to the site where it will multiply.

Because smallpox vaccination is essentially a dermal infection, it is best inoculated into the superficial layers of the skin by multiple puncture or pressure techniques. The intradermal route is also used to forestall the systematic effects of influenza or typhoid vaccines. This route is purported to allow the establishment of immunity with smaller doses of antigen than are effective subcutaneously. However, virtually all comparative studies of the relative efficacy of the intradermal and subcutaneous routes of injection have not used identical dose schedules. Because small doses intradermally may apparently induce the same response as larger subcutaneous doses, it has been frequently and erroneously concluded that intradermal inoculation is superior to subcutaneous in immunizing efficacy. Such conclusions have been derived from studies in which

1. Immunization was not truly primary.
2. The antigenic mass used subcutaneously was larger than necessary for optimal response.
3. The efficacy of several small doses intradermally was compared with that of a single subcutaneous injection.

In 1957, when suboptimal and identical doses of Asian influenza A2 vaccine were given by identical schedules to members of a population without any possible prior experience with the antigen, no significant differences were noted in response to subcutaneous or intradermal injection (McCarroll and Kilbourne, 1958).

The Role of Artificial Immunization in Public Health: Specific Vaccines for Specific Purposes

Vaccines for the Prevention of Mortality.   The decrease of the killing infectious diseases of man (with their major impact in infancy and childhood) is due principally to environmental sanitation rather than to artificial immunization. But several vaccines—two of them the earliest known—are important methods of control for diseases with high mortality rates. Immunization against smallpox and rabies antedates the recognition of their viral etiology. The principles established over a century ago by Pasteur (with rabies) and Jenner (with cowpox) have been the basis for all subsequent vaccines. These principles include the concept of reducing virulence by "attenuation" or passing or deriving the vaccine strain in or from a different (non-human) host.

The diseases that contribute importantly to mortality but are preventable by vaccination include

Smallpox.
Rabies.
Yellow fever (jungle type).
Diphtheria and pertussis (to a lesser extent).
Measles (particularly in primitive communities).

Although usually considered as causes of general morbidity, diphtheria, pertussis, and measles may cause significant mortality in infants and young children.

Tetanus, although uncommon, can kill as many as 40 per cent of its victims, so that vaccination should be considered potentially lifesaving with this disease. Similarly, the total mortality from poliomyelitis is small, but the use of vaccine, particularly in adults, has undoubtedly saved lives.

For completeness, the effective vaccine for the prevention of Rocky Mountain spotted fever should be mentioned. The great reduction in mortality in spotted fever through the use of tetracycline antibiotics has, however, almost eliminated the need for vaccination.

Vaccines for the Reduction of Mortality in Special Risk Groups. Certain vaccines that are not widely or routinely employed in the general population have value for the reduction of mortality in groups at special risk of infection or severe disease.

Influenza vaccines have assumed special importance with the recognition that the disease may be fatal in certain patients with cardiac or chronic pulmonary disease or pregnancy. These persons are no more liable than others to acquire the infection but are peculiarly vulnerable to its effects. It is currently recommended by the Surgeon General of the U.S. Public Health Service that such persons receive annual boosters of polyvalent influenza vaccine following primary immunization.

The use of BCG for the prevention of tuberculosis is usually restricted to children in certain crowded, economically deprived populations in which morbidity is predictably high. In such circumstances it is obvious that mortality is also reduced through prevention of miliary and meningitic forms of the disease.

Rabies represents a unique situation in which the incubation period after exposure is so long (14 to 42 days in man) that primary active immunization can be effected in time to prevent the development of disease. The special groups in which mortality may be prevented would therefore include humans bitten by possibly rabid animals in addition to farmers, animal trainers, veterinarians, and others at special risk. Because the case fatality rate of rabies is 100 per cent, reduction of morbidity by immunization is equivalent to reduction in mortality.

None of the rabies vaccines currently available is completely satisfactory. Of the two inactivated preparations (Table 10-11), the traditional Semple vaccine is the most reliable antigenically. Serious hypersensitivity reactions to brain tissue components, however, make it undesirable for wide-scale use. A modification of this vaccine that represents duck embryo passage material is apparently less dangerous in this respect. Two live-virus vaccines have been produced by multiple serial passages of the Flury strain of virus in chick embryos. These vaccines, LEP (low egg passage) and HEP (high egg passage), are now used widely in the immunization of domestic animals. The HEP (less virulent but also less antigenic strain) has recently been used as "base line" immunization of those constantly exposed to animals. Because antibody measurements are not easily or reliably correlated with immunity in rabies, the immune status of individuals so vaccinated is somewhat unpredictable. In cases of actual specific exposure, booster injections of living or inactivated vaccine may be given—often supplemented by injection of specific immune serum.

In the case of dog-bite victims who have not previously received primary immunization, the live virus vaccines are not relied upon for the "emergency" induction of primary immunity.

Vaccines As Supplements to Environmental Sanitation. The basic control of yellow fever as an arthropod-borne disease and of typhoid as an enteric infection depends on sanitation of the environment. In a sense, rabies also is similarly controlled in most countries by immunization and regulation of the domestic canines, which comprise the important reservoir of infection.

Nevertheless, vaccines for these three diseases, together with the vaccines less commonly used for plague, the rickettsial diseases, and the arthropod-borne encephalitides, are valuable adjuncts for disease control. Although control of the urban dwelling mosquito vector is the key to control of urban yellow fever, similar environmental control of jungle mosquitoes and animal reservoirs is a virtual impossibility with the jungle form of the disease. In the latter case, specific immunization of residents of and visitors to the endemic areas is the only feasible control method.

Although the efficacy of typhoid vaccination still remains in dispute, several carefully controlled studies, including one in Yugoslavia (Cvjetanovic, 1957), suggest its value for those who have not acquired natural immunity from childhood exposure in an endemic area. Certainly, the severity of the disease is less in those who have received specific immunization (Turner, 1959).

Vaccination As a Quarantine Procedure. It is paradoxical that the countries of Asia in which yellow fever has never occurred nevertheless require proof of vaccination for yellow fever from foreign travelers. This measure is obviously not for the protection of the traveler but for the protection of the countries visited, especially if the traveler has recently gone through an area (South America or Africa) in which yellow fever is endemic. In this instance, specific immunization is in effect a quarantine procedure to prevent the importation of the infection into areas in which there are potential vectors for the transmission of disease to the susceptible population. Without this precaution, in these days of swift air travel, persons incubating yellow fever could easily pass from yellow fever zones to any part of Asia in considerably less time than the three- to six-day incubation period of the disease and thus disembark as unrecognized reservoirs of infection. This possibility is forestalled by the requirement that a traveler carry a certificate as evidence of anti-yellow fever vaccination at least ten days before arrival.

The United States and many other countries require smallpox vaccination within a three-year period before citizens are permitted to leave the country. Again, in this case the vaccine is not primarily for the protection of the individual traveler, but for the protection of the country to which he will return—by preventing his acquisition of the disease abroad. The following brief note published in the "Morbidity and Mortality Report" of the U.S. Public Health Service (March 10, 1961) epitomizes the problem involved in the air age:

> The Division of Foreign Quarantine has informed us that recently smallpox was imported to Madrid, Spain by a child who flew from Bombay to Rome on TWA flight #809, January 26 and from Rome to Madrid on Alitalia #346, January 27. Diagnosis was made on February 6 and death occurred on February 14.
> A secondary case in Madrid was confirmed on February 23, and 13 additional cases were reported for the week ending March 4.

The infections other than yellow fever and smallpox that are susceptible to international quarantine regulations are cholera, plague, louse-borne relapsing fever, and louse-borne typhus. For none of these are vaccines important as quarantine measures, although certain Asian countries require cholera vaccination of travelers prior to their entry into the country.

Vaccines for the Reduction of Morbidity in Certain Groups at High Risk. Young adults when crowded together in schools or military camps seem to be particularly susceptible to epidemic infection with respiratory viruses. Vaccines are available for the control of certain of these infections, namely those caused by influenza and adenoviruses. Both the influenza and adenovirus vaccines are polyvalent and contain the viral strains most commonly encountered in epidemic form: influenza A and B and adenoviruses 3, 4, and 7. Extensive studies by the Commission on Influenza of the Armed Forces Epidemiological Board have proved the efficacy of these vaccines under field conditions.

In times of widespread prevalence of influenza when all members of the population are at risk, the general use of vaccine may be considered with special reference to such key personnel as policemen, firemen, physicians, and nurses, in whom simultaneous illness (no matter how benign) may jeopardize the public safety.

In contrast, the use of currently available adenovirus vaccines for other than the special military or school situations seems completely unwarranted because there is no evidence that the virus types in the vaccine cause epidemic disease in the general population.

The Problems and Future of Artificial Immunization—Summary. In principle, artificial immunization is an ideal approach to the prevention of infectious disease. In a "dirty" world saturated with microbial pathogens, the concept of universal environmental sanitation is obviously unrealistic and untenable as a method of controlling all infections. Immunization, in contrast, creates in the recipient a selective "built-in" and mobile shield that under favorable conditions provides lifelong protection in almost all environments. Why not, then, simply capture all the infectious agents of man, produce vaccines from them, and thereby conquer all infectious diseases? After the foregoing discussion this question may seem facetious. In Chapter 3 the varied and subtle hazards experienced in the production of viral vaccines have been considered in some detail. Discussion of currently accepted vaccines in the present chapter has emphasized their limitations. The multiplicity of viral agents has been stressed. It should be clear, therefore, that there is a great gap between any goal of universal artificial immunization and the current practice of the art. In part the problem is a scientific one (see Chapter 3). We do not yet understand sufficiently the nuances of microbial genetics or enough of the basis of immunologic response to operate intelligently (i.e., free of empiricism) in the designing of vaccines. Despite the great successes of this empirical approach it must be confessed that even problems of long standing, such as antigenic variation of influenza virus, cellular immunity in tuberculosis, and the role of local antibody response in immunity, are still not understood. Many infective agents, including the viruses of hepatitis, have defied isolation in the laboratory. When new vaccines are introduced we must view them with caution until they have been tested in the field under natural conditions; there is no reliable method at present for predicting the immunizing potency of a vaccine.

At times the problems are technologic or logistical—a failure to produce enough vaccine or high quality vaccine or a failure in supply or administration. After all, the vaccine has to get from the shelf into the arm of the recipient to be effective. In this connection, the critical point of public acceptance ultimately determines the success of any immunization program—no matter how brilliant the scientific background of the discovery. The imaginative use of communications media may be as vital as the antigenic testing of the vaccine (Figure 10-10).

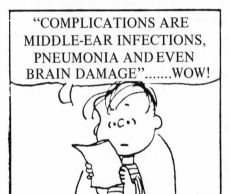
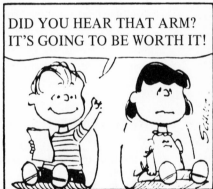
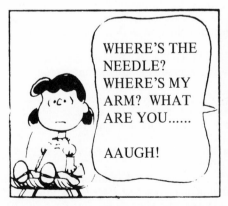
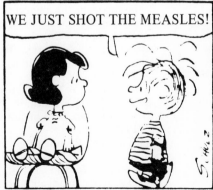

January 6, 1967 PEANUTS cartoon. © 1967 United Feature Syndicate.

FIGURE 10-10. The success of artificial immunization depends ultimately on public acceptance.

The question of "immunization for what?" can be answered: *Immunization for those diseases of public health importance that cannot otherwise be contained (and for which the antigen is available)*. But, it is not always clear what is important or at least what is *most* important. Priorities are sometimes established by emotion and by public demand. Otherwise a vaccine for measles, which produces far greater morbidity and even mortality than poliomyelitis, might have been developed before polio vaccine. Then, too, a lack of knowledge of the natural history of disease may create an error of omission. Failure to appreciate the significance of infection with respiratory syncytial (RS) virus as a cause of pneumonia in children has undoubtedly delayed the development of an effective vaccine.

Finally, the price of success must be considered. In 1963 there were no deaths from smallpox in the United States, but 18 deaths and 3,000 complications were attributable to smallpox vaccination. When do we stop or curtail successful immunization programs? When is herd immunity adequate? (See Chapter 7.) The success of poliovirus vaccine has virtually eliminated wild type polioviruses in some Western countries and immunity induced by diphtheria toxoid has reduced the colonization of human respiratory tracts by *C. diphtheriae*. If cryptic and continual reinfection with the natural prototypes of these agents is necessary to maintain immunity and if they are not completely eradicated—then a new threat to public health may be forthcoming. In the meantime, it is reasonable and essential to pursue our semi-empiric way, to utilize vaccines as they are developed, but to do so with care and with a scientifically based consideration of the consequences. Nonspecific immunization offers another approach —as yet little exploited—for the control of these "inevitable" infections.

REFERENCES

ALLEN, J. C., and KUNKEL, H. G.: Antibodies to genetic types of gamma globulin after multiple transfusions. *Science*, **139**:418–19, 1963.

AYCOCK, W. L., and MUELLER, J. H.: Meningococcus carrier rates and meningitis incidence. *Bact Rev*, **14**:115–60, 1950.

BLACK, P. H., KUNZ, L. J., and SWARTZ, M. N.: Salmonellosis—A review of some unusual aspects. *New Eng J Med*, **262**:921–27, 1960.

BLUMENFELD, H. L., KILBOURNE, E. K., LOURIA, D. B., and ROGERS, D. E.: Studies on influenza in the pandemic of 1957–1958. I. An epidemiologic, clinical and serologic investigation of an intrahospital epidemic, with a note on vaccination efficacy. *J Clin Invest*, **38**:199–212, 1958.

BUDD, M. A., SCHOLTENS, R. G., MCGEHEE, R. F., JR., and GARDNER, P.: An evaluation of measles and smallpox vaccines simultaneously administered. *Amer J Public Health*, **57**:80–86, 1967.

CVJETANOVIC, B. B.: Field trial of typhoid vaccines. *Amer J Public Health*, **47**:578–81, 1957.

ENDERS, J. F., WELLER, T. H., and ROBBIN, F. C.: Cultivation of the Lansing strain of poliomyelitis virus in cultures of various human embryonic tissues. *Science*, **109**:85–87, 1949.

HAMRE, D.: Rhinoviruses. In Melnick, J. L. (ed.): *Monographs in Virology*, Vol. 1. S. Karger, Basel, Switzerland, 1968.

HENNEY, C. S., and ELLIS, E. F.: Antibody production to aggregated human γG-globulin in acquired hypogammaglobulinemia. *New Eng J Med*, **278**:1144–46, 1968.

KILBOURNE, E. D.: Influenza—The cryptic killer. *Amer Rev Resp Dis*, **83**:265–66, 1961.

KOENIG, M. G., SPICKARD, A., CARDELLA, M. A., and ROGERS, D. E.: Clinical and laboratory observations on type E botulism in man. *Medicine (Balt.)*, **43**:517–45, 1964.

Levine, L., Ipsen, J., Jr., and McComb, J. A.: Adult immunization. Preparation and evaluation of combined fluid tetanus and diphtheria toxoids for adult use. *Amer J Hyg*, **73**:20–35, 1961.

McCarroll, J. R., and Kilbourne, E. D.: Immunization with Asian-strain influenza vaccine; Equivalence of the subcutaneous and intradermal routes. *New Eng J Med*, **259**:618–21, 1958.

Melnick, J. L.: A water-borne urban epidemic of hepatitis. In Hartman, F. W., Lo Grippo, G. A., Mateer, J. G., and Barron, J. (eds.): *Hepatic Frontiers*. Henry Ford Hospital, International Symposium, No. 6. Little, Brown and Company., Boston, 1957.

Mosley, J. W.: Water-borne infectious hepatitis. *New Eng J Med*, **261**:748–53, 1959.

Poskanzer, D. C., and Beadenkopf, W. G.: Waterborne infectious hepatitis epidemic from a chlorinated municipal supply. *Public Health Rep*, **76**:745–51, 1961.

Quilligan, J. J., Jr., Minuse, E., and Francis, T., Jr.: Homologous and heterologous antibody response of infants and children to multiple injections of a single strain of influenza virus. *J Clin Invest*, **27**:572–79, 1948.

Rogers, D. E.: Botulism, vintage 1963. Editorial. *Ann Intern Med*, **61**:581–87, 1964.

Salk, J. E., Preconceptions about vaccination against paralytic poliomyelitis. *Ann Intern Med*, **50**:843–61, 1959.

Schluederberg, A., Karelitz, S.: Suppression of measles 19S antibody formation as evidence of immunity. *JAMA*, **191**:86–92, 1965.

Smith, C. B., Purcell, R. H., Bellanti, J. A., and Chanock, R. M.: Protective effect of antibody to parainfluenza type 1 virus. *New Eng J Med*, **275**:1145–52, 1966.

Turner, R.: Vaccination against typhoid fever. *South African Med J*, **33**:639–40, 1959.

U.S. Public Health Service: *Morbidity and Mortality Report of the United States Public Health Service*. Mar. 10, 1961. Government Printing Office, Washington, D.C.

World Health Organization: *WHO Chron*, **14**:297, Geneva, Switzerland, 1960.

———: *WHO Techn Rep Ser*, no. 191, 98, *Insecticide Resistance and Vector Control*. Geneva, Switzerland, 1960.

11

Malnutrition

Nevin S. Scrimshaw and Moises Béhar

INTRODUCTION

Advances in public health and parallel social and technological changes paradoxically have increased the prominence of malnutrition in both less developed and industrialized countries. In the less-developed countries, control of the mass diseases that once decimated whole populations has left evident the underlying malnutrition, particularly among young children, that retards growth and development and increases the severity of common infections (Scrimshaw and Béhar, 1965).* It has also contributed to the higher rates of population increase, which, in turn, have led to an actual decrease in *per capita* food availability in some countries. In the industrialized countries prosperity and an abundance of food have resulted in the rise of obesity as a public health problem and contributed to the increase in coronary heart disease.

NUTRITIONAL PROBLEMS OF LESS-DEVELOPED COUNTRIES

Protein-Calorie Malnutrition

Various degrees of protein and calorie malnutrition are universal among the lower income populations of the less developed countries (Scrimshaw and Béhar, 1961). They are a major factor in the high infant and preschool child mortality in these countries. Protein-calorie malnutrition is more than a medical problem. In those countries where large proportions of the population are living under conditions of limited social and economic development, malnutrition arises from a combination of two main factors: a diet that is quantitatively and qualitatively inadequate, and

* Parts of this chapter are adapted from N. S. Scrimshaw, and M. Béhar: Malnutrition in underdeveloped countries. *New Eng J Med*, **272**:137–144, 193–198, 1965.

superimposed stress, commonly of infectious origin. The deficient diet results in turn from various combinations of low food production, inadequate preservation and distribution of foods, restricted purchasing power, poor food habits, and deficient knowledge of the relation between diet and health. The excessive incidence of infectious disease is consequent to a lack of environmental sanitation, and to poor personal hygiene, inadequate control of vectors, insufficient health services, and lowered resistance due to malnutrition.

The two main factors are, therefore, interrelated and act synergistically to the detriment of nutritional status (Scrimshaw, *et al.*, 1968). Their relative influence determines the clinical results. Of particular significance are the severity and duration of the nutritional deficiencies of protein and calories, and the extent to which protein is deficient relative to calories, the nature and severity of other associated nutritional deficiencies, the age and physiological state of the person affected, and other diseases that have preceded or are concurrent. The mild and moderate forms of protein-calorie malnutrition are frequently unrecognized because they are characterized primarily by retarded physical growth and development (NAS–NRC: *Pre-school Child Malnutrition* ... 1966). Unfortunately, at early ages mental development and subsequent learning and behavior can be affected as well (Scrimshaw and Gordon, 1968).

Mild and Moderate Forms.   In underdeveloped countries the average weight and length of children at birth are close to the values for North American or European children. Most infants grow normally during the first four months of life because they are breast fed. Beginning as early as the fourth month, however, rates of growth decrease and height and weight values depart progressively from established values for well-nourished children. During the second and third years, growth and maturation may be almost at a standstill. Only after this crucial weaning and postweaning period do children partake sufficiently of the family food and acquire enough resistance to infectious diseases so that their growth rate again approaches that of well-nourished children. During the school years rates of growth generally parallel those of well-nourished children, but lost ground is not recovered.

In some populations this amounts to a retardation of two to four years in bone age at the time of entering school, at about age seven. Consequently, when growth stops with the closing of epiphyses the final stature is smaller. Epiphyses seem to close at much the same chronological age despite the lesser size of the child. It is mainly for this reason that adults in underdeveloped countries tend to be smaller than those in industrialized ones. Genetic differences in growth potential are probably of lesser importance.

The period of retarded growth coincides with the increasing inadequacy of breast milk as the sole source of protein and other nutrients and insufficient or improper supplementation of the breast-feeding regimen (Jelliffe, 1955). After full weaning, which may not occur until the third year, the diet given the young child in less-developed countries is still commonly cereal gruels, starchy roots, overdiluted milk, and even cornstarch, with no opportunity provided the child to share in the full adult diet. In most cases this regimen not only fails to provide the needed protein and calories but is deficient in other essential nutrients. Legumes, vegetables, and occasional meat, cheese, or other animal products are usually too few to provide the additional proteins needed. Only toward the latter part of the preschool period, when the child is permitted an adult type of diet, does protein-calorie malnutrition become less common.

Unfortunately, this period of greatest dietary inadequacy coincides with a high exposure to an unsanitary environment at a time when passive immunity from the mother has been largely lost, and acquired immunity is limited. This is the age of highest frequency of diarrheal, respiratory, and parasitic diseases as well as the common communicable diseases of childhood: measles, whooping cough, chicken pox, rubella, and mumps. The second year death rate in a country is the best single index of the extent of malnutrition among young children (Gordon, *et al.*, 1967). The adverse consequences of infectious disease on nutritional status are described later in this chapter.

Because stunting during the period of malnutrition is most marked in those parts of the body that normally grow faster, disproportion develops in anthropometric measures. The shorter limb-to-trunk ratio observed in some poorly nourished population groups is largely from this cause. Moreover, 80 per cent of adult brain growth is achieved before three years of age. It is not surprising, therefore, that early malnutrition has been shown in many less-developed countries to be associated with a smaller permanent head circumference.

The common assumption that genetic factors are responsible for a substantial part of the size differences among adult populations is untenable. Well-nourished children in a healthy environment usually follow the growth patterns of well-fed North American or European children, regardless of their genetic origins. Conversely, children of European racial origins living under adverse conditions consistently show reduced growth.

Adult Protein-Calorie Malnutrition.   The consequences for adult populations of predominantly cereal diets low in protein quality have been little studied. It is presumed that such diets reduce resistance to stress, particularly that resulting from infectious disease and trauma. Calorie deficiency seriously reduces work capacity and thereby interferes with social and economic development, but there is little evidence that many adult males require more protein than they now receive.

For pregnant women and lactating mothers, however, there is widespread indication of a progressive nutritional depletion with repeated reproductive cycles (WHO: *Nutrition in Pregnancy and Lactation*, 1965). Many women fail to gain a normal amount of weight during pregnancy and therefore suffer a net loss of weight after parturition, though the average weights of children at birth are not much affected. A further loss of weight is associated with the usual prolonged breast feeding, largely because body protein is consumed to supply the protein in breast milk. The consequences of repeated pregnancy and lactation on poorly nourished mothers have received far too little attention. It is noteworthy that such women look much older than their chronological age by the standards of more privileged populations.

Marasmus.   Marasmus in children is the result of insufficient food and is therefore a form of starvation (Scrimshaw and Béhar, 1961). The extreme low-calorie diets responsible for the syndrome are obviously also markedly deficient in protein and many other essential nutrients. To compensate for the lack of food, the child utilizes the stress mechanism to mobilize, for gluconeogenesis, amino acids from the skeletal muscle and other tissues, and these essential amino acids are also available for necessary protein synthesis in the liver. Fat stores are also used maximally as an energy source until they are exhausted. Growth stops, but the amino acids and other nutrients liberated from the child's tissues make possible a continuing synthesis of serum albumin, enzymes, and other essential metabolites. For this reason, no serious bio-chemical changes are observed until fat stores and available tissue amino acids have been exhausted. The child with marasmus becomes, however, extremely emaciated owing to a loss of subcutaneous fat, severe muscle wasting, and atrophy of most organs and tissues (Figure 11-1). Despite the apt description of being reduced to "skin and bones," the child remains clinically alert and has a good appetite.

Infantile marasmus is generally associated with early weaning. It is increasing in

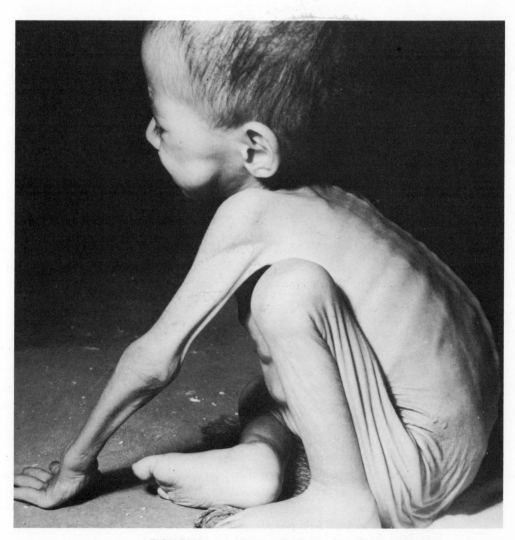

FIGURE 11-1. Moderate marasmus in a Guatemalan child.

frequency as the urban populations of developing countries grow disproportionately. Under urban circumstances, the mothers frequently wean their infants when they are very young, either in imitation of the practice of women of upper socioeconomic status, or in order to work. In either case, the substitute for breast milk is likely to be a watery gruel, thin cornstarch beverage, or overdiluted milk, all extremely deficient in both calories and protein.

Because children under one year grow more rapidly and require more calories and protein per kilogram of body weight than later, marasmus is particularly likely to develop under these circumstances. Later, if more calories are given without added protein, kwashiorkor is likely to be superimposed on a varying degree of marasmus, especially when infectious diseases further increase protein needs and induce a decrease in protein intake.

Kwashiorkor. In contrast to marasmus, there is a lack of essential amino acids available to the liver in kwashiorkor (Scrimshaw and Béhar, 1961; Viteri *et al.*, 1964). When dietary protein is deficient relative to calories, the mechanism that maintains blood glucose levels through amino acid mobilization for gluconeogenesis in the liver does not function. This results in profound physiologic and pathologic alterations.

Clinically, the kwashiorkor syndrome is characterized by edema of varying degree, from a mild form limited to the feet and ankles to severe and generalized, with eyelids swollen shut (Figure 11-2). Movement of the extremities may be limited by the fluid accumulation. Children with kwashiorkor are usually extremely apathetic, with a weak and monotonous cry if disturbed. They may be quite irritable when aroused. Anorexia is usually present and is frequently profound. Diarrhea is an almost constant finding.

The characteristic alterations of the skin resemble the dermatoses of pellagra with which they have often been mistakenly identified. The lesions are pigmented, dry, hyperkeratotic, and often desquamating, varying in size from punctiform to large confluent areas. They are most numerous on those parts of the body most subject to irritation, particularly the perineal region, trunk, and buttocks, although they frequently occur on the extremities and may extend to the face. In severe cases the skin of the entire body is involved.

The hair becomes discolored, dry, fine, and brittle (Figure 11-3). It is generally easily and painlessly pulled out, or may even fall out. In Negro children it may become reddish, but in Indian children, both Asiatic and American, whose hair is normally black, it becomes pale and even white. Successive periods of normal and abnormal growth of the hair can produce pigment changes in stripes. The extremities are frequently cold and cyanotic. The abdomen may be distended owing to flaccid abdominal muscles and to fluid accumulation.

The principal biochemical characteristics relate to alterations in protein metabolism. Low serum concentrations of albumin, β globulin, β lipoproteins and cholesterol, and the carrier proteins, transferrin and ceruloplasmin are found. As a consequence, serum iron and copper concentrations are lowered as well as serum levels of vitamin A, zinc, magnesium, and phospholipids. The activities of pepsin, trypsin, and amylase in samples of duodenal fluid are reduced to nearly zero, although upon feeding these increase immediately. Serum levels of amylase, lipase, pseudocholinesterase, and

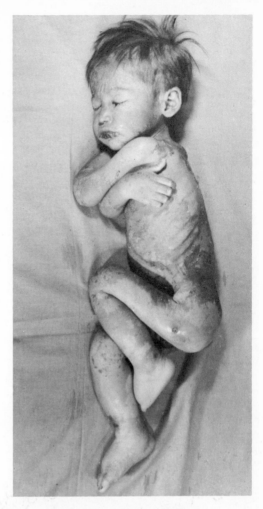

FIGURE 11-2. Kwashiorkor with characteristic skin lesions and edema in a Guatemalan child with some previous marasmus.

alkaline phosphatase are also markedly lowered. While the most essential liver enzymes are resistant to protein depletion, the activities of xanthine oxidase, D-amino acid oxidase, phenylalanine hydroxylase, and urokinase are depressed. Reduced succinate and glycolic oxidase activity, together with decreased oxidative phosphorylation and increased nucleic dehydrogenase, indicate disturbances in carbohydrate metabolism, and fatty acid synthesizing enzymes are also depressed.

The essential amino acids in plasma are consistently and markedly decreased, especially the branched chain amino acids, valine, leucine, and isoleucine. The total free amino acid level is less altered, however, because nonessential amino acids tend to increase. Advantage has been taken of this observation by Whitehead and Dean (1964) to develop a simple test for protein malnutrition utilizing the ratio of several key essential amino acids to selected nonessential ones measured by paper chromatography.

Abnormal nitrogen metabolites, such as B-amino isobutyric acid and ethanolamine, suggestive of alterations in amino acid metabolism, are also found in the urine. Concurrent with the cessation of growth in kwashiorkor and in other malnutritional states, the urinary excretion of hydroxyproline falls. Diminution of muscle mass also results in lowered creatine excretion. Both urinary creatinine and hydroxyproline relative to appropriate standards can be used as indices of malnutrition. Low plasma

289

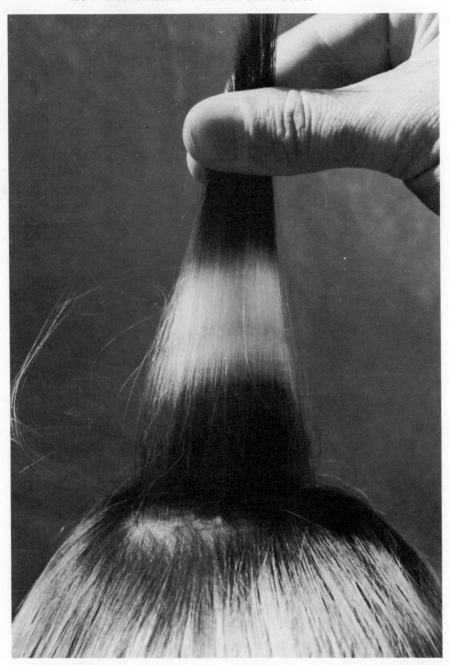

FIGURE 11-3. Extreme example of the hair depigmentation associated with severe protein malnutrition in a child recovering from kwashiorkor as the result of appropriate dietary treatment.

urea values correlate with a low urinary excretion of this substance, and both reflect reduced dietary protein intake.

An increase in total body water with sodium retention and potassium depletion is a constant occurrence, and magnesium deficit has been reported. Reduced basal metabolism, renal plasma flow, glomerular filtration rate, and low electrocardiographic voltages are other physiological changes.

The main pathologic alterations include extensive accumulations of fat in the liver, beginning in the periportal portions of the lobules and extending progressively to the central vein. The pancreas and other exocrine glands become atrophic and the marked atrophy of the intestinal mucosa leads to symptoms resembling those of primary malabsorption. The skin shows atrophy of the epidermis with varying degrees of hyperkeratosis and parakeratosis.

The initial management of kwashiorkor requires correction of dehydration and electrolyte imbalance. Serious complicating infection is also likely to be present despite the absence of fever, leukocytosis, and other common diagnostic signs. For this reason, an antibiotic should generally be administered. The basic requirement, however, for both kwashiorkor and marasmus is a diet providing sufficient protein and all other essential nutrients.

Care and patience are required to administer a satisfactory therapeutic diet in the treatment of the severe protein-calorie malnutrition of the kwashiorkor type in children because of the severe anorexia and vomiting associated with the condition. In the ordinary overcrowded and understaffed hospital ward in the areas where the syndrome is common, the food ordered by the physician frequently is not actually consumed by the child. Also, the child is exposed to multiple cross-infections at a time when he is highly susceptible to them. Under these circumstances, recovery may take many months or not occur at all. If adequate food can be administered with regularity, the anorexia soon disappears and food is well accepted thereafter.

Although the edema and most of the biochemical abnormalities disappear within about two weeks, intestinal absorption of lipids improves more slowly and complete recovery usually requires at least three months. When comparison is made with the creatinine excretion of a well-nourished child of the same height, the daily excretion of creatinine provides the basis for a more reliable indication of recovery than the usual weight-to-height ratio.

Vitamin Deficiency Diseases

The clinical manifestations of protein-calorie malnutrition are frequently complicated by the presence of other nutritional deficiencies. Vitamin A deficiency with serious eye lesions is frequent in both marasmus and kwashiorkor. In kwashiorkor serum vitamin A levels are low and intestinal absorption of vitamin A extremely reduced, even when liver stores of vitamin A are adequate, because of a deficiency of carrier protein.

The diet responsible for protein-calorie malnutrition is also likely to be deficient in B vitamins, particularly riboflavin. The mild normocytic, normochromic anemia attributable to protein deficiency is often complicated and more severe because of simultaneous deficiencies of iron, vitamin E, folic acid, and possibly other hematopoietic factors.

Avitaminosis A.   Vitamin A deficiency is responsible for thousands of cases of blindness in young children in South and East Asia, Africa, and the Middle East (Kinney and Follis, 1958, pp. 103–143). Furthermore, children with such a deficiency suffer an exceedingly high mortality owing to the increased susceptibility to infections, especially bronchopneumonia. In some areas as many as 1 per cent of all children have residual corneal damage sufficient to interfere with vision, and about one fourth of the children in whom xerophthalmia develops do not reach adulthood because of death from secondary infections. Loss of dark adaptation appears widespread among adults in the same areas, although the condition has not been systematically studied.

Wille (Kinney and Follis, 1958, p. 112) describes the

... too, too frequent case in which a mother, after long hesitation, ventures to the doctor, because her small child did not open his eyes for 10 days. The doctor then finds two corneas irretrievably gone. But xerophthalmia is also seen in the case of the school child, ... with a big contusion on his forehead. He ran into a pole the preceding evening at dusk, because he is night-blind, and he has Bitot spots on his eyes.

Much the same conditions that are responsible for the world-wide occurrence of kwashiorkor and marasmus also account for the geographic distribution of xerophthalmia and their often simultaneous presence in the same child. Supplementary foods for young infants are prepared from rice or other cereals deficient in β-carotene and vitamin A as well as protein. Families of unskilled laborers without land, whether urban or rural, tend to subsist on satiety-producing cereals to the neglect of vitamin-containing vegetables and fruits. Vitamin A deficiency occurs in some of the greenest places on earth, where carotene-containing leaves should be readily available, but the end result is the same as in arid rural areas with a sheer lack of carotene sources for most of the year. Parts of North Africa and northeast Brazil are examples of the latter.

Clinically, xerophthalmia is an affection of the conjunctiva and the cornea. A fatty dryness of the conjunctiva is typical, with thickened wrinkles at the corners and hyperpigmentation. Thick, whitish flecks may be seen on the surface, where they accumulate as the frothy-appearing Bitot spots. With adequate vitamin therapy the conjunctiva at this stage can again become transparent and moist within a few days, but the Bitot spot, lacking living cells, may remain for weeks and the hyperpigmentation may become even more pronounced.

Involvement of the conjunctiva is often accompanied by xerosis of the cornea, which becomes hazy, rough, dry, and sensitive. Punctate, superficial infiltrations or small surface erosions may lead, within a day or so, to protrusion of the iris and even prolapse or expulsion of the lens. The late stages are accompanied by inflammatory symptoms.

Keratomalacia, a colliquative necrosis of the whole cornea, follows xerosis. A rather sudden spongy swelling and melting down of the cornea progresses to eventual shrinkage of the eyeball. Because corneal changes are minimal in the germ-free rat with vitamin A deficiency, it may be inferred that secondary infection probably plays a part in the later stages of the disease in man.

Rickets and Osteoporosis.   Rickets develops in growing children as a result of vitamin D deficiency. Because vitamin D is supplied both by breast milk and the action of sunlight on the skin, it has been rare in tropical countries except for occasional children kept from the sun either because of illness or accompanying their mothers, who work all day in covered markets. Urbanization of tropical populations, however, is increasing the frequency of rickets because children get less direct exposure to the sun and air pollution cuts down its effectiveness. There are also reports of osteoporosis in adult Moslem women whose clothing shields them completely from sunlight and whose diet is poor in vitamin D.

Beriberi. Beriberi is almost entirely limited to underdeveloped areas of the Far East, where highly milled rice is the principal food staple (Kinney and Follis, 1958, pp. 3–56). In Japan, rice enrichment and a more diversified diet have virtually eliminated the disease. In the Philippines and Indonesia the incidence has also decreased, probably owing to an increase in variety of diet. In Thailand, Malaysia, and Vietnam, however, beriberi has increased as more efficient small mechanical mills replace hand pounding, which left some of the germ and hull. Moreover, most of the increase has been in infantile beriberi, with its high fatality.

Beriberi in both adults and older children is of three main types. The chronic, dry, atrophic form and the acute, fulminating type are more serious and dramatic, but most cases are mild and subacute. The chronic, dry, atrophic type, with wrist and foot drop, is generally found only in the older adult, often associated with prolonged consumption of alcohol.

The third type, the mild and subacute form, has characteristic nervous manifestations, including alterations in tendon reflexes. Paresthesia is common. The extent of muscular involvement relates to length of the nerve, amount of work done by the muscle group involved, and possibly the blood supply. Sensations of fullness or tightening of the muscles and muscle cramps are common at night. Cardiovascular signs and symptoms range from breathlessness on exertion and palpitation to tachycardia, cardiac dilatation, and some degree of congestive heart failure. Coexisting deficiencies of ascorbic acid, riboflavin, niacin, and vitamin A are common.

The development of infantile beriberi is due to low thiamine levels in breast milk. Among all deficiency diseases it is one of the most dramatic, for a child may be apparently well and yet die from this condition a few hours later. Recovery with parenteral administration of thiamine is equally dramatic. The initial stage is characterized by vomiting, restlessness, pallor, anorexia, and insomnia. In acute infantile beriberi cyanosis, dyspnea, and death ensue rapidly. In the subacute form vomiting, puffiness of the face and extremities, oliguria, abdominal pain, dysphagia, aphonia, and convulsions may appear. This type may go on to a fatal acute episode or may become chronic.

Chronic infantile beriberi sometimes evolves from the initial state without an intervening subacute stage. Vomiting, inanition, anorexia, aphonia, neck retraction, opisthotonus, edema, oliguria, constipation and meteorism are variously seen. There need be no signs of beriberi in the mothers of infants affected. To contract beriberi or to transmit it to a nursing child, a mother must generally derive a high proportion of calories from polished rice.

Pellagra. Pellagra is still found seasonally in Egypt, Yugoslavia, and some parts of Africa, where corn supplies more than 60 per cent of the daily calories. Because of the niacin supplied by beans and coffee, as well as the increased availability of tryptophan from lime-treated corn, it is not seen in Mexico and Central America, even among populations deriving up to 80 per cent of their calories from corn. Persons whose diets are deficient in niacin and contain no excess of tryptophan acquire, on exposure to the sun, a scaly, pigmented dermatitis over the uncovered areas of skin (Goldsmith, 1964). Depending on the type of clothing and occupational activities, the areas most affected are the face, neck, back of the hands, knees, and front of the ankles. Patients with severe cases have atrophy and thinning of mucosal surfaces, leading to sore mouth and diarrhea.

Dementia, one of the classic "three Ds" of pellagra, along with dermatitis and diarrhea, is rarely seen today. Anemias are frequent, presumably owing to associated deficiencies of other components of the vitamin B-complex and/or iron. The so-called "infantile pellagra" once reported from Yucatan and Africa is now recognized as kwashiorkor, the similarity of the skin lesions having led to the confusion.

Ariboflavinosis.   Clinical deficiency signs of riboflavin deficiency of mild degree are common in developing countries, particularly in association with other deficiency diseases of the vitamin B group and with various forms of protein-calorie malnutrition. Glossitis and ocular changes are seen in patients with riboflavin deficiency, but the signs are neither constant nor specific to riboflavin deficiency alone.

Lesions of the lips begin with redness and may develop to shallow ulcerations and crusting. Sore, reddened fissures and encrustations of the corners of the mouth, the so-called angular stomatitis, are classically attributed to riboflavin deficiency, but may also result from deficiency of niacin or iron and may occur idiopathically in well-nourished individuals. A seborrheic dermatitis is also common in this deficiency, characterized by a greasy appearance with erythema at the nasolabial and nasomalar folds, the alae nasi, vestibule of the nose, or around the outer and inner canthi of the eyes, and on the ears.

The swollen, reddened tongue seen in riboflavin deficiency is not clearly separable from that caused by lack of niacin, folic acid, or vitamin B_{12}, and the scrotal and vulval dermatitis is seen in niacin deficiency as well. The circumcorneal vascularization, once considered pathognomonic of riboflavin deficiency, can be produced by many other factors as well. So can such symtoms as soreness and burning of the lips, mouth and tongue and visual symptoms such as photophobia, lacrimation, and burning and itching of the eyes.

Aside from the physical discomfort of ariboflavinosis, the most serious consequence is a decreased resistance to common infection. In the industrialized countries clinical signs attributable to riboflavin deficiencies are often seen in alcoholics along with other B vitamin deficiencies, and in some food faddists.

Consequences of Mineral Deficiencies

Endemic Goiter.   Until recent years, endemic goiter was primarily a place disease, peculiar to areas where geologic factors resulted in a lack of sufficient iodine in the local water and food supply (WHO: *Endemic Goiter*, 1960). Historically, endemic goiter has occurred on every continent and in most countries. In the developed countries, however, it has largely disappeared, in part because of the widespread availability and use of iodized salt, compulsory in many countries, and also because of the increasingly heterogenous origin of the food supply from iodine-rich as well as iodine-poor areas. In most goitrous areas of the underdeveloped countries neither of these factors has yet come into play.

In surveys, goiter is classified as Grade 3 if the thyroid enlargement is visible at a distance, Grade 2 if it is visible on close inspection with the head in a normal position, and Grade 1 if it is smaller, although more than four or five times the normal size. The presence of nodules suggests fetal deprivation of iodine. Most goiters in school children are Grade 1, but Grade 2 and even Grade 3 goiters occur in older children. Rarely is there a suggestion of thyroid dysfunction; in children, at least, enlargement of the gland seems to be a successful compensatory hypertrophy. Goiter may become progressively larger in adults to the point where it is disfiguring, interferes with respiration, and becomes so fibrotic that it cannot be eliminated by iodine therapy. In children simple goiter usually disappears some weeks after iodine administration, but will reappear if iodine is no longer supplied.

Preventive action is desirable in areas where goiter is prevalent. Cosmetic reasons are minor compared to the increased frequency of cretinism, and evidence that an increase in feeble-mindedness and deaf-mutism can be associated with endemic goiter. Furthermore, thyrotoxicosis parallels endemic goiter in most such areas. A relation to thyroid carcinoma is less certain.

The relative contributions to the frequency of endemic goiter of primary iodine lack and the presence of goitrogenic factors in food and water are not well defined. The thiocyanates and thiocyanate precursors present in many members of the cabbage family are known food goitrogens, and a wide variety of other foods, including peaches, pears, strawberries, spinach, and beans, have goitrogenic activity in laboratory animals. Hardness of the water, vitamin A deficiency and polluted water supply have been reported to be goitrogenic in man. The combination of environmental iodine lack and the monotonous, mainly vegetarian diet of foods with goitrogenic activity is sufficient to explain the high prevalence of endemic goiter in so many of the underdeveloped countries.

Other Consequences.   Of the trace minerals, only zinc, magnesium, and copper deficiencies have been specifically identified. Recent studies in the Near East report zinc deficiency to be a responsible factor in a syndrome of dwarfism and hypogonadism in male adolescents. The deficiency of zinc may result either from a low intake or from impaired absorption due to a high dietary content of phosphates and phytates, as in diets predominantly of cereal grains. Similar syndromes in other areas have been attributed to anemia, to liver dysfunction caused by schistosomiasis, or to general undernutrition. Because these factors do not always provide a satisfactory explanation, further studies on zinc deficiency in representative areas are needed.

Iron and copper deficiencies are discussed under Anemias of Nutritional Origin, and calcium deficiency is referred to under "Rickets and Osteoporosis."

Synergism of Malnutrition and Infection

The role of infectious diseases in precipitating kwashiorkor, marasmus, and keratomalacia in children consuming diets of borderline adequacy has already been emphasized. Diarrheal diseases are especially frequent in underdeveloped countries because of poor environmental sanitation and deficient personal hygiene (Scrimshaw *et al.*, 1968). Respiratory infections are also common and tend to be more severe than in more favored regions. These infectious diseases, along with the common communicable diseases of childhood, decrease appetite and cause extra metabolic loss of nitrogen and a number of other essential nutrients. Equally important, attendants commonly reduce the food intake of persons who are ill, especially children, by substituting thin carbohydrate gruels or cereal infusions for the usual solid food. The frequent administration of strong purgatives to children with diarrhea adds to the disastrous nutritional consequences.

Of equal or greater concern is the fact that malnutrition severe enough to interfere with growth and development is also able to interfere with resistance to infections. The common childhood diseases, rarely fatal in well-nourished children and scarcely requiring medical care, are major causes of death in areas where malnutrition prevails in childhood. Despite incomplete reporting of such deaths, mortality from measles in 1962, for example, was approximately 255 times higher in Guatemala, 155 times higher in the United Arab Republic, and 140 times greater in Chile than in the United States (WHO: *World Health Statistics Annual*, 1965). Nevertheless, measles caused no special problems among the better nourished children of families with middle and upper incomes in the same countries.

An analysis of the deaths of children in four Guatemalan highland communities in a two-year period indicated that diarrheal disease and common childhood infections were apparently responsible for nearly two thirds of the mortality in the group from one to five years of age (Béhar, *et al.*, 1958). Few of these infections would have been fatal in well-nourished children. Conversely, approximately two fifths of the children of this age group who died during the period of observation had symptoms of kwashiorkor, but the syndrome appeared to have been precipitated in every case by a preceding episode of diarrhea, measles, or other infection. Over-all mortality in children of this age in the four communities, as in Guatemala as a whole, was over 40 times higher than in the United States and Western Europe, and the difference could be accounted for largely by the synergism of nutrition and infection.

In a five-year study by the Institute of Nutrition of Central America and Panama (INCAP) in the rural Guatemala highland village of Santa Catarina Barahona, children under five years and all pregnant and nursing mothers were offered a supplement providing 15 gm of protein and 450 calories five days a week. No medical care was given. Mortality of preschool children decreased as compared with preceding years, whereas no change occurred in the control village of Santa Cruz Balanyā (Ascoli *et al.*, 1967).

It is now increasingly recognized that the acute diarrheal disease of infants and young children so common in developing countries during and shortly after weaning is microbiologically nonspecific and constitutes an epidemiologic entity to which the name "weanling diarrhea" has been applied (Gordon *et al.*, 1963). Throughout the world a known pathogenic agent can be identified in only about 20 to 30 per cent of cases of weanling diarrhea. The remainder defy expert microbiologic investigation, including a search for causative enteroviruses. Infectious agents identified are mainly various strains of enteropathogenic *Escherichia coli*, shigellas, and occasional salmonellas.

The hypothesis is advanced that many weanling diarrheas are the consequence of organisms not normally pathogenic in a well-nourished child. Even those strains of *Escherichia coli, Shigella,* and *Salmonella* with accepted pathogenic properties are known to invade the well-fed nursing infant under four months of age without necessarily causing diarrhea. The incidence of diarrhea is relatively low at this time, as is the mortality rate. After the mother's milk is no longer a sufficient source of protein, the same organisms may then be associated with diarrheal disease. Cases and deaths increase, and rates continue high throughout the long weaning period and for the months immediately thereafter. It is noteworthy that weanling diarrhea is spread by direct and indirect contact rather than by food or water of common origin.

Progress in identifying the mechanisms whereby malnutrition exaggerates infection has been slow (Scrimshaw *et al.*, 1968). It is well known from studies in laboratory animals that a variety of nutritional deficiencies will interfere with antibody formation and with leukocyte response and activity. In kwashiorkor the antibody response is inhibited. This has also been observed in malnourished patients with chronic infections and in experimental pantothenic acid and pyridoxine deficiency in human volunteers. Children with kwashiorkor may show no febrile or leukocytic reaction to infection. Nothing is known, however, of the extent of involvement of any of these mechanisms in the lowered resistance of subclinical deficiency states.

Alterations in tissue integrity, especially of mucous membranes and other epithelial structures, so characteristic of kwashiorkor, vitamin A deficiency, scurvy, pellagra, ariboflavinosis, and some other deficiencies, also are partly responsible for increased susceptibility to some infections. Other potential but unproved means by which resistance is decreased in malnourished inhabitants of underdeveloped countries include interference with general resistance factors such as lysozymes, interferon, and properdin, decreased nonspecific resistance to bacterial toxins, endocrine imbalances, and altered intestinal flora.

Nutritional Anemias

Nutritional anemias due to insufficient intake of hematopoietic factors, to their poor absorption, or to increased demands because of abnormal blood losses are frequent in tropical and subtropical areas (International Symposium on Vitamin-Related Anemias, 1968). Pregnant women, infants, and small children are most seriously affected in the areas where the problem exists. Mild-to-moderate cases in the general population are often highly prevalent and yet unrecognized. A deleterious effect of anemia on work performance and general well-being is suspected but not quantitatively determined.

Iron deficiency anemia is the most common type in tropical and subtropical areas. A good correlation is found between the number of worms and the level of hemoglobin in heavy hookworm infections. In a significant number of cases, however, the same type of anemia is observed without hookworm disease, and similarly, although less frequently, in areas where hookworm does not exist. Venezuelan studies suggest that less than a third of the iron deficiency anemias observed in hookworm-infested areas are due solely to the parasites.

Increased loss of iron by sweat and dermal desquamation is a factor of unknown significance in areas where environmental conditions favor profuse sweating. Other possible factors interfering with iron absorption and requiring further study are the frequently associated infections and protein deficiency.

Total iron intake, as estimated by dietary surveys, is usually within recommended amounts or even higher in areas where iron deficiency anemia is prevalent, either with or without hookworm disease. The extent of absorption of the iron contained in the diets is less well known. Diets in developing countries ordinarily include a large proportion of cereal grains and legumes as the principal sources of iron. Recent studies suggest that the iron of cereals is not well absorbed, at least by anemic persons.

Megaloblastic anemias are less common than the microcytic hypochromic type associated with iron deficiencies. They are reported particularly in pregnant women and in severely malnourished children. Folate deficiency, either of dietary origin or from other factors interfering with its metabolism, seems to be a frequent cause. Vitamin B_{12} deficiency has also been reported, particularly in populations with a predominantly vegetarian diet, and in pregnant women. In addition, anemias responding to vitamin E have been described in several developing countries. The anemia of kwashiorkor has been mentioned earlier.

Malnutrition, Learning, and Behavior

There is increasing evidence that the degree of malnutrition responsible for the early retardation of growth and development among infants and preschool children in developing countries is sometimes also sufficient to interfere with brain development, learning, and behavior (Scrimshaw and Gordon, 1968). Data from many investigators indicate that such children have a smaller head circumference at maturity than do those who have not experienced such early malnutrition. Although differences in head circumference are of little significance among well-nourished individuals, the smaller head circumference associated with early malnutrition does indicate smaller brain size. Recent work has shown that the number of brain cells is reduced as well (Winick, 1968).

In addition, several field studies have shown that preschool children who are most retarded in height and weight for age also tend to have the lowest scores on tests of intersensory perception and cognitive behavior. Because the social deprivation so commonly associated with malnutrition in underprivileged populations may have similar effects, the relative importance of these two major factors is still to be determined and indeed must vary with the circumstances. Nevertheless, the implications are clear. There is a risk that early malnutrition of children in the first one to two years of life today may adversely influence the capacity of this generation upon whom developing countries must count for future progress.

Caries and Periodontal Disease

Dental caries is exceedingly prevalent in most of the underdeveloped countries (Scrimshaw and Béhar, 1965). Comparatively young persons with teeth broken off at the gums or entirely absent are a common sight. Tooth decay is presumably not more active in such areas than in many highly developed countries, but because of the lack of dental care, its consequences are more serious. Indeed, some malnourished populations enjoy remarkably good teeth, particularly when the natural fluoride content of soil and water reaches prophylactic levels. Periodontal disease is also a serious public health problem, again owing more to poor dental hygiene and lack of dental care than to malnutrition.

NUTRITIONAL PROBLEMS OF INDUSTRIALIZED COUNTRIES

In industrialized countries, malnutrition due to nutritional deficiency is rare, but obesity is very common (Van Itallie, 1960). Whether or not obesity is regarded as a disease state, it has a direct relationship to the development of cardiovascular disease. It is also clear that the combination of a high proportion of calories from fat in the diet and limited physical exercise make for a relatively early development of atherosclerosis and a relatively high prevalence of coronary heart disease.

In countries like Japan, where many of the foods are very high in salt content, this is a distinct factor in producing a high national incidence of hypertension. There is also a relationship between the high intake of calories, particularly from carbohydrates, and the relatively greater frequency of diabetes in the industrialized countries. Finally, as already mentioned, diets high in refined carbohydrates are conducive to the development of dental caries.

In addition to these diseases of dietary excess, nutritional anemias are also much more prevalent in industrialized countries than is generally realized (International Symposium on Vitamin-related Anemias, 1968). They are particularly associated with faddist diets, teen-age neglect of nutrition or adoption of bizarre diet patterns, and self-prescribed reducing regimens. Two periods are particularly vulnerable to anemia: infancy and pregnancy. Because few infants are breast fed in the industrialized countries and because cow's milk is much lower in iron, anemia has been fairly common. There is now a growing concern for the prevalence of microcytic, hypochromic anemia in infancy associated with cow's milk formulas that are not enriched with iron. In addition, the diets of some women are apparently inadequate in folic acid for the demands of pregnancy and lactation, and they develop a megaloblastic anemia for this reason.

FACTORS RESPONSIBLE

The public health approach to the causes of malnutrition must be an ecological one, taking into account the interaction of host, agent, and environment (Scrimshaw, 1964; Scrimshaw and Béhar, 1964). This approach permits the selection of those preventive measures that are most likely to be successful. Moreover, effective prevention of most malnutrition requires attention to several factors concurrently.

In the case of nutritional disease the agent must be thought of as either the deficiency or the pathological excess of a specific nutrient or nutrients. Environmental factors are those of the physical, biological, and social environment, and each may affect availability, consumption, or host requirement of a nutrient.

To the extent that the availability of food is the limiting factor, measures must be those that will increase the production of food from plant and animal sources or increase its availability through storage and handling practices that will reduce unnecessary losses to rodents, insects, mold, and spoilage. The problem may be primarily one of distribution and marketing rather than total production. On the other hand, actual production may be so inadequate that food will need to be imported in order to avert widespread malnutrition.

Most often, malnutrition is caused not by an absolute scarcity of food but by social and economic factors that result either in inadequate knowledge of proper food selection or insufficient purchasing power to acquire the foods needed for optimal nutrition. It is not just lack of knowledge that results in malnutrition, but also belief in food practices that are nutritionally unsound. As mentioned earlier, a major factor in the occurrence of protein-calorie malnutrition in children is the tendency to give watery or starchy gruels of little or no protein content to the young child who develops diarrheal disease (Jelliffe, 1955). Meat and eggs are often thought "too strong" for the weanling infant and cow's milk is believed dangerous because it results in diarrhea or "causes the worms to rise." Added to the effect of less nourishing diets is the administration of strong purgatives, which accentuate the diarrhea and worsen the nutritional situation. Similarly, various prejudices and taboos relating to the diet during pregnancy and lactation contribute to malnutrition.

The role of infection in producing the degree of malnutrition characterizing the majority of children in developing countries has already been discussed along with the frequency with which clinical nutritional disease is precipitated by an episode of acute infection. It follows, then, that lack of environmental sanitation and personal hygiene are major factors in the occurrence of malnutrition because they contribute so importantly to the high frequency of diarrheal disease in less-developed countries. Similarly, physical, biological, and social circumstances that favor the occurrence of malaria, schistosomiasis, cholera, hookworm, and other mass diseases significantly increase the frequency of malnutrition. Conversely, the relatively good environmental sanitation characterizing most populations in the industrialized countries has contributed to the virtual disappearance of malnutrition.

Another reason for the prevalence of malnutrition in developing countries is the limited degree to which medical and public health services reach the majority of the populations. Effective maternal and child health programs can do a great deal to reduce the frequency of severe malnutrition by their educational impact, their roles in the prevention of diseases, and by direct nutritional measures such as supplementary feeding or nutritional rehabilitation where these are required.

The physician dealing with underprivileged populations in private or public health practice also has an opportunity to recognize the possible development of specific and dangerous nutritional disorders such as marasmus, kwashiorkor, xerophthalmia and keratomalacia, pellagra, beriberi, rickets, and scurvy and to see that proper treatment is instituted promptly. It is where the population does not have access to medical services that these diseases so commonly go on to their tragic consequences of disability or death.

Unfortunately, medical practices sometimes have their adverse effects on nutritional status. For example, food is withheld from children with diarrhea as a temporary therapeutic measure and this is interpreted by the mother as the proper treatment for the symptom. Pediatricians must also share some of the responsibility for the over-feeding of children in more favorable social and economic conditions.

In the industrialized countries members of the medical and public health professions have a special obligation to promote those measures that will contribute to improved nutritional status, such as a moderate food intake to avoid obesity, and regular physical exercise, as a preventive measure for both obesity and coronary heart disease. They should also oppose harmful faddist diets and nutritional quackery of all types. In both industrialized and developing countries they have an obligation to support administrative measures that will contribute to the nutritional health of the population, such as fluoridation of water, iodization of salt, and fortification of cereals.

Finally, the importance of medical and public health support in the promotion of family planning can scarcely be overestimated. The health implications of present rates of population increase are discussed in Chapter 1. It is sufficient here to point out that *per capita* food supplies are actually decreasing in many developing countries as population increases faster than food supply. Furthermore, rapid urbanization with its disruption of traditional food practices is creating nutritional problems that have reached alarming proportions in some countries. The problem of malnutrition is inseparable from that of population growth. It is not sufficient for food supplies to match population growth; they need to exceed it in most developing countries in order to improve present diets and to meet the rising expectations for more and better foods as improved economic and social status is achieved. Moreover, the problem is not just one of food production; distribution to and consumption by vulnerable population groups must be assured.

CONTROL AND PREVENTION

Emergency or Palliative Measures

A common response to the existence of malnutrition is the initiation of a supplementary feeding program. This may or may not alleviate the immediate problem, but it is seldom a satisfactory long-term solution. Participation in such programs by those most in need, even when the programs are free, is usually far from satisfactory. They tend not to reach the most vulnerable group, preschool children, because the mother is too busy to bring the child regularly to a feeding station or is unconvinced of its importance. Distributing food for the mother to take home also has its limitations because it is generally shared with the family or even sold. Moreover, termination of the program results in a return to the original conditions unless it is used for nutrition education and arrangements are made for nutritious foods within the purchasing power of the people to be available on a permanent basis.

Two kinds of successful supplementary food distribution deserve special mention. One is providing sufficient food, to be taken home every one or two weeks, for poorly nourished children, or preferably, for all young children in a family, combined with instruction in nutrition and personal hygiene and accompanied by periodic visits to the home to see that the food is being used properly. Such programs have been effective in improving growth and development and decreasing disease morbidity of poorly nourished young children. A second is the association with a health center of a nutritional rehabilitation unit where a child with malnutrition who might otherwise need hospitalization can be left each day to receive two or three complete meals. The mothers are expected to participate in the running of such a center primarily as a means of educating them as to the benefits of a proper diet for their children.

Corrective Specific Measures

Sometimes specific measures will effectively wipe out a nutritional disease in a manner analogous to that which can be achieved by immunization or vector eradication for the control of some infectious diseases. These measures generally consist of enrichment or fortification of a basic food staple. Endemic goiter, even where it is severe, can be effectively eliminated as a public health problem among children and young adults in a few months if effective iodization of all salt for human consumption is introduced. Because this measure can be introduced by administrative action, adds only negligibly to the cost of the salt, and does not require education of the public, there is little justification for the continued persistence of endemic goiter in many countries.

Enrichment of rice with thiamine and other essential nutrients is an effective and economical way of preventing beriberi (Williams, 1961). Unfortunately, political and economic obstacles have prevented the widespread adoption of this measure in rice-eating countries. Increasing the thiamine content of milled rice by parboiling is feasible but increases the hazard of producing the potent toxin aflatoxin from the growth of *Aspergillus flavus*. The technique involves coating some of the rice grains with a mixture of riboflavin, thiamine, niacin, and calcium. This combination of nutrients can be added to corn where this cereal is the staple and has been demonstrated to be effective in preventing pellagra. The enrichment of wheat in this manner serves to eliminate the likelihood of deficiencies of such nutrients in populations consuming significant quantities of wheat.

The main factor in the disappearance of beriberi from regions in which it was once highly prevalent is the introduction of greater variety into diets that were previously based largely on rice. To the extent that beriberi in industrialized countries is associated with alcoholism, parenteral thiamine may be required therapeutically and the excessive use of alcohol terminated.

Recently the addition of the essential amino acid lysine has been recommended as a means of improving the protein quality of wheat and lysine fortification of wheat bread and flour has already begun in India on a substantial scale. Amino acid fortification of corn with lysine and tryptophan could double the protein quality of this cereal, but with the present high cost of tryptophan, the introduction through cross-breeding of one of the genes opaque-2 or floury-2 seems a more promising way of achieving this end (Mertz and Nelson, 1966).

There have been recent spectacular increases in cereal yields in a number of developing countries through the use of improved varieties of seeds combined with the necessary fertilizer and pesticides (*Strategy for the Conquest of Hunger*, The Rockefeller Foundation, 1968). Because these varieties are not improved in protein quality, it is still important to improve protein value of diets based on these cereals through appropriate fortification and supplementation.

In most industrialized countries the irradiation of cow's milk serves to increase its vitamin D activity and this measure is sufficient to prevent rickets in children. Vitamin A and D concentrates are universally prescribed by pediatricians and health centers for children under one year of age. In the tropical countries adequate vitamin D has in the past been supplied by breast milk and by exposure of the child to sunshine. In view of growing urbanization, which leads to earlier weaning and less exposure to sunshine, specific ways need to be found to add vitamin D to the diets of mothers and children in tropical cities NAS–NRC: *Progress in Meeting Protein Needs of Infants and Preschool Children*, 1961).

Simultaneous administration of capsules containing vitamins A and D is now standard policy of the United Nations Children's Fund (UNICEF) for milk distribution to children in areas with possible vitamin A deficiency. Alternatively, powdered milk for use in such circumstances can be enriched with water-miscible synthetic vitamin A. In many tropical areas, red African palm oil is readily available as a rich source of carotenes with vitamin A activity. Nutrition education programs in such countries place particular stress on green and yellow vegetables and on certain fruits, such as mangoes, papaya, squash, and melons as important sources of active carotenes in a balanced diet.

There are specific as well as general nutritional measures that can contribute directly to the reduction of dental caries (Nizel, 1966). The addition of fluoride to water supplies of communities without natural fluorine in the water to levels of about one part per million generally reduces caries in children by at least half. Not only is dental caries in adults also reduced to some extent by fluoridation, but there is also suggestive evidence that osteoporosis is decreased. Some recent experimental studies suggest that phosphate enrichment of cereal staples or other foods may have an effect additive to fluoride and bring about further caries reduction. Diet patterns relatively high in soluble carbohydrate promote dental caries.

In areas where no low-cost protein-rich food is already available that is suitable for the supplementary feeding of young children during and after weaning, the production and marketing of such a protein source can be an important specific measure in reducing the incidence of protein-calorie malnutrition (UN: *International Action to Avert the Impending Protein Crisis*, 1968). These are usually based on a combination of an oilseed meal and a staple cereal such as corn or wheat. A meal containing approximately 50 per cent protein is left after the oil is extracted from soy beans, peanuts, or cotton, sesame, and sunflower seed. Examples are Incaparina in Latin America, Bal-Ahar in India, and ProNutro in South Africa.

Bland, deodorized fish protein concentrates containing approximately 80 per cent protein can be produced from fish not otherwise valued for human food, but have not yet been utilized to a significant degree. Such concentrates are highly effective in improving the protein value of cereal-based foods and will eventually be widely used.

Food yeast grown on molasses or sulfite liquor and containing approximately

50 per cent protein is already used to a limited degree in a wide variety of processed foods, including those for infants and young children. Other single-cell sources of protein produced on petroleum fractions as an energy source are under development, utilizing ammonia-nitrogen fixed from the air. Single-cell organisms have the great potential of growth in enormous quantities without the use of agricultural land and they contain protein of demonstrated usefulness. If, however, they are to be used in large quantities in order to supply a major proportion of the dietary protein, their high nucleic acid content will need to be reduced somewhat in order to avoid the possibility of producing abnormally high serum uric acid levels, and extensive biological testing will be required.

General Measures

Because the causes of malnutrition are multiple, general control measures are equally broad and must involve social and economic as well as medical and public health improvements. Some malnutrition is due to a primary lack of available foods of sufficient nutritive value. Therefore, increased agricultural production of food crops may be necessary (UN: *International Action to Avert the Impending Protein Crisis,* 1968). It is necessary to distinguish, however, between human need for food and what the economists call effective demand for it. More often malnutrition results from lack of resources for the purchase of protective foods. The solution is either to make available foods of adequate nutritive value at lower cost, or to improve the purchasing power of the family. In either case nutrition education is essential so that the right foods will be chosen, especially for the feeding of the young child during and after weaning.

The extent to which ignorance of nutritional principles and food values is responsible for malnutrition, even among the low-income populations of developing countries, should not be underestimated. It is exceedingly common for kwashiorkor to occur primarily because the food available for the rest of the family is not shared with the young child because it is thought inappropriate or even dangerous for him. The most valuable type of nutrition education for mothers in developing countries stresses the appropriate and increasing supplementation of breast milk beginning at about the fourth month of life. For the older child and adult, emphasis is on a balanced diet each day, incorporating protein foods, green and yellow vegetables, and fruits, as well as the cereal or root staples commonly making up the bulk of the diet.

For the industrialized countries the problem is quite different. For most of the population food is available in abundance and purchasing power allows them to buy more of it than is really needed. Even children are given the money to buy candy and soft drinks that replace nutritious foods with "empty calories" and contribute to the incidence of dental caries. For this group also education in nutrition must emphasize a balanced diet containing a supply of each of the basic food groups every day. It must also include the undesirability of overweight for both children and adults and its control by appropriate caloric intake and physical activity. The taking of vitamin concentrates should not be encouraged, because this is generally a waste of money as well as a poor substitute for a proper diet.

Because a major factor in the occurrence of malnutrition in less developed countries is the high incidence of acute and chronic infections, it follows that measures to control infection have an important place in the prevention of malnutrition. As already indicated, diarrheal disease is probably the single most debilitating factor for the preschool child, and measures to reduce its incidence include constructing privies and toilets, improving the quality of the water supply and, desirably, supplying adequate water for sanitary purposes directly to each household.

These measures will also reduce the burden of intestinal parasites, which are almost universal among rural children in developing countries and are common in the poor urban districts as well. The specific burden of hookworm disease can be largely eliminated by the wearing of shoes.

Health education can help to encourage sanitary disposal of feces, to reduce the numbers of flies and their contact with feces and food, and perhaps most important of all, to improve personal hygiene. The agents of diarrheal disease are most commonly spread by the mother's hands from feces to food, nipple, and the child's mouth. Personal cleanliness including appropriate washing of hands would help to reduce weanling diarrhea.

Other infections that serve to precipitate acute nutritional disease in chronically malnourished children are the common communicable diseases of childhood: measles, whooping cough, chicken pox, rubella, and mumps. The first two can and should be prevented by immunization. To the extent that respiratory disease and tuberculosis are associated with overcrowding, better housing can be a factor in reducing the frequency of respiratory infections in children. Where major endemic diseases such as malaria and schistosomiasis are a factor, campaigns for their prevention will have favorable repercussions on the nutritional status of the population.

Role of Medical Services

Medical care is important in the treatment of individuals with severe malnutrition and in reducing mortality from this cause, but medical treatment is a poor approach to malnutrition. To an even greater extent than with infectious disease, the emphasis must be on prevention. When cases of malnutrition do come to the physician for treatment, he has a particular obligation to use the opportunity to explain the cause and prevention of the condition.

In less-developed countries the role of the public health center and clinic is primarily one of promoting better nutritional practices, especially for the growing child and the pregnant and lactating mother. Many cases of malnutrition will be observed that will not require later nutritional rehabilitation or hospitalization if the public health physician and nurse are alert and properly discharge their obligation for nutritional counseling.

Although education should be the main reliance, it may also be desirable for maternal and child health centers in developing countries to make food available for malnourished children at a reduced price or without charge. Otherwise these children progress to require more costly rehabilitation or hospitalization, or may suffer permanent damage. Moreover, the future social and economic development of all countries depends upon the adequate physical and mental development of their young children.

REFERENCES

Ascoli, W., Guzmán, M. A., Scrimshaw, N. S., and Gordon, J. E.: Nutrition and infection field study in Guatemalan villages, 1959–1964. IV. Deaths of infants and preschool children. *Arch Environ Health* (*Chicago*), **15**:439–49, 1967.

Béhar, M., Ascoli, W., and Scrimshaw, N. S.: An investigation into the causes of death in children in four rural communities in Guatemala. *Bull WHO*, **19**:1093–1102, 1958.

Goldsmith, G. A.: The B vitamins: thiamine, riboflavin, niacin. In Beaton, G. H., and McHenry, E. W. (eds.): *Nutrition, A Comprehensive Treatise*, Vol. II. Academic Press, New York and London, 1964.

Gordon, J. E., Chitkara, I. D., and Wyon, J. B.: Weaning diarrhea. *Amer J Med Sci*, **245**:345–77, 1963.

———, Wyon, J. B., and Ascoli, W.: The second year death rate in less developed countries. *Amer J Med Sci*, **254**:357–80, 1967.

International symposium on vitamin-related anemias. In Harris, R. S., Wool, I. G., and Loraine, J. A. (eds.): *Vitamins, Hormones*, **26**:313–719. Academic Press, New York, 1968.

Jelliffe, D. B.: Infant Nutrition in the Subtropics and Tropics, *WHO Monogr Ser*, no. 29. Geneva, 1955.

Kinney, T. D., and Follis, R. H., Jr. (eds.): *Nutritional Disease*. Proceedings of a Conference on Beriberi, Endemic Goiter and Hypovitaminosis A, Held at Princeton, N.J., June 1–5, 1958. *Fed Proc*, 17, Suppl no. 2, 1958.

Mertz, E. T., and Nelson, O. E. (eds.): *Proceedings of the High Lysine Corn Conference*, June 21–22, 1966, Purdue University, Lafayette, Indiana. Published by Corn Industries Research Foundation, a division of Corn Refiners Association, Inc. 1001 Connecticut Avenue, N. W., Washington, D.C., 1966.

National Academy of Sciences–National Research Council: *Pre-school Child Malnutrition, Primary Deterrent to Human Progress*. An International Conference on Prevention of Malnutrition in the Pre-school Child, Washington, D.C., Dec. 7–11, 1964, Pub. no. 1282, NAS–NRC, Washington, D.C., 1966.

———: *Progress in Meeting Protein Needs of Infants and Preschool Children*. Proceedings of an International Conference held in Washington, D.C. Aug. 21–24, 1960. Pub. no. 843, NAS–NRC, Washington, D.C., 1961.

Nizel, A. E. (ed.): *The Science of Nutrition and Its Application in Clinical Dentistry*. W. B. Saunders Company, Philadelphia and London, 1966.

Rockefeller Foundation: *Strategy for the Conquest of Hunger*, Proceedings of a Symposium convened by the Rockefeller Foundation, April 1 and 2, 1968, at The Rockefeller University, New York.

Scrimshaw, N. S.: Ecological factors in nutritional disease. *Amer J Clin Nutr*, **14**:112–122, 1964.

———, and Béhar, M.: Causes and prevention of malnutrition. In Beaton, G. H., and McHenery, E. W. (eds.): *Nutrition, A Comprehensive Treatise*, Vol. II. Academic Press, New York and London, 1964.

———, and ———: Malnutrition in underdeveloped countries. *New Eng J Med*, **272**:137–144, 193–198, 1965.

———, and ———: Protein malnutrition in young children. *Science*, **133**:2039–47, 1961.

———, and Gordon, J. E. (eds.): *Malnutrition, Learning and Behavior*. Proceedings of an International Conference, Co-sponsored by the Nutrition Foundation, Inc., and the Massachusetts Institute of Technology, held at Cambridge, Mass., Mar. 1–3, 1967. The MIT Press, Cambridge, Mass., and London, England, 1968.

———, Taylor, C. E., and Gordon, J. E.: *Interactions of Nutrition and Infection, WHO Monogr Ser no. 57*, Geneva, 1968.

United Nations: *International Action to Avert the Impending Protein Crisis*. Report to the Economic and Social Council of the Advisory Committee on the Application of Science and Technology to Development, E/4343/Rev. 1. UN, New York, 1968.

Van Itallie, T. B.: Obesity. Symposium: Nutrition: Current advances with clinical applications. *Modern Medicine*, 100–7, Aug. 1, 1960.

Viteri, F., Béhar, M., Arroyave, G., and Scrimshaw, N. S.: Clinical aspects of protein malnutrition. In Munro, H. N., and Allison, J. B. (eds.): *Mammalian Protein Metabolism*, Vol. II. Academic Press, New York and London, 1964.

Whitehead, R. G., and Dean, R. F. A.: Serum amino acids in kwashiorkor, I. Relationship to clinical condition. *Amer J Clin Nutr*, **14**:313–19, 1964.

———: II. An abbreviated method of estimation and its application. *Ibid.*, 320–30.

Williams, R. R.: *Toward the Conquest of Beriberi*. Harvard University Press, Cambridge, Mass., 1961.

Winick, M.: Nutrition and cell growth. *Nutr Rev*, **26**:195–97, 1968.

World Health Organization: *Endemic Goiter. WHO Monogr Ser*, no. 44, Geneva, 1960.

———: *Nutrition in Pregnancy and Lactation.* Report of a WHO Expert Committee. *WHO Techn Rep Ser*, no. 302. Geneva, 1965.

———: *World Health Statistics Annual*, Vol. I, 1962, *Vital Statistics and Causes of Death.* Geneva, 1965.

12

New
and Emergent
Diseases

Eric J. Cassell

INTRODUCTION

We are going to look at some of the diseases that have emerged to prominence in the United States as major causes of death or disability: arteriosclerotic heart disease, automobile accidents, chronic obstructive pulmonary disease, and iatrogenic disease. In some ways they are new diseases, and of course, in other ways they are not at all new. John Hunter, in the 1700's said, referring to his angina, "I am at the mercy of anyone who angers me." (Considering his legendary hot temper, he was at the mercy of many.) But it is only since the 1920's that coronary artery disease has been considered a clinically important disease. Now, one out of three die of it.

The first death from a motor vehicle was registered in the United States in 1899, but in the last few years we have begun to recognize that these deaths, now in the many tens of thousands each year, are not chance occurrences but have many of the characteristics of a disease: predictable age and sex distribution, populations of increased susceptibility, precipitating factors, and the like. But even as we look at some of these diseases in depth, we will see that their presence among us is not a chance occurrence. They are part of a pattern of disease that is almost inevitable at this time in a society and culture like ours. Just as there are water-borne and air-borne diseases, these are culture-borne diseases. In our culture, a disease pattern has emerged to whose over-all form genetics has contributed, as well as diet, medical care, societal norms and values, industrialization, and many other factors. Although it may seem obvious that in these major public health problems the determinants are multifactorial, a full realization of the need to deal with all these complicating elements is relatively recent. The increased sophistication of the present is due in part to the fact that we have not been able to understand the causes of these particular diseases as simply as it appeared that we understood the causes of the microbial diseases. (It is now apparent that one-cause–

308

one-disease concepts of the microbial era were oversimplifications even for the bacterial diseases.) It cannot be stated too often that one can no more understand a disease apart from the society in which it occurs than one can treat the disease apart from the individual in whom it is seen.

Certain gross differences between the patterns of disease in the so-called developing areas of the world and the developed areas may lead to simplistic views of the reasons for the differences. For example, malaria was a common disease in the upper Mississippi Valley in the late eighteenth and nineteenth centuries. The anopheline mosquito vector was widespread. Despite apparently equal susceptibility and access to the disease, malaria was very much more common among the American settlers than among the French. Planned antimalarial measures were nonexistent for both groups and so could not have accounted for the difference. The classic American pattern of individual homesteads with one clearing in the wilderness, in which both the agricultural lands and the buildings stood, provided ideal breeding grounds for the mosquitos. The roughly finished log cabin—hallmark of the frontier—provided easy access to the human host for the hungry mosquito. The French pattern was to provide separate clearings; one for a tightly knit village of sturdy homes and another, at a distance, for the jointly worked agricultural lands. This effective, though unplanned, antimalarial measure among the French arose solely from their basic cultural differences from the susceptible Americans. Malaria subsided in the region by the end of the nineteenth century. The decrease was secondary to changes in transportation, a shift to dairying, modifications in settlement patterns, and improved houseforms (Ackerknecht, 1945).

During the great cholera epidemics in the United States, much simplistic moralizing was based on the observation that the poor, the "shiftless," and the "intemperate" appeared to bear the brunt of the disease and its mortality. In one Mississippi river village the reverse occurred. The several wealthy homes on the bluff suffered decimating mortality while the poor, living on the banks of the river, had little disease. The wealthy homes all drew their water from a creek that ran behind them on whose banks perched their outhouses.

No medical sophistication is required to realize how widespread protein-calorie malnutrition could be expected to be in the developing nations solely on the basis of the ratio of the growing populations to available foodstuffs. There is little doubt that differences in local culture influence the incidence and severity of the expression of this malnutrition. The important cultural variables include local agricultural practices and the use of foodstuffs; the place of cattle and milk in religious beliefs and traditions; child spacing; practices and schedules of weaning; and distribution of foodstuffs within the family.

That malnutrition is intimately bound with culture and society has been made abundantly clear by the difficulties that have been met in attempts to introduce new, protein-rich foodstuffs into traditional societies. Because of the resistance to change, supplying protein in an innovative form to an area of deprivation is by no means the equivalent of increasing the protein intake of the population. The influence of malnutrition on the ecology of disease and the disease patterns of an area extends beyond its ability to produce the reddened hair and swollen belly of classical kwashiorkor. Malnourishment is one of the underlying factors in the marked differences in mortality from the common contagious diseases of childhood in different regions. Malnourishment changes measles, for example, from an annoying disease of children in the United States to a major killer in other nations (Table 12-1; see also Chapter 11).

TABLE 12-1
Case Rates and Death Rates from Measles in Selected Countries, 1964*

Nation	Population (1964)	Reported Cases of Measles	Reported Deaths from Measles
United States	192,120,000	458,083	421
United Arab Republic	28,900,000	14,177	3,420
Mexico	41,253,000	73,180	7,908

* Vital statistics of World Health Organization—United Nations.

Culture may thus influence the ecology of disease merely by bringing a susceptible host into contact with disease agents or changing the susceptibility of the host. That the patterns of action and interaction within communities and their environments are influential in determining the profile of disease will become more apparent as we look at diet and heart disease, and at automobile accidents.

It is not uncommon for recent graduates or students in their clinical years to want to leave their dull wards and go to Africa or India where there is still "real" disease. They want to share in the excitement of caring for smallpox or cholera, rather than the routine cases of their own hospital. A short time in any of these areas and a new monotony would be discovered. The monotony of endless cases of smallpox, typhoid, or cholera. And so it goes, with each place, culture, or society having its own monotony of disease—its own distinct pattern or profile of morbidity and mortality. This last point is not easily appreciated by even the most itinerant of physicians, and it is here that epidemiology makes its major contribution.

To understand a disease, to get "a feel for" the behavior of any particular disease, is essential to the proper diagnosis and therapy of individual cases. When seeing the disease in a patient, to have the feeling that one is confronting an "old friend" (or "old enemy," depending on how you feel about these things), helps immeasurably in the evaluation of severity, course, and therapeutic response. The bedside study of disease is essential to that close understanding. But, as epidemiologic methods have made patently clear, disease is poorly understood if it is conceived simply as a series of contests between germs on the one side and susceptible humans on the other. To us the question can no longer be whether culture influences the ecology of diseases, but how. For us the interactions between culture and disease give a way of understanding how diseases become "new" and emerge to dominance in a society, of why the "monotony of disease" occurs.

Culture not only influences the objective profile of disease in communities, but the subjective picture of health and disease as well; the way communities perceive their own health. As noted earlier, our own extended community has only recently begun to view automobile accidents as a health problem. Certainly, each individual accident victim was seen as having an injury, but the society as a whole did not view automobile accidents in totality as a disease entity. The reasons for the obscurity of an etiology that had produced a million deaths by 1951 are complex. For example, in 1964 the leading cause of death in the age group 15–44 for Colombia, Mexico, and Nicaragua was homicide. Death rates were between 40 and 50/100,000, and homicide accounted for between 11 and 17 per cent of all the deaths in the age group. Yet in a discussion of their leading public health problems by these three nations in the World Health Situation Report for 1964, the homicide problem is not mentioned. Certainly, both of these causes of death—automobile accidents and homicide—are a part of the fabric of the societies in which they occur. In a manner of speaking, they are not diseases, they are the society. They have been given moral overtones that tend to remove them from considerations as diseases.

Those factors that we will note to be important in coronary artery disease, such as diet, exercise, and cigarette smoking, also have moral nuances quite apart from their physical effects. We should expect that, as the disease pattern of a society begins to change, the passing of the old diseases will be heralded long before there is an awareness of the emergent ones.

PATTERNS OF DISEASE

The Developing Nations

The cruelest monotony of the developing nations is premature death. Death of infants is commonplace, death of children is ordinary, and death of young adults is not uncommon. Table 12-2 shows the death rates of several countries.

TABLE 12-2

Death Rates per 100,000 for Selected Countries, 1962 *

Country	All Ages	Infant Mortality Per 1,000 1963	Age 1–4	Age 5–14	Age 15–44	Age 45–64
Canada	774	24.7	112	47	146	947
Guatemala	1,550	87.9	3,322	603	610	1,919
Mexico	1,082	64.5	1,093	192	391	1,336
Sweden	1,015	14.2	39	39	113	758
Taiwan	628	23.9	541	85	246	1,236
United States	945	24.8	98	44	181	1,152
United Arab Republic	1,885	118.6	4,233	211	326	1,235

* Vital statistics of World Health Organization—United Nations.

It is clear from the table that one of the major effects on health from increasing development in nations is the protection of the young. Between the ages of 1 and 14, one child out of 5 will die in the United Arab Republic, one child out of 16 will die in Mexico, and one child out of 130 will die in the United States. The mode of death is instructive.

Table 12-3 lists the leading causes of death in the young in the several countries selected.

TABLE 12-3

Five Leading Causes of Death, Ages 1–4, in 1962 for United Arab Republic, Mexico, and the United States*

Cause	Rate/100,000	Per cent of Each Cause to All Causes
United Arab Republic		
1. Gastritis, duodenitis, colitis, enteritis	2658	62.8
2. Bronchitis	761	18.0
3. Influenza and pneumonia	210	4.9
4. Measles	190	4.5
5. Accidents	66	1.6
All other causes		7.5
Per cent of the 10 leading causes of death due to infectious diseases		91.0
Mexico		
1. Gastritis, duodenitis, colitis, enteritis	315	28.8
2. Influenza and pneumonia	208	19.0
3. Measles	64	5.8
4. Whooping cough	46	4.2
5. Bronchitis	39	3.6
All other causes		38.6
Per cent of the 10 leading causes of death due to infectious diseases		55.6
United States		
1. All accidents	31	31.1
2. Influenza and pneumonia	14	14.0
3. Congenital malformations	11	11.6
4. Malignant neoplasms	10	9.9
5. Gastritis, duodenitis, colitis, enteritis	3	3.1
All other causes		30.3
Per cent of the 10 leading causes of death due to infectious diseases		23.6

* Vital statistics of World Health Organization—United Nations.

From these data it is apparent that not only is early death part of the pattern of the developing countries, but that death in the young is most frequently due to infectious agents. The continued high rate of death from infectious disease in older groups is equally striking. Here, death is primarily due to tuberculosis and influenza/pneumonia.

Parenthetically, the countries chosen to represent the pattern of developing nations were chosen primarily because of the availability of their statistics, rather than because of being the most extreme examples. It would not be surprising to see the point made even more dramatically in other parts of Africa or even in India where, in 1964, there were 53,000 reported cases of cholera with 17,000 deaths and 37,000 reported cases of smallpox with 10,000 deaths.

It is not necessary to visit Africa or Asia to see the pattern of disease we have shown in the less-developed nations. The American Indian and the Alaskan Eskimo continue to present the pattern of premature death from primarily infectious diseases.

Navajo (Deuschle and Adair, 1960) present an example of an underdeveloped island in the middle of great affluence. Shortened life expectancy and an infant death rate three times the general United States rate, combined with a high birth and fertility rate, provide a population growth rate of 4 per cent; twice that of the United States as a whole and higher than those of Ceylon and India. The disease pattern is also similar. Seventy per cent of the health problems found during one survey were caused by or the consequence of microbial disease. The prevalence rate for all forms of tuberculosis was 9 per cent. Thirty-three per cent of tuberculosis-tested children less than twelve years of age had a positive test. This is at least ten times the tuberculosis infection rate in children of comparable age in non-Indian communities.

And so it goes from one developing area to another. And, as has been indicated in the case of the Navajo, an area of backward development may exist as an island within the pattern of affluence. Areas of intense poverty within cities of the United States also show the disease pattern of medical retardation; high birth and death rates; a shift toward premature death; increased rates of death from infectious diseases (including a rise in tuberculosis rates); an increase in the percentage of death due to microbial disease, and in the American Continents, an increase in death from homicide.

It must be clear from what has already been discussed that these patterns are a biologic phenomenon with intertwined and complex causes as well as effects.

The Developed Nations

The pattern of death and disease in the developed nations is not merely what is left over when a society protects itself from the ravages of infectious diseases.

Just as when the infectious diseases have full head, societies have characteristic patterns, so too is this true of those societies where the infectious diseases are well controlled. Certain generalities are apparent. (These generalities are drawn from the death rates of Canada, United States, Austria, Belgium, Denmark, Finland, France, West Germany, Greece, Hungary, Iceland, Italy, Netherlands, Norway, Poland, Sweden, Switzerland, United Kingdom [England and Wales, Northern Ireland, Scotland], Australia, and New Zealand.)

Heart disease has been the leading cause of death for many years. The rates per 100,000 ranged between 151 and 397 and averaged 303 in 1964.

This cause of death was responsible for an average of 32 per cent of all deaths. The comparable figure in the developing nations is about 8 per cent. In 1954 heart disease accounted for 29 per cent of deaths in the developed nations and about 7 per cent in the less developed.

Malignant neoplasms accounted for 19 per cent of all deaths in 1964, and this figure represents a slow rise in both absolute and relative rates over the previous ten years. Concealed in these figures are considerable variations in the rates from individual cancers from nation to nation.

Vascular lesions of the central nervous system are the next most frequent cause of death, accounting for about 13 per cent of deaths. This figure has not changed appreciably over the last several years. Heart disease and vascular lesions of the central nervous system together account for about 45 per cent of all deaths. When to those are added malignant neoplasms, then about 64 per cent of all deaths are accounted for. And thus, the familiar monotony of the American hospital: heart disease, cancer, and stroke. Within this broad outline, however, are differences that make it clear that individual societies influence the mode of death of their individuals.

From Table 12-4 it is clear that rates of death at different ages vary widely from one developed country to another although they all share the same pattern of cause. Included in the table are the rates for the diseases that make up the pattern.

One may speculate endlessly on the reasons for these variations, including factors as disparate as the use of grain whiskeys and welfare programs, but the answers are not clear. It seems most doubtful, however, that chance alone makes Sweden and France and the United States all different.

Some facts and much myth have associated certain causes of death with certain nations. Suicide has popularly been thought the province of Sweden (20/100,000) although it is common to many nations (United States 11/100,000, Austria 23/100,000, Hungary 29/100,000, West Berlin 42/100,000). It is among the ten leading causes of deaths in many of the developed and developing nations alike. Similarly cirrhosis of the liver is popularly associated with France (32/100,000), but is commonly found in a number of European and South American countries with similar frequency. Patterns are subject to change, and in the United States, the rate of cirrhosis has fluctuated with law and war and is gradually increasing (1964—12.1/100,000).

On occasion a disease is seen to emerge to prominence apparently by accident of geographic isolation. Such an example is the death rate from diabetes on Malta; at 43/100,000 it is more than double the rate in any other country (U.S. 17/100,000). (Although there are several important environmental determinants of diabetes [Levin and Recant, 1966].)

In the United States the pattern is similar to that of the other developed nations, heart disease, cancer, stroke, and accidents accounting for almost three quarters of all deaths. This has been our pattern for more than a generation, with the death rate from all causes falling as the infectious diseases fell away. It is our heritage of death, and as will be clearer when the diseases are discussed, it is a heritage that we have created.

DETERMINATION OF DISEASE TRENDS—VITAL STATISTICS

Disease and illness frequencies, prevalence, incidence, and trends tell us about the health of our world in statistical terms. They underlie the entire discussion of this chapter and our appreciation of emergent diseases. They allow us to know where we have been and sharpen our insights into where we are going. They are made possible by the collection of vital statistics.

Consideration of the health of a society requires more than merely a knowledge of the number of individuals with illness (the numerator). There are so many different features of individuals that affect their illness that the numerator is meaningless without precision in the denominator. The denominator is the population at risk. Knowledge of age, sex, marital status, occupation, race, and so forth, help put precision in the denominator. The more precise it is, the more precise will be conclusions drawn from vital statistics. (It goes without saying that precision is equally important in the numerator.)

TABLE 12-4

Death Rates per 100,000 at Selected Ages and for Selected Causes in six Developed Nations, 1964*

Cancer	Hyper-tension	Arterio-sclerotic H.D.	All Heart Disease	Stroke	Nation	10–14	20–24	40–44	50–54	60–64	70–74
203	9.7	80	366	128	France	30	110	310	750	1,750	3,970
220	27.9	306	574	156	England Wales	30	80	260	720	1,960	4,760
226	26.0	352	637	194	Scotland	40	80	330	890	2,350	5,440
191	29.7	306	525	120	Sweden	30	80	210	540	1,430	4,080
133	18.0	241	379	78	Canada	40	120	280	730	1,890	4,290
151	36.4	313	508	103	United States	40	130	370	910	2,070	4,540

* Vital statistics of World Health Organization—United Nations.

The basic element in vital statistics is the census. This is a massive undertaking, which, though subject to some errors, is an extremely sound source of information.

Increasingly our concern is with health trends that cross international boundaries. As we cross them the difficulties in estimating the precision of both numerator, the disease in question, and denominator, the population at risk, are greatly increased. With the establishment of the World Health Organization as a specialized agency of the United Nations, efforts to establish a single world body concerned with health matters were culminated. The World Health Organization now publishes important vital statistics publications such as the *Epidemiological and Vital Statistics Report*, the *Weekly Epidemiological Record*, and the *World Health Statistics Annual*. In addition, the Statistical Office of the United Nations publishes *Statistical Papers* including *Population and Vital Statistics Report*. These reports and publications make careful note of the conditions of data collection and publication that affect validity and comparability. The wealth of available information has made possible greatly increased understanding of health trends and public health problems. Thus, there are available for much of the world, as well as for the United States, detailed statistics on populations, mortality, and increasingly, morbidity. Although the enumeration of the census has been a relatively recent event, registration of births, deaths, and marriages has a long history.

The form of the death certificate has been established by international agreement and generally is arranged as follows.

Disease or condition directly leading to death   a_____

                                                       b_____

Conditions giving rise to the above   c_____
Other significant conditions   d_____

Vital Statistics in the United States

The National Office of Vital Statistics publishes a number of current reports. *Morbidity and Mortality Report* arises from the Communicable Disease Center and contains the incidence of reported communicable diseases state by state; in addition, certain summary reports of selected subjects are included where pertinent. *Monthly Vital Statistics Report* contains monthly and cumulative data on births, marriages, deaths, and infant deaths by states and selected cities.

Vital Statistics of the United States, Annual Report, Volume I, contains statistics on marriage, divorce, births, fetal mortality, infant mortality, and total mortality for the United States and possessions. Statistics are given in considerable detail by age, sex, state, metropolitan areas and nonmetropolitan areas, and so on. The report contains summaries of the information obtained by marriage, divorce, birth, and death registration.

Vital Statistics of the United States, Annual Report, Volume II, contains detailed statistics on mortality data by region, age, sex, cause, race, and so on.

In addition, the National Center of Health Statistics publishes periodic reviews, life tables, and vital and health statistics derived from the National Health Survey.

Mortality

Death is not only "nature's way of telling you to slow down." It is also the end result of a long series of events, only some of which may be evident at the time of its occurrence. Despite the fact that all its operands are not obvious, the fact of death itself is so undeniable that it is often used in epidemiologic studies beyond its actual usefulness.

The risk of dying varies with factors inherent to the individual and over which he has no control, such as age, sex, physical constitution, inheritance; factors in which he takes an active part, such as marital condition, occupation, locality of residence; and factors apart from himself over which he has no control, such as the physical environment.

To be meaningful, methods of analysis should be designed to differentiate or control the influence of these various factors, as well as distinguish the contribution of the different medical causes of death.

Certain cautions must be exercised for the fruitful use of mortality data. Although death may occur in one location, the operating factors in the production of the death may have occurred at another site. For example, the person with severe chronic lung disease may, because of this disease, go to live in another climate and die there. In the United States, mobility of the aged and diseased is increasingly common, and some areas, such as Florida and California, may be overrepresented in mortality statistics. (For example, in Tucson, Arizona, the death rate from bronchitis is five times the national average.)

Considerable fluctuations of numbers of deaths may occur over short periods of time giving the misleading appearance of undue change and prompting the assignment of specific reasons. For example, in New York City, where the average number of deaths per day is about 240, the day to day fluctuation can be considerable. Numerous investigators have been tempted to assign specific environmental causes, such as air pollution, to the fluctuations. Figure 12-1 shows a one-month, then one-year, then three-year view of a mortality graph drawn to the same scale for New York City. What appears to be extreme variability in the short view is seen to be remarkably stable in the long view. Only the most potent environmental influences disturb this uniformity in any obvious manner. This fact is demonstrated by the spike that is easily seen in both the one- and three-year views. The spike corresponds to a period of extreme heat and humidity between June 27 and July 3, 1963 (Cassell *et al.*, 1968).

Variability can be even more misleading where fewer numbers of deaths are involved. Consequently, when populations are small it is advisable to base calculations on a number of years in the determination of rate.

As noted earlier, the form of the death certificate, and the assignment of cause of death, are based upon international agreement. Cause of death on death certificates, however, continues to be considered a major source of inaccuracies. Although the *International Statistical Classification of Diseases, Injuries and Causes of Death* has brought uniformity to international comparisons and increased the specificity of diagnosis, it has by no means solved all the problems. (The International Statistical Classification is less refined in assignment of cause than the *American Standard*

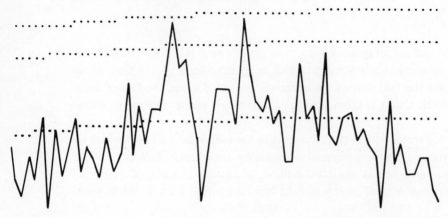

Total deaths, all ages, New York City, December 1, 1963 - January 31, 1964

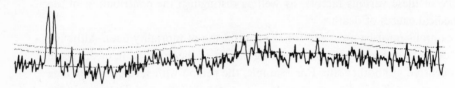

Total deaths, all ages, New York City, June 1, 1963 - July 1, 1964

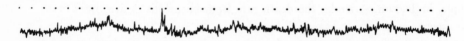

Total deaths, all ages, New York City, July 1, 1962 - June 27, 1965.

FIGURE 12-1. A graphic perspective of mortality in New York City (all age groups) showing marked variability when looked at closely (2-month period) but increasing uniformity when viewed over greater periods (1 year, then 3 years). (Reproduced from E. J. Cassell *et al.*: *Am J Public Health*, **58** : 1655, 1656, 1968.)

Nomenclature of Disease. It is precisely its lesser degree of refinement that makes the International List a more useful statistical tool.)

The accuracy of the death certificate diagnosis is adversely affected by (1) changing diagnostic fashions [which not only change from time to time, but vary from place to place at the same time]; (2) variations in the knowledge of the signatory physicians; and (3) limitations that arise from the form of the death certificate and the understanding of its intent.

The effect of the changing diagnostic fashion is greatest where death occurs outside of the hospital and cause is not accurately known. (In the United States it is now common to assign the diagnosis "arteriosclerotic heart disease" if the deceased is old and cause is not well known.)

For the purpose of comparing mortality trends over long periods of time, or for widely separated areas, the disadvantages of death certificate diagnosis are minimized by using broad groups of causes. Thus, for example, by grouping together all heart disease, other diseases of the circulation, and intracranial lesions of vascular origin, a general picture of trend may be obtained of the degenerative vascular diseases. If nephritis and bronchitis were added (in the developed countries) a general picture of all degenerative disease would be obtained. It is doubtful if greater refinement would add to the meaning.

Death Rates

Death rates measure the relative frequency of death in a population over a specified interval. They may be general, encompassing the entire population, or specific, encompassing a specified portion of the population, or specified disease. Death rates are generally expressed as a number per 100,000 or a number per 1,000 whichever is more convenient, but it is important to be sure that when rates are compared the denominators are the same. As noted earlier, accuracy in the denominator, or risk population, is as important as accuracy in the numerator, or disease. A death rate must always include a time unit such as 24/100,000 per year or per month. In published tables of death rates for large populations, the population providing the denominator is generally taken as the mean population during the unit of time.

Considerable information on death rates and life tables are contained in standard textbooks on statistics and vital statistics. The proper use of mortality information can be extremely rewarding, as we have seen, in understanding the effect of a place, culture, or society upon trends in death and disease.

THE EMERGENT DISEASES

Arteriosclerotic Heart Disease and Coronary Artery Disease

In the early 1920's myocardial infarction was not considered to be of major clinical significance. During the same period, the first papers appeared showing that it was possible to diagnose it before death. From the life tables of 1959–61 it is apparent that the average American at birth has a one in three chance of dying of arteriosclerotic heart disease. The picture has obviously changed, and a major disease has emerged. We have seen previously that the United States shares this trend with other developed nations. It is not merely the result of stripping away the infectious diseases with a resultant increase in population age. It is a disease with determinants that arise from our way of life; our activity, diet, habits, and the types of people we are. As such, it might have been predicted, and as such, we might be able to predict that it will diminish in importance as our values and habits change.

From the National Health Survey of 1960–62 it was apparent that of the 111.1 million adults in the United States aged 18–79 years, 3.1 million had definite coronary artery disease and 2.4 million had suspected coronary artery disease. More than 1.5 million adults had definite angina pectoris and more than 2.3 million had suspected angina pectoris. Definite myocardial infarction was present in 1.4 million adults.

The incidence of heart attacks appears to be rising, and almost 600,000 Americans died of them in 1964. All these figures justify our belief that this is not only an emergent disease but that it has reached almost epidemic proportions.

The basic disease responsible for these deaths and manifestations is arteriosclerosis, and there is every indication that its prevalence in the United States is rising. Comparison of autopsied cases for the degree of atherosclerosis in two periods, 1931–35 and 1951–55, has shown that, whereas in the earlier period only 1 in 50 had more than minimal coronary arteriosclerosis, in the recent period, more than minimal coronary arteriosclerosis was found in 26 out of 50 males under the age of 45 (Spain, 1960). An autopsy study of all the unexpected and sudden deaths from coronary artery disease reported to the Medical Examiner's Office in Westchester, New York, revealed that in 1949 only 1 out of 7 was under the age of 45, but that by 1959 this number had increased, so that 1 out of 4 cases was under the age of 45. Similar changes have been reported in other countries. Spain (1960) has likened the difference in degree of coronary arteriosclerosis over the twenty years of his study period to the difference between the South African Bantu males and metropolitan New York males. Other autopsy studies (White *et al.*, 1950) have shown that the degree of arteriosclerosis of coronary arteries increases rapidly in the age period 30 to 49 years.

Epidemiologic Determinants

Age.   As has been noted earlier, coronary arteriosclerosis occurs commonly in young males and has been found to a surprising degree in autopsied soldiers in their twenties. However, the disease does not usually manifest itself clinically under the age of 45 and is rare under the age of 25.

TABLE 12-5

Death Rates per 100,000 from Arteriosclerotic Heart Disease,
United States 1964, by Sex, Rate and Age*

Age	Sex M	F	Age	Sex M	F	Age	Sex M	F
20–24	1.9	1.1	45–49	257.8	53.6	70–74	2,457.7	1,296.3
25–29	5.9	2.0	50–54	457.5	113.9	75–79	3,430.6	2,207.1
30–34	18.1	5.1	55–59	756.7	212.6	80–84	5,152.9	3,840.8
35–39	54.6	11.5	60–64	1,138.9	417.6	85+	8,720.8	7,936.4
40–44	133.3	26.3	65–69	1,754.9	764.0			

* Vital statistics of World Health Organization—United Nations.

Table 12-5 makes clear the rapid rise with age in both males and females. There appears to be little significant difference between the effect of age in Negros and whites. **Sex.**   Males have rates exceeding those of females at all ages, and the differences are marked. The male-female ratio of deaths varies, however, with age, with a peak in the age group 30–35, and a gradual decline thereafter. The male-female ratio is not nearly as striking among American Negroes as among American whites. (There is also considerable variation in ratio among different countries.) There is some indication that the male-female ratio has been increasing in recent years.

Speculation about the falling male-female ratio in older groups has centered upon the effect of menopause, and has even led to the use of estrogens in males as a therapeutic regimen (with unimpressive results). Careful analysis of the data tends to diminish the impression that the effect is menopausal (Tracy, 1966). The same sex differentials have been found by virtually every study method in coronary artery disease. It is important that there is some evidence of a recent increase in the autopsy incidence of coronary artery disease in women (Parrish, 1966).

Race. Although some mortality studies have shown an increased rate of arteriosclerotic heart disease among whites as compared to Negroes, the National Health Survey was unable to find such a difference. As noted above, however, the sex ratio is different for the two groups. There has been some suggestions that the rates for Northern Negroes approximate the white death rate (Stamler, 1959) but that Southern Negro death rates are lower (Lillienfeld, 1956). In view of what will be presently said of the effect of social and geographic mobility (Syme, 1966), these discrepancies may not be surprising. Negroes, both male and female, have very mich higher rates of both hypertension and hypertensive heart disease than do whites.

Socioeconomic Status and Occupations. A popular myth has been attached to myocardial infarctions. A hard-driving, wealthy executive clutches his chest and falls to the floor—obviously the victim of a heart attack. (But if a shop foreman clutches his chest and falls to the floor, it is probably an Indian arrow.) Coronary artery disease has frequently been associated with higher levels of management and upper socioeconomic levels. The earlier studies of Logan (1952) in England and Wales seem clearly to indicate that death from coronary artery disease was a distinction of the British upper class. More recently the trend has changed. By 1949–53 the gradient had disappeared for women and was much diminished for men. There appears to be a cohort effect. That is, men born before, say, 1900 have a positive relationship between socioeconomic group and prevalence, whereas for men born after that time, the relationship is not present. It is not sure whether such a changing relationship is present in the United States. However, for men 55–64 years of age in 1950, a positive association with social class was present; for men in the youngest group an inverse relationship between coronary artery disease and social class seemed present.

A number of more recent studies (Pell and D'Alonzo, 1963; Kent et al., 1958; Stamler et al., 1960; Bainton and Peterson, 1963) have pointed to a reversal of the myth: with lower rates appearing among the more educated and higher rates among those with less education. The lowest rates were found among the professional-managerial and subprofessional levels; highest for clerical workers, then foremen, and clerical supervisors; intermediate rates among the skilled, semiskilled, and unskilled workers.

In general the upper executive group has had less disease than expected, and the lower, more. In New York City there was a tendency toward inverse association between median family income and death rates from coronary artery disease. The National Health Survey also confirmed the inverse relationship between income and the prevalence of coronary heart disease. (To strengthen this inverse relationship it is necessary to exclude from consideration those in agriculture, forestry, and fisheries.)

If this disease is derivative from the changing way of life in the United States; the changing diet, habits, activity, and other attributes of affluence, then we would expect the rate to be initially higher in higher social classes and gradually to extend down as the fruits of affluence are enjoyed by an increasing number.

That the rate should reverse in recent years points to further trends in society away from those factors contributing to the excess mortality. They should allow us to predict that the total rates will begin to fall within a period of time, related not so much to change in therapy as to changes in the culture.

Geographic Distribution.   The world-wide distribution of arteriosclerotic heart disease has already been described. In the United States, as in other nations, an urban-rural difference has been described for coronary heart disease with the preponderance of the disease in urban areas. Although not a consistent finding, the fact of lower rates among farm, fishery, and agricultural persons and their families seems undisputed. The 1950 death rates for coronary heart disease present an interesting geographic pattern (Enterline, 1956). The death rate for coronary heart disease was roughly twice as high in some states as in others. In New Mexico, Arkansas, and Kentucky the age-adjusted death rates among white males were 191.1, 201.2, and 211.2 respectively as compared with death rates in New York, Rhode Island, and the District of Columbia of 393.8, 364.3, and 344.3. (It is of some interest that the states making up the original thirteen colonies have rates comparable to those of England and Wales, Scotland, Australia, and New Zealand.)

TABLE 12-6

Crude Death Rates per 100,000 for U.S. Regions (Arteriosclerotic Heart Disease) *

	Year	
Region	1954	1965
New England	317.4	365.1
Middle Atlantic	302.6	358.9
East North Central	246.9	314.5
West North Central	238.0	318.9
South Atlantic	172.7	240.0
East South Central	157.6	241.5
West South Central	173.3	233.0
Mountain	175.7	202.5
Pacific	252.1	240.2

* Vital statistics of National Center for Health Statistics.

Table 12-6 shows that geographic variables still remain in mortality statistics although morbidity surveys have not shown the same differences.

From time to time so-called "favored areas" are found with what seem to be inordinately low rates of disease. Keys' (1966) discussion of the report on one such area is valuable for the insights it gives into the pitfalls of mortality studies.

Cigarettes.   It is generally appreciated that cigarette smoking is a hazard to health. The increase in mortality attributed to cigarette smoking in other diseases is also found in coronary heart disease. It is interesting that a hazard that now seems so clear should have been obscure to us for so long. In part the reason stems from the fact that the total duration of cigarette smoking is one of the factors that increases risk. However, some of the obscurity is because the mechanism by which cigarette smoking induces its effects is still unclear.

Data from both morbidity and mortality sources have confirmed the association between cigarette smoking and both increased morbidity and mortality from coronary artery disease. The risk increases with the amount smoked and the duration of smoking. The added risk is not a feature of pipe or cigar smoking, and diminishes or disappears after cigarette smoking has been stopped (Hammond and Horn, 1958).

Generally little information is available, but what is present (Shapiro *et al.*, 1965) indicates that women's risk for arteriosclerotic heart disease is also increased by cigarette smoking.

One paradoxical and important finding is that in the Albany and Framington studies of heart disease risk (Doyle *et al.*, 1962), as well as in others, no association between smoking and angina pectoris appears. Similarly odd is the failure to find an increased risk for subsequent infarction among cigarette smokers. It might be fruitful at this point to speculate on the processes involved. The effect of cigarette smoking on the circulation is thought to be due to nicotine. This substance regularly increases blood pressure and heart rate and reduces skin flow. Some individuals show substantial increases in the work of the left ventricle after smoking, and in sensitive subjects rhythm and T-Wave changes have appeared in the electrocardiogram. Nicotine also causes the discharge of catecholamines from the adrenals. Some recent, careful studies have shown that an increase in blood coagulation is related to the nicotine dose time. Coagulation is quickened when high nicotine cigarettes are smoked rapidly but not when the same dose of nicotine is spread over a longer period (Cliffton *et al.*, 1968).

In addition to nicotine effects, cigarette smoking increases blood carbon monoxide with consequent increases in carboxyhemoglobin. The richness of the speculation points to the lack of real knowledge about the mechanisms involved but in no way detracts from the very firm observation of the increased risk for coronary heart disease attributable to cigarette smoking.

Diet. Perhaps none of the apparent determinants in arteriosclerotic heart disease has aroused as much controversy as diet. Americans have seen themselves gulping down oils they had never previously heard of, and swinging their diets this way and that, in tune to the changing pronouncements on risk reduction.

In the beginning of this century, Ignatowski (1933) observed that Russian Army officers on a meat diet had more arteriosclerosis than the peasants on a vegetable diet. He succeeded in producing arteriosclerotic changes in the aorta of the rabbit by feeding animal proteins. In 1913 Anitschkow (1933) fed rabbits cholesterol and produced hypercholesterolemia and arteriosclerotic changes. Since those early experiments the debate had raged over the role of dietary lipids in the production of atheromata.

It is natural that diet should have been explored because the basic lesion of arteriosclerotic heart disease, the atheromatous plaque, starts off as an accumulation of lipid-laden foam cells on the arterial wall. Developing into a grossly recognizable lipid streak or plaque, it is the organization of such plaques that leads to the typical disease described in textbooks of pathology.

The clear-cut relationship of serum cholesterol level to the risk of myocardial infarction further stimulated interest in the serum lipids and their relation to diet, and there is no question that the diet can have a profound effect on serum lipids. Naturally, initial interest, and the most attention, have centered on dietary fat. Until recently it was believed that the total quantity of fat consumed in the diet was the major exogenous factor affecting serum lipids. The dietary effect of increasing affluence would seem to be increased consumption of meat, fat, and refined sugar. (You may remember the headmaster of the orphanage in Dickens' *Oliver Twist* showing how well he fed his boys by pointing out how greasy they were.) The American diet, at its most uncontrolled, provides 40 to 45 per cent of its calories from fat. This is in marked contrast to areas of chronic want where only 20 to 28 per cent of calories may be supplied by fat.

Interest shifted from the total amount of fat ingested to certain of the properties of dietary fat, such as chain length and saturation, after it was shown that diets containing abundant quantities of vegetable oil as their source of fat were able to substantially lower serum cholesterol. It is now clear that the fatty acid compositions of the fat in the diet, rather than the absolute quantity of fat, is of greatest importance in determining the pattern of serum lipids. Serum levels of cholesterol and low-density lipoproteins can be changed significantly when the pattern of fatty acids in the diet is rearranged. When the glycerides of dietary fat contain predominantly long-chain saturated fatty acids, serum cholesterol and low-density lipid proteins rise. When dietary fat is made up of an appreciable portion of polyunsaturated fatty acids, serum cholesterol and low-density lipoproteins tend to fall (Felch and Van Itallie, 1960; Van Itallie and Felch, 1960). It must be pointed out that individual variations in response to diet may be great. Other elements of diet, such as refined sugars, have been shown by some workers to have a major effect on serum cholesterol and lipoproteins with considerable rises in serum cholesterol occurring in some individuals on diets high in refined sugars.

It is appropriate and important at this juncture to point out another of the paradoxes of coronary heart disease. The level of serum cholesterol seems to be related to the risk of myocardial infarction, a disease arising on the basis of atheromatous disease of the coronary arteries. Indeed diseases in which cholesterol levels are frequently elevated, such as diabetes, have an increased risk for coronary thrombosis. However, the South African Bantu and the Japanese, both with characteristically very low levels of serum cholesterol and very infrequent myocardial infarction, have very high rates of cerebral vascular accidents—a disease arising on the basis of atheromatous disease of the cerebral circulation. Similarly, familial hypercholesterolemia is very commonly associated with heart attacks but does not seem to be associated with higher than usual rates of cerebral or peripheral vascular disease. From several points of view coronary heart disease distinguishes itself as a special manifestation of arteriosclerosis, which has its own biochemical pathology and pathophysiology as well.

It is possible to produce a "prudent" diet conforming to the American pattern but supplying equal quantities of saturated, polyunsaturated, and monosaturated fats for a total of 30 to 32 per cent of calories (Jollife *et al.*, 1959). Middle-aged men on this diet have shown sustained lowering of their serum cholesterol as well as a reduced incidence of coronary heart disease compared to a control group consuming the usual American diet (Christakis, 1966). These obviously important findings have received some confirmation (Leren, 1966), but require further support. They do, however, point in the needed direction; a clear demonstration that a reversion to a "less" affluent diet will decrease the risk of myocardial infarction.

Personality and Stress. One phone in each hand, two others ringing, and a million dollars hanging on every decision, is the popular picture of the coronary-prone individual. The influence of personality and stress on the development of coronary heart disease has received much attention but is an area where little hard information exists. We have already seen that the disease is at present perhaps inversely related to executive responsibility, although, as noted earlier, it may have been the province of higher socioeconomic groups earlier in the century. Few heart attacks occur during heavy physical activity. The majority occur during sleep in the early hours of the morning and a lesser number at rest but during waking hours. That extreme exertion is considered to be a precipitating factor is reflected in Workmen's Compensation decisions. When an attack occurs during the performance of the usual activity for the occupation it is not compensable, but should it occur during unusually heavy labor it may be compensable.

One of the writer's patients customarily carried one large crated tape recorder up the stairs to the storage area of his place of work. On the occasion of carrying two such crates up the stairs, he developed chest pain and the subsequent infarct was declared compensable. Over the ensuing years, before his sudden death from a final coronary, this patient had several other infarcts. All were ruled to be related to the first myocardial infarction. It is thus obvious that the economic ramifications of such decisions can be considerable. Nonetheless, coronary thrombosis under such circumstances is apparently uncommon. The effect of stress has been studied from several viewpoints, however (Chapman *et al.*, 1966; Wolf *et al.*, 1962; Peterson *et al.*, 1962), and the findings justify continued inquiry.

The early attempts in the field of psychosomatic medicine to fit a specific personality to a specific disease was carried over into coronary artery disease. Dunbar (1954) described the coronary personality as one of surface calm concealing underlying aggression and resentment. Typically hard-working, the patient had great compulsive strivings and urges to "get to the top." In general, this one-to-one, personality-to-disease approach has fallen into disfavor in psychosomatic medicine because its overly simple constructs have too often been contradicted by individual patients. However, interest in the personality of patients with coronary artery disease has continued to evoke lively discussion (Wardwell *et al.*, 1963; Mordkoff and Parsons, 1967). In some cases, findings have been confused by the obvious effects of a myocardial infarction on subsequent emotions (Miller, 1965; Friedman and Rosenman, 1959).

The so-called type A behavior pattern described by Rosenman and his group (1964) is a complex composed primarily of competitiveness, excessive drive, and an enhanced sense of time urgency. This personality pattern has also been found associated with several of the other apparent determinants of coronary artery disease, such as elevation of blood cholesterol, beta lipoproteins, and triglycerides.

Despite the vagaries that plague the attempt to find personality attributes associated with coronary artery disease, the pursuit seems reasonable. It is a particularly hard kind of thing to study because of the action and interaction of other variables such as age, sex, and socioeconomic status.

Exercise.   In numerous epidemiologic investigations it has been shown that coronary artery disease occurs more commonly in the habitually sedentary than in the habitually active. Often this relationship is hard to find because of the difficulty in finding a group of sufficient numbers in modern times who are habitually active. Probably there has been no more profound alteration in habits in recent times in this country than in our occupational (and other) physical activity. Field studies have revealed that the daily physical expenditure of even many laborers and modern farmers remove them from the category of heavy workers. As with the alterations in our diet, the diminishing physical activity is one of the hallmarks of affluence. Even in the face of the investigational difficulties, the relationship between inactivity and the disease persist, although Spain (1960) was unable to demonstrate a difference in the degree of underlying atherosclerotic change at autopsy in individuals of differing activity. Some physiologic basis for the correlation is found in animal experiments (Eckstein, 1957), which have shown that following experimental partial coronary occlusion the development of intercoronary collateral anastomosis was significantly greater in the dogs exercised following the occlusion than in the animals that were not exercised. Further support comes from the demonstration of the therapeutic efficacy of exercise in individuals with existing coronary artery disease.

The Determination of Risk.   One of the most interesting by-products of all the work on arteriosclerotic heart disease and myocardial infarction has been the assessment of risk for disease in the healthy individual. Material for the prediction of risk has emerged from the several prospective studies of coronary heart disease of which the Framingham Study is perhaps the best known. The Framingham Study has been following a sample of 5,127 adults in the town of Framingham, Massachusetts, since 1949 (Dawber et al., 1963; Friedman et al., 1967). After an initial examination, participants have been followed primarily by biennial examinations, but other sources of information, such as death certificates, private physician reports, and hospital records, have been used to determine whether coronary heart disease developed. The findings of the Framingham Study are typical and reveal many of the factors already discussed to be associated with the risk of coronary disease (Dawber, 1963; Kannel et al., 1966; Kannel et al., 1962). Figures 12-2 to 12-11 illustrate the magnitude of risk of several factors found in the Framingham experience. Some notes of caution in literal interpretation are warranted. It is common experience for certain statistical analyses to better fit the data from which they were derived than new data. In other words, the ability to predict future risk with any accuracy for new populations or even for future experience in the same population is far different than the ability to expose the risk factors in the original data. The traditional analytic method of epidemiologists, multiple cross-correlations, is impracticable in the face of large numbers of interrelated or even separate risk factors. The exploration and development of more complex analytic tools has been one of the salutory benefits of studies such as the Framingham Study. Nonetheless, such analytic methods are in their infancy in the accurate prediction of risk. The advantages of being able accurately to predict the risk of an individual's developing coronary heart disease would be of inestimable value, and it is probable that future investigations will bring that ability closer. That will not solve the equally important problem of changing the risk even when the factors that make it up are known.

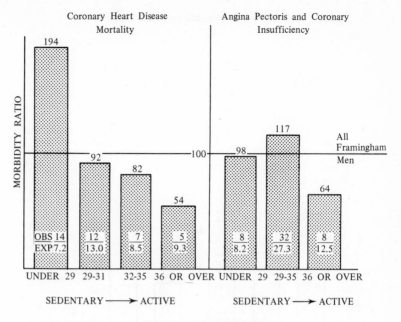

PHYSICAL ACTIVITY INDEX

FIGURE 12-2. The association of physical activity with heart disease risk. (Reproduced from *U.S. Public Health Service Publication* no. 1515, National Heart Institute, 1966.)

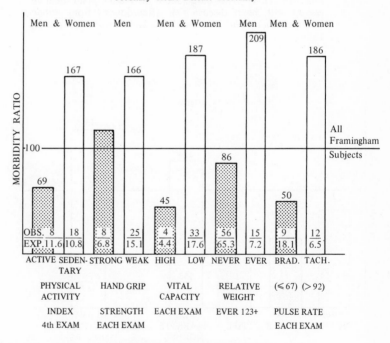

MEASURE OF PHYSICAL ACTIVITY

FIGURE 12-3. The association of measure of physical activity with heart disease risk. (Reproduced from *U.S. Public Health Service Publication* no. 1515, National Heart Institute, 1966.)

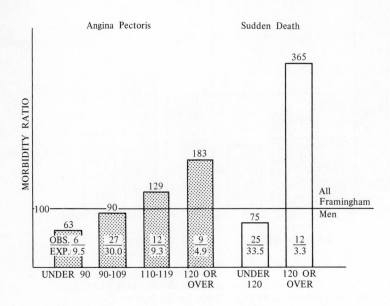

FRAMINGHAM RELATIVE WEIGHT

FIGURE 12-4. The association of Framingham relative weight with heart disease risk. (Reproduced from *Public Health Service Publication* no. 1515, National Heart Institute, 1966.)

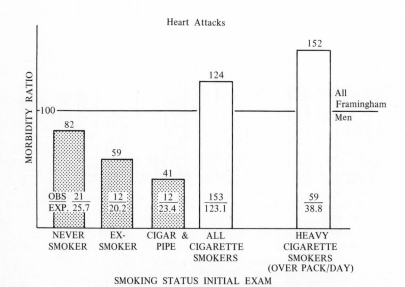

SMOKING STATUS INITIAL EXAM

FIGURE 12-5. The association of smoking status with heart disease risk. (Reproduced from *U.S. Public Health Service Publication* no. 1515, National Heart Institute, 1966.)

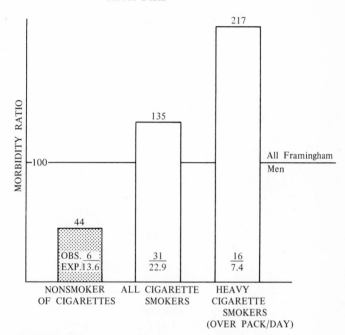

FIGURE 12-6. The association of smoking with heart disease risk. (Reproduced from *U.S. Public Health Service Publication* no. 1515, National Heart Institute, 1966.)

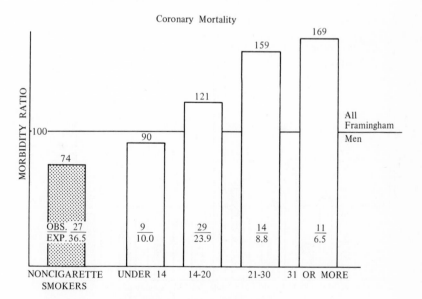

NUMBER OF CIGARETTES PER DAY

FIGURE 12-7. The association of number of cigarettes per day with heart disease risk. (Reproduced from *U.S. Public Health Service Publication* no. 1515, National Heart Institute, 1966.)

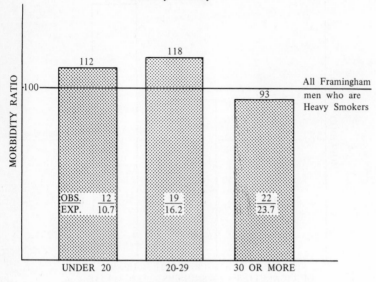

YEARS DURATION

Heavy Smokers - Over Pack/Day of Cigarettes

FIGURE 12-8. The association of years' duration of cigarette smoking with heart disease risk. (Reproduced from *U.S. Public Health Service Publication* no. 1515, National Heart Institute, 1966.)

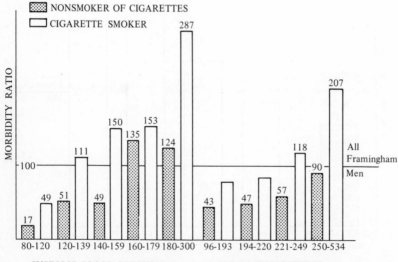

FIGURE 12-9. The association of cigarette smoking at levels of blood pressure and serum cholesterol with heart disease risk. (Reproduced from *U.S. Public Health Service Publication* no. 1515, National Heart Institute, 1966.)

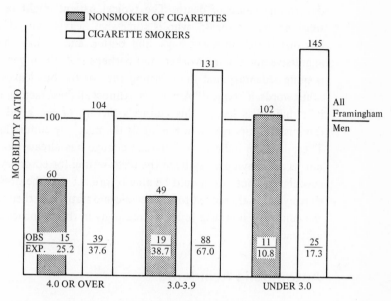

FIGURE 12-10. The association of cigarette smoking at levels of vital capacity with heart disease risk. (Reproduced from *U.S. Public Health Service Publication* no. 1515, National Heart Institute, 1966.)

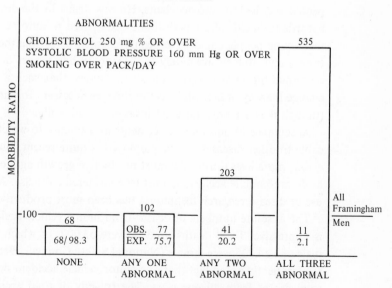

FIGURE 12-11. The effect of combinations of abnormalities on heart disease risk. (Reproduced from *U.S. Public Health Service Publication* no. 1515, National Heart Institute, 1966.)

The Total Picture. Within the last two generations in the United States and other parts of the Western World, a disease has emerged from relative obscurity to become the leading cause of death. The typical patient might be described as a cigarette-smoking male, over 45, who is somewhat heavy, and perhaps slightly hypertensive. His diet is rich in meat, eggs, and butter, and he likes his dessert. Although he is aggressive and a hard worker, and perhaps feels the urgency of time pushing him, he is quite sedentary and the morning run for the bus leaves him breathless. He is, in other words, a "typical" American. Almost all these factors are signs that he has "made it"; that he is leading his culture's picture of the good life. For these factors to diminish in importance in the life of the man, the culture and its values must change. There is some indication that such change has already started and that the cultural norms are moving away from the ideal setting for coronary heart disease. It is purely speculation, but one should be able to predict that the disease will become first more sharply inversely related to socioeconomic status and then tend to subside throughout the culture as it is then found increasingly in the countries and cultures emerging into affluence.

Automobile Accidents

Once the writer was waiting to testify at a hearing on the effects of air pollution on health in one of our Western states. The levels being discussed in purple prose as possible hazards were ridiculously low and would have been considered pristine in New York. To pass the time, he read the local newspaper, including the obituaries. There had been three deaths the preceding day: one older than seventy and the other two younger than twenty. It was statistically probable, and true, that the two young people had died in auto accidents. He was struck by the disparity of concern over the hazards to health of air pollution as compared to auto accidents. The deaths of the two young people could have been prevented by raising the minimum driving age to twenty-one. But so intimately is the automobile a part of the physical, social, and economic life of that state and all the states, that such a change would drastically change the way of life, whereas the changes necessary for air pollution control seemed (though they are not) quite extrinsic to everyday life.

Acceptance of automobile accidents as a disease to which research methods applicable to other diseases can be employed is quite recent. But certainly any cause that claims more lives during the most productive growth ages of 15 to 44 than any other, as do automobile accidents, must be considered a disease. As will be noted below, the use of disease research techniques has been most productive.

The absolute numbers of deaths from motor vehicle accidents in the United States is impressive. Total deaths in 1966 were 53,000, of which 38,316 (72 per cent) were male and 14,725 were female (National Safety Council, 1968). And, of course, there is the frequently noted fact that our motor vehicle accident deaths exceed the combined total deaths from all our wars. The tragedy of road accidents is that they involve mostly the young, especially males, 15 to 30. In the developed countries, this cause of death exceeds the combined deaths from all infectious and communicable disease. Disability and economic loss are also staggering. The problem is by no means confined to the United States, but is, rather, an increasing international public health problem. Table 12-7 shows rates from several countries and demonstrates the increase in deaths in some areas as opposed to apparent control in others.

TABLE 12-7

Death Rates per 100,000 from Motor Vehicle Accidents 1950–1952 Compared to 1960–62 in Selected Countries*†

	Death Rates/100,000 Population	
	1950–52	1960–62
United States	23.8	21.3
Canada	18.8	21.8
Venezuela	9.3	16.6
Japan	4.1	14.0
France	8.6	19.4
United Kingdom	9.8	14.1

* Vital statistics of World Health Organization— United Nations.

† A note of caution is necessary in interpreting motor vehicle accident rates. Three denominators are commonly used: rates per 100,000 population, rates per 100,000,000 miles driven, and rates per 10,000 registered vehicles. These denominators express different dimensions of the problem, which may give different meanings to the rates. Unless the traffic density (vehicles per mile of road), vehicles per population, or number of miles driven annually are known, it is difficult to compare rates. The definition of fatal accident also varies from country to country.

The Epidemiology

Age and Sex. At all ages, except under one, and in all nations, motor vehicle fatalities are primarily male. The age pattern is also different in males and females (Figure 12-12). Table 12-8 gives the United States breakdown by age for fatal and nonfatal accidents for 1967. The same pattern, though less marked, is present for women. For males, married men have the lowest death rates per 100,000 population. The rates generally increase through the single and widowed, with the highest rates among the divorced.

Geographic Variation

Urban-rural. More motor vehicle deaths occur in rural area, but for specific types of accidents the proportions vary considerably. For example, two thirds of pedestrian deaths occur in urban places, but only one quarter of the vehicular collision deaths occur in urban sites. In general, fatal accidents occur more commonly on rural roads

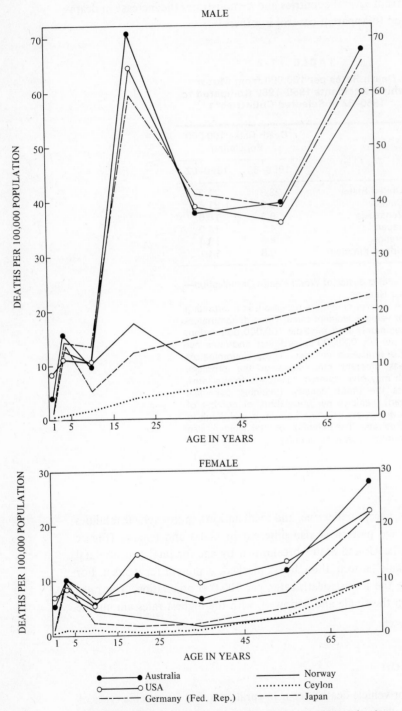

FIGURE 12-12. Mortality in motor vehicle accidents in three highly motorized and three less motorized countries, 1954–58. (Reproduced from L. G. Norman: *Road Traffic Accidents.* Public Health Papers, no. 12, WHO, Geneva, 1962.)

TABLE 12-8

Age of Drivers—Total Number and Number in Accidents, 1967*

| Age Group | All Drivers | | Drivers in Accidents | | | | | |
| | | | Fatal | | All | | Per No. of Drivers | |
	Number	Per Cent	Number	Per Cent	Number	Per Cent	Fatal†	All‡
Total	103,000,000	100.0	64,500	100.0	24,300,000	100.0	63	24
Under 20	10,500,000	10.2	10,300	16.0	4,200,000	17.3	98	40
20-24	11,000,000	10.7	11,400	17.7	4,200,000	17.3	104	38
25-29	10,100,000	9.8	7,200	11.2	2,800,000	11.5	71	28
30-34	9,700,000	9.4	6,200	9.6	2,200,000	9.1	64	23
35-39	10,600,000	10.3	5,300	8.2	2,200,000	9.1	50	21
40-44	11,100,000	10.8	5,300	8.2	1,900,000	7.8	48	17
45-49	10,100,000	9.8	4,700	7.3	1,850,000	7.6	47	18
50-54	8,800,000	8.6	3,700	5.7	1,450,000	6.0	42	16
55-59	7,000,000	6.8	2,900	4.5	1,250,000	5.1	41	18
60-64	5,400,000	5.2	2,450	3.8	900,000	3.7	45	17
65-69	4,000,000	3.9	1,950	3.0	700,000	2.9	49	18
70-74	2,800,000	2.7	1,500	2.3	350,000	1.4	54	13
75 and over	1,900,000	1.8	1,600	2.5	300,000	1.2	84	16

* Reproduced from *National Safety Council Accident Facts*. Chicago, Illinois, 1968. Source: Drivers in accidents based on reports from 23 state traffic authorities. Number of drivers by age are NSC estimates based on reports from state traffic authorities, research groups, and the U.S. Bureau of Public Roads.
† Drivers in Fatal Accidents per 100,000 drivers in each age group.
‡ Drivers in all accidents per 100 drivers in each age group.

and nonfatal accidents more commonly on urban roads. The distribution of deaths by state in the United States varies considerably as can be seen in Table 12-9. The distribution is affected by rurality, minimum driving age, law enforcement, and also by the local significance of the automobile in the economic and social life of the state. Data are not available directly relating socioeconomic status to accident or fatality rates.

Contributory Factors

Vehicle Design.   Considerable controversy has erupted in recent years over the safety of modern vehicle design. As a result of experimental accident studies, the sources of injury or death once an accident has occurred are better understood. The wide advocacy and increased use of seat belts are an example and have resulted from aware-ness that the unrestrained occupant of a vehicle in a crash becomes a projectile, striking exposed projections with incredible force. Seat belts plus improved door locks decrease driver ejection with its attendant high mortality. The pace of improved safety design appears to be increasing as a result of enlarging public pressure. It is of some interest to our general thesis that an attempt to use safety as a major selling point for automobiles was notably unsuccessful a number of years ago. A point appears to be reached by a society when it begins to accept a public health problem as just that and lends support to its eradication. That time seems to have begun in the United States.

A similar process has occurred in the control of environmental pollution. These changes in public acceptance are part of the complex situation in which consumer demand acts both directly on the manufacturer and indirectly in the form of an

TABLE 12-9

Death Rates per 100,000 from Motor Vehicle Accidents by State, 1967*

	Deaths	Rate		Deaths	Rate
Alabama	1,226	34.6	Nebraska	464	32.3
Alaska	26	14.3	Nevada	338	43.7
Arizona	615	37.6	New Hampshire	161	23.5
Arkansas	669	34.0	New Jersey	1,206	17.2
California	—	—	New Mexico	460	45.9
Colorado	614	31.1	New York	2,900	15.8
Connecticut	462	15.8	North Carolina	815	36.1
Delaware	128	24.5	North Dakota	210	32.9
Dist. of Columbia	159	19.7	Ohio	2,436	23.3
Florida	1,834	30.6	Oklahoma	—	—
Georgia	1,121	29.8	Oregon	687	34.4
Hawaii	150	20.3	Pennsylvania	2,493	21.4
Idaho	282	40.3	Rhode Island	111	12.3
Illinois	2,329	21.4	South Carolina	887	34.1
Indiana	—	—	South Dakota	238	35.3
Iowa	836	30.4	Tennessee	1,360	34.9
Kansas	632	30.0	Texas	3,212	29.6
Kentucky	1,009	31.6	Utah	293	28.6
Louisiana	1,256	34.3	Vermont	128	30.7
Maine	261	26.8	Virginia	1,228	27.1
Maryland	795	21.6	Washington	929	30.1
Massachusetts	—	—	West Virginia	513	28.5
Michigan	2,104	24.5	Wisconsin	1,142	27.3
Minnesota	1,008	28.1	Wyoming	152	48.3
Mississippi	938	39.9	Puerto Rico	481	17.8
Missouri	1,371	29.8	Virgin Islands	9	18.2
Montana	338	48.2			

* Reproduced from *National Safety Council Accident Facts.* Chicago, 1968.

increasing constituency in the support of control and safety legislation. Frequently, each group of individuals in the multivariable reaction acts as though it alone were present and acting for change. By virtue of the present attitude, changes and trends, the present increasing safety engineering may well continue.

The Road.   There is a strong association between road traffic accident rates and the design, construction, and surfacing of highways. Recently traffic engineering has taken these factors into consideration and modern highways have lower fatality rates. The turnpike system death rate in 1967 was 2.4 per 100,000,000 vehicle miles of travel. On all the nation's rural roads (including the turnpike system) the rate was 7.6.

Climatic conditions probably affect the incidence of road accidents through their effect on road surface as well as visibility. In the United States in 1967, 66.5 per cent of accidents occurred on dry roads, 22.3 per cent on wet roads, and 10.4 per cent on snowy or icy roads. Disproportionately more fatal accidents occur on dry roads and fewer on snowy or icy roads. The true interpretation of the figures is difficult without some comparison of the number of vehicle miles driven on each surface.

Season, Day, and Hour.   As might be expected, there are differences in accident prevalence from month to month in the United States. Deaths increase during the summer months, and after tapering off slightly in the fall, rise to a peak in December. The lowest rate occurs in February followed by a slow rise toward summer. This kind of seasonal variation is seen in all countries with well-marked seasons.

Monday through Thursday average about the same per cent of vehicular deaths (11 per cent each in 1967), but totals are sharply above that for Friday (16 per cent), Saturday (22 per cent), and Sunday (18 per cent).

The hourly distribution shows that for Monday through Thursday, fatal accidents occur most frequently between 4:00 and 8:00 P.M. On Friday, deaths occur more often during the evening rush hour and then late at night, as might be expected. Saturday, early morning and evening, and Sunday, early morning, have more than their share of fatal accidents. The differences between day and night accident incidence is sharpened when the deaths are related to miles of travel, as is seen in Table 12-10.

TABLE 12-10
Day-Night Accident Deaths*

	Total		Urban		Rural	
	Per cent of Deaths	Death Rate	Per cent of Deaths	Death Rate	Per cent of Deaths	Death Rate
Day	47	3.7	46	2.2	48	5.2
Night	53	9.7	54	6.2	52	13.2
Death Rates = deaths per 100,000,000 vehicle miles						

* Reproduced from *National Safety Council Accident Facts*. Chicago, Illinois, 1968.

The hourly distribution of deaths varies with the category of road user in much the manner one would expect.

The Driver. Although it is true that every accident requires for its occurrence a configuration of road, vehicle, and environmental variables, the driver carries the main responsibility for traffic accidents.

Driving is a skill that must be acquired and maintained through regular practice. It involves the well-coordinated use of the senses and motor dexterity and requires a high level of vigilance for its safe performance. That two vehicles can proceed side by side at 60 or 70 miles per hour as a routine turnpike procedure is a remarkable tribute to the integrative capabilities of the human computer. Platt (in Norman, 1962) has suggested the following rates of occurrences based on observations and published statistics.

Observations	200 per mile
Decisions	20 per mile
Errors	1 per 2 miles
Near collisions	1 per 500 miles
Collisions	1 per 61,000 miles
Personal injuries	1 per 430,000 miles
Fatal accidents	1 per 16,000,000 miles

It is obvious that many factors within the individual and in his environment can contribute to alterations in performance. It was originally suggested by Tillman and Hobbs in 1949 that "a man drives as he lives" and that suggestion is supported not only by our own everyday experience, but by considerable study. But delineating with certainty those factors that enter into "accident proneness" has proven difficult.

The concept of "accident proneness"—the existence of a group of drivers who have a higher frequency of accidents than experienced by the entire universe of drivers— seems to have validity. Strengthening the notion is the fact that relatively few of the drivers who could have accidents (the entire population of licensed drivers) are involved in accidents; i.e., say 4 per cent of drivers have 100 per cent of the accidents. The question is, do the same drivers have the accidents the following year?

Statistical studies of bus and trolley operators (Hääkinen, 1958) in Finland supported the concept that some of the drivers had accident rates consistently higher than others and that the differences seemed to be independent of risk exposure.

Having established that a group of drivers is having more than its share of accidents (and although this appears to be true, it is not universally accepted), it is necessary to see whether it is possible to discriminate between the two groups by tests or other means. Shaw (1965) has used extensively a series of psychological projective techniques in an effort to predict which bus drivers would have high accident rates. From her studies she has evolved a personality picture of the bad accident risk that is markedly variant from the individual with good risk. The high-accident-risk individual was found to be immature, unstable, overambitious, aggressive, impatient, irresponsible, uncooperative, intolerant, as opposed to the mature, stable, even-tempered, responsible, alert driver, who can be expected to have a low accident rate.

Other investigators have reached much the same conclusions (Tillman and Hobbs, 1949; Tillman, 1967; Litman and Tabachnik, 1967; Tabachnik and Tillman, 1966; Schuster, 1968). Although the methods employed have varied quite widely, the consonance of the personality picture that has emerged from different investigations is quite impressive. Hostile, impulsive, rebellious, carping, immature, acting-out, are terms that repeatedly occur in descriptions of the person with high accident risk.

Perhaps the best predictor of subsequent involvement in accidents is an individual's previous record of violations. The greater the number of moving violations the greater the chance that he will be involved in an accident. Psychologic studies of violators as opposed to nonviolators have suggested distinct differences in attitudes between the two groups, differences that will allow predictions of the problem driver (Beamith and Malfetti, 1962).

Thus, although the ability to use psychologic means to predict who will have an automobile accident may still be in question, there is little doubt that there are individuals who use their cars as an extension of themselves in the interplay between their unconscious dynamics and their society.

As in the other diseases under discussion, it is a far cry from the detection of risk to the prevention of accidents. Even brief thought will reveal what hardship would be imposed on those who were deprived of the right to drive because predictive techniques showed them to be a significant highway danger. So much is the automobile a part of the society that certain means of making a living as well as large areas of residence would perforce be denied those who were prevented from driving because of their elevated risk. On the other hand, they continue to constitute a significant danger that, now that it has been identified, requires some remedial action. The development of driver education courses, driver improvement clinics, and similar efforts at reducing identified risk have received considerable attention in recent years (Greenshields, 1966).

With even considerable success of all these approaches, there will remain a group who are at high risk for automobile accidents but do not respond to remedial measures (see the discussion on alcohol). A change in societal values and attitudes will be required before it is possible to deny them the right to drive. Such a change is by no means unthinkable and would represent one of the ways a society adapts to its acceptance of something as a public health hazard.

Physiological Determinants and Drugs. As noted earlier, the task of driving involves the integration of considerable perceptual information, rapid and frequent decision-making, and the exercise of considerable motor skills. Interference with any of these steps can be expected as a result of stress, fatigue, drug ingestion, disease, or other physiologic determinants.

Our own experience suggests to us that perceptual acuity and decision-making ability deteriorate with increasing fatigue, and indeed, studies of driver performance support the belief (Brown, 1967; Rosenow and Watkins, 1967). Motor skills are the least affected. Aging tends to produce the same effect, although the increase in judgment attendant on age offsets some of the accident potential of the physiologic loss. Even menstruation and the premenstrual state have been indicted as causing increased accident liability (Dalton, 1960).

The increasingly common use of psychotropic agents, antihistamines, and other drugs whose side effects include drowsiness, slowed reaction times, and perceptual interferences represent a substantial road hazard. Although the pharmacologic literature suggests caution in taking these medications when driving, the warning is frequently forgotten by both physician and patient alike. The driver may be unaware of the extent of impairment of his driving skills produced by drugs. The use of amphetamines and similar agents to reduce fatigue while driving may be accompanied by a decrease in judgment, as well as subsequent let-down, and therefore constitute a danger of which the driver may be unaware. The extent to which these various physiologic variables and drugs are operative in accident production is receiving increasing attention. As more thorough studies are made of drug levels in the accident victim, the importance of the problem will become clearer.

Alcohol. The dangers of driving under the influence of alcohol are apparent to even the least sophisticated driver. The higher the concentration of alcohol in the blood, the greater are its adverse effects on driving (Drew *et al.*, 1958; U.S. Dept. of Transportation, 1968; Loomis and West, 1958).

The physiologic effects of alcohol in diminishing concentration, coordination, comprehension, judgment, and vision are present at even low blood levels and progressively increase as the blood level rises until the individual is stuporous. The trustworthiness of a man's judgment of his own driving skill may be impaired after even a small quantity of alcohol producing a blood level of less than 50 mg per cent.

Although the effects of alcohol on driving skills vary from person to person and are influenced by the usual drinking habits of subjects, some effects will be present in almost everyone at levels between 50 and 100 mg per cent. The World Health Organization's Expert Committee on Alcohol (1954) noted:

Taking into consideration (1) the investigations performed in recent years on the effect of alcohol on different functions in laboratory experiments, (2) the results of statistically designed practical tests on drivers, air pilots, etc., and (3) the statistical evidence from the few adequate studies existing on alcohol and road accidents, the inference cannot be avoided that at a blood alcohol concentration of about 50 mg/100 ml a statistically significant impairment of performance is observed in more than half the cases examined.

The U.S. Department of Transportation defines the terms "intoxicated" and "under the influence of alcohol" as blood alcohol concentrations of no more than 0.10 per cent by weight, and requires of the states a provision making it either unlawful or presumptive evidence of illegality if the blood alcohol concentration of a driver equals or exceeds the limit so established.

The blood level of alcohol is determined by the amount ingested, but is dependent also on the period of time over which the alcohol was consumed, the characteristics and amounts of other foods or beverages also ingested, and the weight of the individual. In an average individual, ingestion of about five ounces of 80-proof vodka on an empty stomach will produce a blood alcohol of about 100 mg per cent within slightly more than an hour. The blood alcohol will remain above 60 mg per cent for more than five hours. The same amount of alcohol after a meal will produce a concentration of alcohol in the blood that barely reaches 50 mg per cent.

Despite the long-term interest in the contribution of alcohol to traffic accidents, truly controlled studies have been done in only the past few years (McCarroll and Haddon, 1962). In recent years, however, excellent evidence has accumulated that points clearly to the conclusion that alcohol is the largest single factor leading to fatal crashes. Further, it would appear that the higher a driver's blood alcohol concentration, disproportionately greater is the likelihood that he will crash, greater is the likelihood that he will have initiated any crash in which he is involved, and greater is the likelihood that the crash will be severe.

Various studies (Holcomb, 1938; Lucas et al., 1955; Borkenstein et al., 1964) have shown that between 70 and 90 per cent of drivers not involved in crashes (random surveys, noncrash drivers tested at sites and times of crashes, and so forth) have not been drinking; between 5 and 20 per cent have blood levels below 100 mg per cent; and between 1 and 4 per cent have levels in the range of intoxication (greater than 100 mg/100 ml).

By contrast, some 48 to 57 per cent of drivers fatally injured in single vehicle crashes had blood alcohol concentrations of 100 mg per cent or higher. Similarly high concentrations were found in about 45 per cent of fatally injured drivers in multiple vehicle accidents. These results and others are summarized in Figure 12-13. As is seen in Figure 12-14, alcohol figures heavily in pedestrian fatalities. Of pedestrians stopped at random at the time and place of fatal pedestrian accidents, only about 10 per cent have blood alcohol levels in excess of 100 mg per cent. Thus, the conclusions noted earlier on the magnitude of the contribution of alcohol to automobile accidents seem justified.

Of considerable interest in terms of the problem of alcohol as well as the problem of "accident-proneness" are the findings on the drinking driver. Drivers involved in crashes or citations associated with alcohol have been found to possess substantial histories of social, medical, and legal problems related to alcohol. They are frequently already known to community agencies because of their drinking. Figures 12-15 and 12-16 demonstrate this. From the foregoing and other evidence, the drinking driver

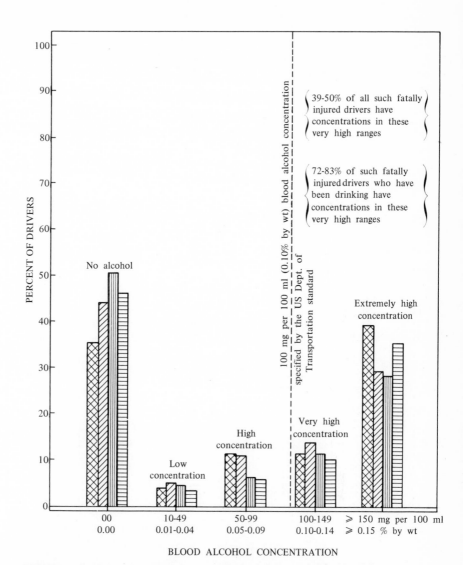

39-50% of all such fatally injured drivers have concentrations in these very high ranges

72-83% of such fatally injured drivers who have been drinking have concentrations in these very high ranges

100 mg per 100 ml (0.10% by wt) blood alcohol concentration specified by the US Dept. of Transportation standard

No alcohol

Extremely high concentration

Very high concentration

High concentration

Low concentration

| | 00 | 10-49 | 50-99 | 100-149 | ≥ 150 mg per 100 ml |
| | 0.00 | 0.01-0.04 | 0.05-0.09 | 0.10-0.14 | ≥ 0.15 % by wt |

BLOOD ALCOHOL CONCENTRATION

PERCENT OF DRIVERS

FIGURE 12-13. Blood alcohol concentration among drivers fatally injured in nonpedestrian crashes—results of four different studies. (Reproduced from U.S. Department of Transportation: *Alcohol and Highway Safety*, August 1968.)

involved in an accident is not likely to be merely a run-of-the-mill driver who happened to be drinking, but an individual in whose life the abuse of alcohol has already played a major part. The similarity to other forms of violence is obvious.

The Total Picture.   The automobile accident, major category of accidental death, is, as we have seen, a disease with multiple and complex contributions to its total picture. The automobile has made possible the sprawling cities and even the unbroken megalopolis. But those sprawling cities have made the automobile indispensable. The structure of our society and many of our values are so intimately bound with the automobile that we are even unaware of the extent. Just as our diet and exercise patterns have

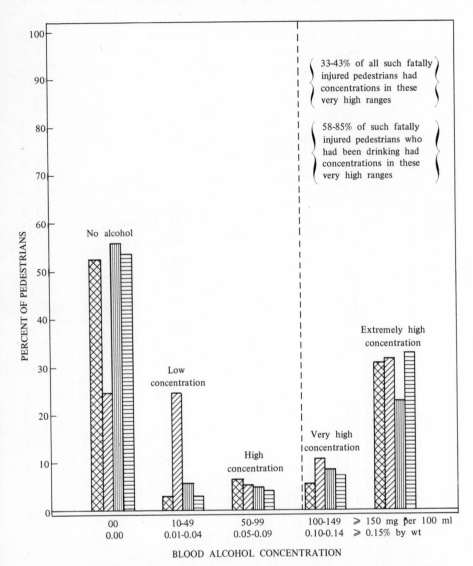

FIGURE 12-14. Blood alcohol concentrations among adult pedestrians fatally injured in crashes—results of four studies. (Reproduced from U.S. Department of Transportation: *Alcohol and Highway Safety*, August 1968.)

changed because of increasing affluence without our awareness, so does the full meaning of the automobile surpass our comprehension.

For some, the automobile is an extension of themselves, and their unconscious dynamics are played out in the manner in which they drive. An accident is an event that occurs because of a configuration of factors in the vehicle, road, and driver. As we have seen, there has been much progress toward better roads and beginning progress toward safer automobiles. The driver, most important of all, remains the element about which we have done the least. Typically, the victim of this disease is a young male, hostile, immature, and impulsive, who uses alcohol to abuse and who has demonstrated his sociopathy by previous contact with community agencies. Unfor-

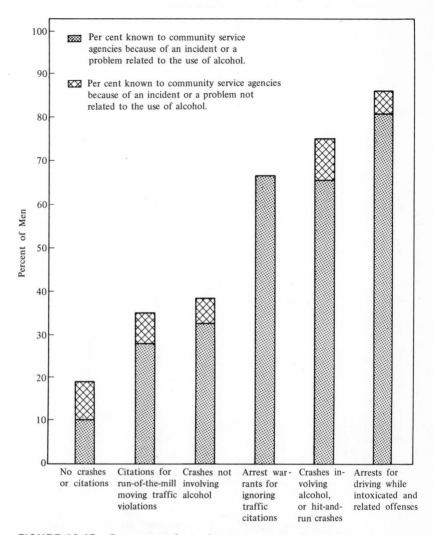

FIGURE 12-15. Percentage of men known to community service agencies because of an incident or a problem related to the use of alcohol, or because of other reasons among men with no crashes or traffic citations, with citations for run-of-the-mill moving traffic violations, with crashes not involving alcohol, with arrest warrants for ignoring traffic citations, with crashes involving alcohol or which were "hit and run," and with arrests for driving while intoxicated and related offenses. (Reproduced from U.S. Department of Transportation: *Alcohol and Highway Safety*, August 1968.)

tunately, of course, other crash victims may result who are free of these characteristics but whose demise or injury followed the initiation of the accident by another. The situation is somewhat analogous to that of coronary artery disease. Improved intensive care and resuscitation and other therapeutic measures may decrease the mortality rate somewhat, but major improvement will only follow the preventive steps that appear to require modification in the modern way of life. Improved vehicular design, highway construction, and emergency medical care, among other measures, will reduce traffic

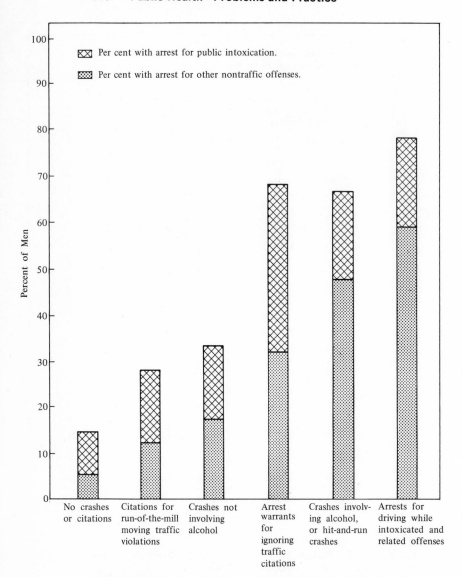

FIGURE 12-16. Percentage of men with previous nontraffic arrests and with previous arrests for public intoxication among men with no crashes or traffic citations, with citations for run-of-the-mill moving traffic viola- tions, with crashes not involving alcohol, with arrest warrants for ignoring traffic citations, with crashes involving alcohol or which were "hit and run," and with arrests for driving while intoxicated and related offenses. (Reproduced from U.S. Department of Transportation: *Alcohol and Highway Safety*, August 1968.)

fatalities, but major reduction in death rates will only come about through preventive programs primarily aimed at the drinking driver. Because the identification of the problem in such specific terms is a relatively new phenomenon, insufficient time has passed for major legislative or education programs to evolve. Clearly, however, such programs will tend to alter the traditional views of the society toward the automobile, the right to drive, and drivers' rights.

A similar process is occurring in the other industrialized nations as automobile ownership becomes increasingly widespread. The data in Table 12-7, though difficult to interpret because of the lack of a meaningful denominator, indicate an increasing death rate from automobiles in other nations. Because the factors involved in these high death rates are so intertwined with social values, it can be anticipated that there will be a considerable lag before the changes necessary to reduce the death rate are brought into force.

Chronic Bronchitis and Emphysema

Chronic bronchitis can hardly be called a new or emergent disease. First described by Bodham in 1808, it has had a place of honor among causes of death in England for many, many years. In the United States, though not considered as usual as in Britain, it has been a common condition, stirring little interest until recently. What is new is our recognition of its rising toll and its relationship to our habits and our environment.

One would certainly think that a disease that had been described 160 years ago would be simple to define, but that is not the case. The title of this section could have been, as well, "Chronic Obstructive Pulmonary Disease," "Chronic Lung Disease," or even "Respiratory Symptoms Complex" without drawing criticism for inaccuracy. Therefore, one of the first things that this disease or symptom complex has shown us is how difficult and important it is to standardize our definitions before we can begin to understand the epidemiology of a disease. The disease became a subject of considerable interest when it was seen to have strikingly different mortality rates in England and Wales as compared to other countries in Europe and North America (Reid, 1956). Its possible relationship to air pollution heightened interest and led to the many studies that have since contributed to its understanding. Tables 12-11, 12-12, and 12-13 give a picture of the mortality from bronchitis.

From Table 12-11 it can be seen that mortality rates from bronchitis differ strikingly among the nations listed. Generally, after a slow fall in mortality over the years (accentuated in the beginning of the antibiotic era), death rates have recently started to rise again. In Table 12-12, it is seen that the fall in rates is universal among the young in all nations and is accounted for by the decrease in acute bronchitis. (As mentioned earlier, acute bronchitis is an important cause of death among children in developing nations.) Our concern here is with chronic bronchitis, and it is this disease, occurring in older groups (but not the very old), that has seen rising death rates within the last decade or so in several countries. The change is striking in the United Kingdom, but is also seen, in Table 12-12, in Canada. The change is not apparent in the United States until the death rates are separated by sex as well as age as displayed in Table 12-13. There the important fact of the much greater frequency of the disease among males is seen, as well as the fact that deaths from the disease continue to drop among females but are rising among males in both countries. Displayed in this manner, the reason for the great concern with this problem, especially in Britain, is obvious.

The reasons for the apparently different mortality rates in different nations are far from obvious. Although the *International Statistical Classification of Disease, Injuries, and Causes of Death* is used by all these countries in coding causes of death, there are

TABLE 12-11

Death Rates per 100,000 from Bronchitis in Selected Countries from 1921–62*

	1921–25	1926–30	1931–35	1936–40	1941–45	1946–50	1951–55	1956–60	1961	1962
Canada	10.2	5.2	3.8	2.9	3.6	3.2	3.6	4.8	4.6	5.0
United States	8.1	5.2	3.4	3.0	2.7	2.2	1.9	2.2	2.2	2.5
United Arab Republic	—	229	215	191	272	197	197	180	150	—
Japan	7.3	50	41	35	31	34	15.7	9.5	7.9	8.4
Sweden	21	17	8.8	8.1	5.8	3.8	4.2	4.0	4.3	—
United Kingdom	94	71	49	84	71	66	68	63	68	71
Netherlands	24	24	16	15	14	9.7	10.6	11.4	10.2	11.7
France	—	32	21	—	10.4	6.4	4.9	3.4	3.9	4.9

* Vital statistics of World Health Organization—United Nations. The statistics refer to the international classification of disease diagnosis—bronchitis (B32).

346

TABLE 12-12
Death Rates per 100,000 from Bronchitis by Age for Selected Countries, 1931–35 and 1957–61 *

		All Ages	0–1	1–4	5–14	15–24	25–44	45–64	65–74	75+
Canada	1931–35	3.8	37.7	3.4	0.2	0.3	0.4	2.1	12.6	94.4
	1957–61	4.8	21.5	1.9	0.3	0.1	0.4	5.8	24.4	63.3
United States	1931–35	3.2	26.7	2.4	0.3	0.4	0.7	2.8	12.0	73.01
	1957–61	2.2	14.0	2.0	0.2	0.1	0.3	2.3	9.1	17.5
U.A.R.	1931–35				N O D A T A					
	1957–61	180.7	1509	800	19.5	4.0	8.9	38.8	215.5	632.3
Japan	1931–35	40.6	13	3.4	4.3	11.9	10.1	31.0	154.8	404.5
	1957–61	9.1	68.0	4.0	0.5	0.3	0.6	4.2	45.9	251.6
Sweden	1931–35	8.8	172.9	9.8	0.7	0.2	0.8	3.1	15.5	65.9
	1957–61	4.1	10.5	2.4	0.4	0.4	0.3	2.3	10.9	56.0
United Kingdom	1931–35	49.2	280.7	18.9	1.5	2.1	5.4	40.1	213.1	978.8
	1957–61	63.1	45.7	4.9	0.5	0.5	2.8	62.3	272.9	579.2
Netherlands	1931–35	15.8	61.9	4.8	0.7	0.9	1.5	10.6	114.2	693.6
	1957–61	11.1	3.7	1.2	0.1	0.2	0.5	12.9	50.1	173.9
France	1931–35	21.3	162.1	13.1	1.6	3.3	5.2	21.7	110.4	
	1957–61	4.3	5.6	0.6	0.0	0.1	0.1	2.2	13.5	55.6

* Vital statistics of World Health Organization—United Nations.

TABLE 12-13
Death Rates per 100,000 from Bronchitis by Age and Sex, United States and United Kingdom for 1931–35 and 1957–61 *

		All Ages	0–1	1–4	5–14	15–24	25–44	45–64	65–75	75+
United States 1931–35	Male	3.3	30.0	2.5	0.3	0.4	0.8	3.5	12.1	69.3
	Female	3.1	23.1	2.3	0.3	0.3	0.6	2.0	11.9	76.3
1957–61	Male	3.1	19.4	2.3	0.2	0.1	0.3	3.8	15.9	25.2
	Female	1.4	13.8	1.7	0.2	0.2	0.2	1.0	3.3	11.7
United Kingdom 1931–35	Male	52.0	313.0	19.2	1.5	2.3	7.3	56.5	247.4	1045.2
	Female	46.6	247.1	18.6	1.4	1.8	3.6	25.8	183.0	937.0
1957–61	Male	92.0	51.1	4.5	0.6	0.6	3.6	108.0	510.0	954.2
	Female	36.2	40.0	3.3	0.5	0.5	2.0	20.9	111.0	373.0

* Vital statistics of World Health Organization—United Nations.

differences in the practice of coding and classification that affect considerably the comparability of official mortality statistics on bronchitis (Mork, 1964). In addition, and of greater importance, medical traditions vary from place to place and markedly affect the diagnoses on medical certificates. There is certainly more chance that a British physician will diagnose chronic bronchitis as the underlying cause of death than would an American or Japanese physician in the same patient.

Underlying all these problems is the fact that there is no general agreement on definitions and terminology in the disease. It must be stressed that these difficulties are not present only across national boundaries, but are also present within different parts of the same country. Nonetheless, differences as striking as those displayed in Tables 12-11 to 12-13 call for further investigation because they seem to promise some understanding of the relationship between this disease and patterns of living. Despite these ambiguities, it has been possible to designate certain syndromes with explicit criteria whose epidemiology can then be studied (Goldsmith, 1960; Ciba Foundation, 1959; Fletcher, 1959).

A task force constituted by the Public Health Service, in conjunction with the National Tuberculosis Association, adopted the following definition (USPHS, 1967).

> Chronic bronchitis is a clinical disorder characterized by excessive mucous secretion in the bronchial tree. It is manifested by chronic or recurrent productive cough. The diagnosis of chronic bronchitis can be made only if other bronchopulmonary or cardiac disorders are excluded as the cause for these symptoms. The predominant pathologic change is hypertrophy and hyperplasia of the mucous secreting glands in the trachea and bronchi....
> Pulmonary emphysema is an anatomic alteration of the lung characterized by destruction of alveolar walls accompanied by abnormal enlargement of the air spaces distal to the terminal, nonrespiratory bronchiole.

It has not been possible, thus far, to provide a definition of chronic bronchitis that does not require the exclusion of other causes for the symptoms. Reid (1965) has given a useful structural basis to the clinical picture in her description of the alterations in the mucous and the mucous secreting structures of the bronchial tree. The change in the ratio of the diameter of mucous gland to the thickness of its wall has proved extremely reproducible with higher ratios found in chronic bronchitis and even emphysema than in the normal.

For the purposes of epidemiologic studies, the diseases can be defined in terms of the response to a standardized questionnaire as well as alterations in pulmonary function tests. The development of a questionnaire acceptable for use in different countries has represented a major advance in the studies of these diseases as well as a major example of the potential of international epidemiology. Almost universally used at the present time is the questionnaire (or its variant) developed in the United Kingdom by the Medical Research Council (Ashford, 1965).

On the basis of these questionnaires, chronic bronchitis is defined as persistent or recurrent cough and phlegm. Many studies have employed this tool and they form the basis for much of our knowledge of its prevalence in various parts of the United States as well as internationally. In an effort to put greater precision into the assessment of the prevalence of chronic obstructive pulmonary disease, pulmonary function tests have been extensively used in field studies. Pulmonary physiologists have been by no means consonant in their choice of the best measure of airway obstruction. A discussion of the pros and cons of the various techniques is beyond the scope of this chapter, but any investigator would be well advised to be cautious before stepping in the quicksands of choosing the "best," "simplest," or most "objective" measure of airway obstruction. By far the most commonly used pulmonary function test in field studies is the forced vital capacity. Of the numerous methods used to analyze it (Maximum Mid-Expiratory Flow Rate, MMFR; Forced Expiratory Volumes, FEV;

at different time intervals; Peak Flow Rate, PFR, and so on), the FEV 1.0 is perhaps the most frequently employed (Macklen and Mead, 1967). In addition to prevalence studies based on questionnaires and pulmonary function tests, studies on the determinants of these diseases have also been based on changes in morbidity and mortality in groups already diagnosed as having chronic pulmonary disease.

Thus far it has been possible to show a relationship between chronic obstructive pulmonary disease and a number of variables: age, sex, place of residence, socioeconomic status, season (climate), cigarette smoking, air pollution, occupation, and infection. The California Health Survey showed that a higher prevalence of chronic bronchitis was found in association with low family income (Goldsmith, 1965). A similar finding emerged from the Nashville Study on air pollution and health (Kenline and Contee, 1967). It must be remembered that families with low incomes tend to live in areas of higher environmental pollution so that the association could be spurious, but the findings of Winkelstein (1967) make it clear that socioeconomic status, even when it is disassociated from place of residence and degree of exposure to air pollution, is an important determinant in respiratory mortality.

By far the clearest association is between cigarette smoking and obstructive pulmonary disease. In virtually every study, no matter how done, the cigarette stands out as a disease determinant. So strong is the link that it tends to overwhelm other factors in which one may be interested. The relationship is not to cigars or pipes, or even to other peoples' smoke. As in other diseases, the symptoms frequently regress when smoking is discontinued. The effect of the cigarette is present if cough is the only symptom and is even present in the asymptomatic subject as shown by alterations in pulmonary function (Wynder et al., 1965; Zwi et al., 1964; Goldsmith et al., 1962; Densen et al., 1967). The effect of cigarette smoking has been assessed in monozygotic twins and is just as potent a factor as in others, thus distinguishing the effect from heredity (Cederloff et al., 1966).

The effect of climate and season is almost too obvious to require comment. However, the effect of climate is probably dependent in part upon the manner in which a population protects itself from the weather. In the United States, except in low economic groups, the year-round climate is, perhaps, 72°F. In the United Kingdom the situation is very different. There are those who feel that the absence of "adequate" heat and protection from the climate may play a part in what has been called the "English disease."

Since Reid's early studies (1956), the possible relationship between air pollution and chronic respiratory disease has attracted considerable attention. Within limited and climatically fairly homogeneous areas—for example, in London—the distribution of bronchitis mortality has been shown to reflect the varying concentrations of smoke and sulfur dioxide in the local atmosphere. A marked gradient exists between country districts and urban areas, one which correlates well with local pollution levels. Elevated levels of smoke and sulfur dioxide, however, are more than indicators of air pollution. Therefore, it may be unwarranted to assume a cause-and-effect relationship between air pollution and bronchitis. But sophisticated techniques have been used that show a positive correlation between local air-pollution levels and bronchitis death rates that are independent of such social characteristics as population density and income level.

The investigation of industrial cohorts has been widely used to delineate the various factors in the disease. In England studies on occupational groups where job and pay are uniform throughout the area have demonstrated an excess in bronchitis morbidity in the most heavily polluted districts (Reid, 1956; Cornwall and Raffle, 1961; Holland *et al.*, 1965). Postal employees, for example, working outside, have a higher bronchitis morbidity than postal employees who work inside.

Investigations employing the same techniques as those used in England have been carried out in the United States (Holland *et al.*, 1965; Densen *et al.*, 1967). The greater frequency of chronic respiratory disease in Britain as compared to the United States that has been indicated by the differences in death rates was confirmed (though to a lesser degree) in these studies of respiratory symptoms. The results also confirmed previous indications of more respiratory disease in British cities than rural areas. The prevalence of chronic respiratory disease was not as high in the United States as in rural England. In addition, the urban-rural differences were smaller in the United States and the prevalence has not been shown to vary greatly from New York to San Francisco or Los Angeles.

There are several areas in the United States where ambient sulfur dioxide concentrations are as high as those reached in London, although particulate matter is almost invariably very much less. In view of other evidence suggesting that the air pollution effect may result from a synergism between particle and gas, this atmospheric difference may be important (Cassell, 1968).

There may be some question about the role of air pollution in the production of chronic respiratory disease, but there seems to be no question that it is a factor in the aggravation of pre-existing symptoms or disease. It has been repeatedly demonstrated that the state of well-being of groups of patients with chronic pulmonary disease fluctuates in association with fluctuations in environmental pollution (Angel *et al.*, 1965; Lawther, 1958). It must be stressed that studies on the health effects of air pollution show quite convincingly that there is an effect of air pollution as a generality, but that the effect disappears when the role of individual pollutants is examined. The effect of the whole (including weather) appears to be greater than the sum of the parts.

The importance of occupation in diseases of the chest has long been known and many surveys of the prevalence of the pneumoconioses exist. The complex of symptoms that we are presently discussing has also been found in association with certain industries. The effects of cigarette smoking again enter the picture when it is shown that the decrement in pulmonary function in welders is greater if they are also smokers (Hunnicutt *et al.*, 1964). Enterline's (1967) studies on the prevalence of chronic pulmonary disease in miners have shown distinct variations from one mining community to another, although coal miners in general seem to have a far higher prevalence of the disease than the general United States population.

The Total Picture

Here, then, is a disease in which multiple factors are seen to play a role. Separating one factor out as the determinant is difficult, although the cigarette would have to take honors as the most prominent. The reasons for differences between nations, noted initially, have not been clarified. Although the existence and importance of national fashions in diagnosis as a reason for seeming differences in disease rates is apparent, they do not appear to be the sole reason for those differences. Students in this field are brought again and again against societal differences that appear to play a role. Even in cigarette smoking it is apparent that the British smoke differently than Americans (butt length, filters, puffs, and inhalation per minute, and so on). Home heating, open windows, and climate, medical care, and an endless number of other factors that are culturally determined take on meaning in the pattern of the disease. The realization of this immense complexity in the balance between health and disease should stimulate efforts to look beyond the narrow confines of sickness in an individual. It should make clear that an understanding of epidemiology is necessary for the understanding of the disease.

In the United States the individual with chronic obstructive pulmonary disease is a male cigarette-smoking, blue-collar worker over 45 and living in the poorer section of town. His air is dirty and his cough is responsive to the air and the weather. Why there are more of him today than ten years ago is not entirely clear. Whether his numbers will continue to increase, whether the essential determinant is laid down in child-hood is also not known. But he and his fellows have revealed to us the importance of multifactorial research in a manner that will not allow a retreat to more simplistic approaches.

IATROGENIC DISEASE

Iatrogenic disease may be divided into several categories: disease caused by inadvertent error and that due to diagnostic or therapeutic fashion (widespread tonsillectomy or hysterectomy and the treatment of "low blood pressure," as examples) are not new nor specifically the result of the changes wrought in medicine by its technological advances and its existence within the present social milieu. But three other areas remain that are relevant to our discussion.

The first is disease that occurs because of success in the treatment of other disease. The successes of the antibiotics in the treatment of the common bacterial diseases have not, as might have been naïvely expected, eliminated bacterial disease. The effect has been to change the prevalence of infection by various agents. Those organisms origin-ally responsible for many of the deaths from infection that occurred within the hospital, such as the pneumococcus and streptococcus, are replaced as a cause of death by other microbes. First, in the era between the emergence of penicillinase producing staphylo-cocci and their control by the penicillinase resistant penicillins, the staphylococcus came to prominence as a cause of infection and death (Finland et al., 1956). When these staphylococci also fell under the onslaught of effective antimicrobials, the gram-negative bacterial and fungi often replaced them in the lesions of hospitalized patients (Kislak et al., 1964). This evolution of resistant organisms is a dynamic process and it is to be expected that the distribution of organisms cultured from patients will continue to change as their environment changes (see Chapter 3).

What we learn from this is to distinguish between infectious diseases whose charac-teristics are primarily dependent upon the infecting organism and diseases whose characteristics are primarily dependent upon alterations within the host. The importance of the distinction in terms of therapeutic goals is considerable but frequently not reflected in the therapeutic regimen, which may be directed primarily against the organism instead of in support of the host (Cassell, 1962).

Successful maintenance of life by the use of steroids, immunosuppressive agents, radiation, and anticancer agents in patients who might otherwise have died of their basic disease sufficiently alters the host so that sometimes ordinarily benign organisms become pathogenic. The example given in Chapter 3 of the emergence of cytomegalic inclusion disease in the altered host is duplicated by other organisms such as the fungi and other commensals. In some instances these new infectious diseases are the lesser evil and the patient tolerates his new disease as the price of life. On other occasions the emergent infection is overwhelming and uncontrollable. Not all the changes in microbial disease are so easily related to changes in therapeutic agents or known alterations in the host. The change in streptococcal disease noted earlier and, for example, the changing pattern of bacterial endocarditis (Rabinovich *et al.*, 1968) serve to remind us of the dynamism of the interplay between organisms, environment, and host. Although we seem to know some of the determinants such as the use of antibiotics and the intentional alterations in the host, large parts of the picture remain unclear.

A second kind of iatrogenic disease is that which emerges solely as the result of new therapies or technology.

One of the older examples is the hemolytic anemia caused by glucose-6-phosphate dehydrogenase (G6PD) deficiency in the red blood cell. The cause of the anemia of favism, this hemolytic disease is also caused in G6PD-deficient individuals by drugs such as primaquine sulfonamides and other oxidant drugs (Wintrobe, 1967).

The syndrome of immunologic rejection is of major importance in the field of organ transplantation. Rejection crisis is a disease solely dependent on the immunosuppressive measures necessary to insure successful transplantation (Amos, 1968). Cardiac surgery offers another example in the hemolytic anemias attributed to increased intracardiac turbulence that have resulted from the use of artificial heart valves such as the Starr-Edwards ball valve (Brodeur *et al.*, 1965).

Not the least of the new diseases that have emerged as a result of technologic change are the psychiatric complications of organ transplants, the long-term use of the artificial kidney, and the sensory deprivation-like state of intensive care units (Kornfield, 1965). Frequently these emergent iatrogenic diseases have provided invaluable insight into basic pathophysiologic mechanisms.

Finally, iatrogenic disease can result from the unwanted and unexpected side effects of apparently appropriate therapy. Where disease emerged because of therapeutic success, it does not seem realistic to return to the previous era to avoid the new disease. Where disease has been uncovered by technologic advance it is not possible to "unmake" the disease by retreating to previous ignorance (but possibility of the newly emergent disease should become a factor in decision-making).

In the final category it often appears that the iatrogenic disease is a result of inadequate assessment of the risk of adverse reaction in the course of treatment. In part this may be because of poorly conceived therapeutic goals, but is is also because the magnitude of the probabilities of these new diseases is just becoming known to us.

In the past few years there has been increasing interest in the hazards of hospitalization and medical care. A surprisingly high prevalence of adverse episodes occurring in the hospital have been reported from good institutions (McLamb and Huntley, 1967; Schimmel, 1964). An adverse episode is defined as any response to medical care that is unintended, undesirable, or harmful to the patient. These episodes do not include inadvertent error or surgical complication, and thus represent true hazards of medical treatment or hospitalization. They range from reactions to therapeutic drugs through reactions to diagnostic or therapeutic procedures, acquired infections, and miscellaneous hospital hazards. About 20 per cent of patients admitted to hospitals will have such an episode. Of these, perhaps 50–60 per cent will be minor and subside spontaneously or not interfere with the patient's care or prolong his stay. About 30 per cent will be moderate and cause an increase in the length of hospitalization or require treatment. In the reported studies, from 6 to 20 per cent were life-threatening or contributed to death. (In the study of Schimmel, 1965, there were 16 deaths over the eight-month period of observation from a population at risk of 1,014 patients: a death rate of 2,000 per 100,000 per year!)

The populations in whom these episodes occur are similar to the general population of the hospital except that they tend to be slightly (but not greatly) older. Their diseases are the same and their readmission rate is similar. Their primary distinguishing characteristic is their length of hospital stay. It appears that the longer the patient remains in the hospital, the greater is his chance of an untoward episode, and thus the operative etiology seems to be the general hazard of hospitalization.

The greatest single contributor to the hazard appears to be untoward reactions to drugs—causing about 50 per cent of the episodes. Cluff and his group have studied this aspect in detail, using epidemiologic methods (Cluff *et al.*, 1965; Seidl *et al.*, 1966; Smith *et al.*, 1966). They have found that about 14 per cent of all patients develop an adverse reaction to at least one drug during hospitalization.

This expectation is doubled in patients who have been admitted because of a previous drug reaction. The risk is directly related to the number of drugs administered to the patient but cannot be primarily attributed to drug interaction, but to additive risk. Cardiac drugs and antibiotics are most often responsible for the reactions.

Women have a higher incidence of adverse reactions than men, but this is wholly accounted for by a predisposition, particularly in older women, to gastrointestinal side effects. (In white women over 50 years of age the rate of drug reactions approaches 40 per cent and is significantly higher than among Negro women.) The average duration of hospital stay is greater for those in whom a drug reaction occurs. The studies on penicillin reactions reveal the importance of using good epidemiologic methods for problems such as these. Adverse reactions to penicillin were found to occur in 8 per cent of the hospitalized population treated with the drug. That figure is considerably higher than the usually reported incidence of reactions. The higher rate is attributable, at least in part, to the closer observation of the hospitalized patients. (Over 40 per cent of the penicillin reactions in hospitalized patients were manifested by fever only.)

CONCLUSION

It should be apparent by now that the diseases that have been considered here are not the only ones that could have been chosen to show the intimacy of the relationship between society and disease. When any disease emerges to prominence or recedes to obscurity it does so as a result of changes in the host and his physical, medical, and social environment. Because the interrelationships are complex and often obscure is no reason to pretend a simplicity in regard to disease that does not exist.

It is not comprehension of the nature of the relationships that is necessary, but a clear understanding that the relationships exist and are vital to an understanding of health and illness.

And the process is a dynamic one. If the basic social change of the twentieth century is the emergence of disenfranchised peoples (as it may well be), then the emergence of women must certainly be one of the most important extensions of that change in the United States. Such an emergence would be impossible if women were not freed from long years of child-bearing by the low infant and childhood mortality that is our pattern. But what will be the effect of this major cultural change on our future illness pattern? And so it goes on.

REFERENCES

ACKERKNECHT, E. H.: Malaria in the Upper Mississippi Valley 1760–1900. *Bull His Med*, Suppl. no. 4. Johns Hopkins Press, Baltimore, 1945.

AMOS, B.: Immunologic factors in organ transplantation. *Amer J Med*, **44**:767–75, 1968.

ANGEL, H. H., *et al.*: Respiratory illness in factory and office workers. *Brit J Dis Chest* **59**:66, 1965.

APPLE, DORRIAN: How laymen define illness. *J Health Hum Behav*, **1**:219–25, 1960.

ASHFORD, JOHN: *Comparison of Two Symptom Questionnaires in Comparability in International Epidemiology*. In Acheson (ed.): 90–106. Milbank Memorial Fund, New York, 1965.

BAINTON, CEDRIC R., and PETERSON, DONALD R.: Deaths from coronary heart disease in persons 50 years of age and younger. *New Eng J Med*, **268**:569–74, 1963.

BEAMITH, JEROME J., and MALFETTI, JAMES: A psychological comparison of violator and non-violator automobile drivers in the 16–19 year age group. *Traffic Safety*, **6**:12–15, 1962.

BENJAMIN, B.: *Elements of Vital Statistics*. George Allen and Unwin, Ltd., London, 1959.

———: *Social and Economic Factors Affecting Mortality*. Mountain & Co., Hague, Netherlands, 1965.

BLOOM, SAMUEL W.: *The Doctor and His Patient*. Russell Sage Foundation, New York, 1963.

BORKENSTEIN, R. F., *et al.*: *The Role of the Drinking Driver in Traffic Accidents*. Department of Police Administration. Indiana University, Bloomington, Ind., 1964.

BRODEUR, M. T. H., *et al.*: Red blood cell survival in patients with aortic valvular disease and ball-valve prostheses. *Circulation*, **32**:570, 1965.

BROWN, I. D.: Decrement of skill observed after seven hours of car driving. *Psychonomic Science*, **7**:131–32, 1967.

CASSELL, ERIC J.: The tactics of chemoprophylaxis and chemotherapy. *Amer Rev of Resp Dis*, **86**:726–28, 1962.

CASSELL, ERIC J.: The health effects of air pollution and their implications for control. *Law and Contemporary Problems*, 33:197–216, Spring, 1968.

—— *et al.*: Reconsiderations of mortality as a useful index of the relationship of environmental factors to health. *Amer J Public Health*, 58:1653–57, September 1968.

CEDERLOFF, R., *et al.*: Respiratory symptoms and "angina pectoris" in twins with reference to smoking habits. *Arch Environ Health*, 13:726–37, 1966.

CHAPMAN, JOHN M., *et al.*: Relations of stress, tranquilizers, and serum cholesterol levels in a sample population. *Amer J Epidemiol*, 83:537–47, 1966.

CHRISTAKIS, GEORGE, *et al.*: Summary of the research activities of the anti-coronary club. *Public Health Rep*, 81:64–70, 1966.

CIBA FOUNDATION: Report on symposium on terminology, definition and classification of chronic pulmonary emphysema and related conditions. *Thorax*, 14:286, 1959.

CLIFFTON, EUGENE E., *et al.*: Effects of cigarette smoking on the coagulation of the blood. Unpublished data, 1968.

CLUFF, L. E., *et al.*: Epidemiological study of adverse drug reactions. *Trans Ass Amer Physicians*, 178:255–68, 1965.

CONGER, JOHN, *et al.*: Psychological and psychophysiological factors in motor vehicle accidents. *JAMA*, 169:1581–87, 1959.

CORNWALL, C. J., and RAFFLE, P.: Bronchitis sickness absence in London transport. *Brit J Industr Med*, 18:24, 1961.

DALTON, KATHERINE: Menstruation and accidents. *Brit Med J*, 1425–26, Nov. 12, 1960.

DAWBER, THOMAS R.: Coronary heart disease—morbidity, in the Framingham study and analysis of factors of risk. *Bibl Cardiol*, 13:9–24, 1963.

DAWBER, THOMAS R., KANNEL, WILLIAM, and LYELL, LOMA: An approach to longitudinal studies in a community: The Framingham Study. *Anns NY Acad Sci*, Art. 2, 107:539–56, 1963.

DENSEN, PAUL, *et al.*: A survey of respiratory disease among New York City postal and transit workers. *Environ Res*, 1:265, 1967.

DEUSCHLE, KURT, and ADAIR, JOHN: An interdisciplinary approach to public health on the Navajo Indian reservation: Medical and anthropological aspects. *Anns NY Acad Sci*, Art. 17, 84:887–905, 1960.

DOYLE, JOSEPH T., *et al.*: Cigarette smoking and coronary heart disease. *New Eng J Med*, 266:796–801, 1962.

DREW, G. C., COLQUHOUN, W. P., and LONG, H. A.: Effect of small doses of alcohol on a skill resembling driving. *Brit Med J*, II:993–99, 1958.

DUNBAR, HELEN F.: *Emotions and Bodily Change*. Columbia University Press, New York, 1954.

ECKSTEIN, R. W.: Effect of exercise and coronary artery narrowing on coronary circulation. *Circ Res*, 5:230, 1957.

ENTERLINE, PHILIP E.: The effects of occupation on chronic respiratory disease. *Arch Environ Health (Chicago)*, 14:189, 1967.

—— and STEWART, WILLIAM H.: Geographic patterns in deaths from coronary heart disease. *Public Health Rep*, 71:849–55, 1956.

FELCH, WILLIAM C., and VAN ITALLIE, THEODORE B.: Reflections on the pathologic physiology of atherosclerosis. *New Eng J Med*, 263:1243–1246, 1960.

FINLAND, M., and JONES, W. F.: Staphylococcal infections currently in large municipal hospitals. *Anns NY Acad Med*, 65:191–205, 1956.

FLETCHER, C. M.: Chronic bronchitis: Its prevalence, nature and pathogenesis. *Amer Rev Resp Dis*, 80:483, 1959.

FRIEDMAN, GARY, *et al.*: An evaluation of follow-up methods in the Framingham heart study. *Amer J Public Health*, 57:1015–24, 1967.

FRIEDMAN, MEYER, and ROSENMAN, ROY H.: Associations of specific overt behavior pattern with blood and cardiovascular findings. *JAMA*, 169:1286, 1959.

GALDSTON, IAGO (ed.): *Man's Image in Medicine and Anthropology.* Monograph IV, Institute of Social and Historic Medicine. International Universities Press, New York, 1963.

GARTLEY, E. (ed.): *Patients, Physicians and Illness.* JACO, Free Press, Glencoe, Ill., 1958.

GOLDSMITH, J. R.: Epidemiologic studies of obstructive pulmonary disease. A review of concepts and nomenclature. *Amer Rev Resp Dis,* **82**:485, 1960.

———: Epidemiology of bronchitis and emphysema. *Med Thorac,* **22**:1–23, 1965.

——— *et al.*: Pulmonary function and respiratory findings among longshoremen. *Amer Rev Resp Dis,* **86**:867, 1962.

GREENSHIELDS, B. D.: Changes in driver performance with time in driving. *Highway Research Record.* Highway Res Board, Art. **122**:75–88, 1966.

HÄÄKINEN, S.: *Accidents and Driver Characteristics: A Statistical and Physicological Study.* Institute of Occupational Health, Helsinki, Finland, 1958.

HAMMOND, E. C., and HORN, DANIEL: Smoking and death rates—report on forty-four months of follow-up of 187,783 men. *JAMA,* **166**:1159–72, 1958.

HOLCOMB, R. L.: Alcohol in relation to traffic accidents. *JAMA,* **111**:1076–85, 1938.

HOLLAND, W. W., *et al.*: Respiratory disease in England and the United States. *Arch Environ Health (Chicago),* **10**:338, 1965.

HUNNICUTT, T. N., *et al.*: Spirometric measurements in welders. *Arch Environ Health (Chicago),* **8**:661, 1964.

IGNATOWSKI, A.: Cited by Anitschkow in Cowdry, E. V. (ed.): *Arteriosclerosis.* New York, 1933.

JENKINS, C. DAVID: Group differences in perception: A study of community beliefs and feelings about tuberculosis. *Amer J Sociol,* **71**:417–29, 1966.

JOLLIFFE, N., *et al.*: Anti-coronary club: Including discussions on serum cholesterol level of middle-aged men. *Amer J Clin Nutr,* **7**:451–62, 1959.

KANNEL, WILLIAM B., DAWBER, THOMAS R., and McNAMARA, PATRICIA: Detection of the coronary-prone adult: The Framingham Study. *J Iowa Med Soc,* **56**:26–34, January 1966.

——— *et al.*: Epidemiology of coronary heart disease. *Geriatrics,* **17**:675–90, 1962.

———: Risk factors in coronary heart disease. An evaluation of several serum lipids as predictors of coronary heart disease: The Framingham Study. *Ann Intern Med,* **61**:888–899, 1964.

KENLINE, P., and CONTEE, C.: Nashville air pollution and health study—A summary. *Public Health Rep,* **82**:17, 1967.

KENT, ANNE P., *et al.*: A comparison of coronary artery disease (arteriosclerotic heart disease) deaths in health areas of Manhattan, New York City. *Amer J Public Health,* **48**:200–07, 1956.

KEYS, ANCEL: Arteriosclerotic heart disease in a favored community. *J Chronic Dis,* **19**:245–54, 1966.

KING, STANLEY H.: *Perceptions of Illness and Medical Practice.* Russell Sage Foundation, New York, 1962.

KISLAK, J. W., *et al.*: Hospital acquired infections and antibiotic usage in the Boston City Hospital. *New Eng J Med,* **271**:834–35, 1964.

LAWTHER, P. J.: Climate, air pollution, and chronic bronchitis. *Proc Roy Soc Med,* **51**:262, 1958.

LEREN, P.: The effect of plasma cholesterol lowering diet in male survivors of myocardial infarctions. *Acta Med Scand,* **466**:1–92, 1966.

LEVIN, M. E., and RECANT, L.: Diabetes and the environment. *Arch Environ Health (Chicago),* **12**:621, 1966.

LILLIENFELD, ABRAHAM: Variations in mortality from heart disease. *Public Health Rep,* **71**:545–52, 1956.

LITMAN, R. E., and TABACHNIK, N.: Fatal one-car accidents. *Psychoanal Quart*, **36**:248–59, 1967.

LOGAN, W. P. D.: Mortality from coronary and myocardial disease in different social classes. *Lancet*, **262**:758–59, 1952.

LOOMIS, T. A., and WEST, C. A.: The influence of alcohol on automobile driving ability. *Quart J Stud Alcohol*, **19**:30–46, 1958.

LUCAS, G. T., *et al.*: Quantitative studies of the relationship between alcohol levels and motor vehicle accidents. *Proc. 2nd International Conference on Alcohol and Road Traffic, 1953*, 139–42. Garden City Press, Toronto, 1955.

MCCARROLL, J. R., and HADDON, W., JR.: A controlled study of fatal automobile accidents in New York City. *J Chronic Dis*, **15**:811–26, 1962.

MACKLEM, PETER, and MEAD, JERE: The physiological basis of common pulmonary function tests. *Arch Environ Health*, **14**:5–9, 1967.

MCLAMB, J. T., and HUNTLEY, R. R.: The hazards of hospitalization. *Southern Med J*, **60**:469–72, 1967.

MILLER, CLARENCE K.: Psychological correlates of coronary artery disease. *Psychosom Med*, **27**:257–65, 1965.

MORDKOFF, ARNOLD M., and PARSONS, OSCAR: The coronary personality: A critique. *Psychosom Med*, **29**:1–14, 1967.

MORK, TORBJØRN: International comparisons of the prevalence of chronic bronchitis. *Proc Roy Soc Med*, **57**:975–78, 1964.

NATIONAL SAFETY COUNCIL: *National Safety Council Accident Facts*. Chicago, 1968.

NORMAN, L. G.: *Road Traffic Accidents*. Public Health Papers, no. 12, WHO, Geneva 1962.

PARRISH, HENRY M., *et al.*: Increasing autopsy incidence of coronary heart disease in women. *Arch Intern Med (Chicago)*, **118**:436–45, 1966.

PAUL, BENJAMIN D. (ed.): *Health, Culture and Community: Case Studies of Public Reaction, to Health Programs*. Russell Sage Foundation, New York, 1955.

PEARSALL, MARION: *Medical Behavioral Science: A Selected Bibliography of Cultural Anthropology, Social Psychology, and Sociology in Medicine*. University of Kentucky Press, Lexington, Ky., 1963.

PELL SIDNEY, and D'ALONZO, ANTHONY: Myocardial infarctions in a large industrial population. *J Am Cir Assoc*, **185**:831–38, 1963.

PETERSON, J. E., *et al.*: Hourly change in serum cholesterol concentration effects of the anticipation of stress. *Circulation*, **25**:798, 1962.

PLATT, F. N.: As quoted by Norman, L. G., *op. cit.*, 51.

RABINOVICH, SERGIO, *et al.*: The changing pattern of bacterial endocarditis. *Med Clin N Amer*, **52**:1091–1101, 1968.

REID, D. D.: General epidemiology of chronic bronchitis. *Proc Roy Soc Med*, **49**:767, 1956.

REID, LYNNE: Natural history of mucus in the bronchial tree. *Arch Environ Health*, **10**:265–73, 1965.

ROSENMAN, ROY H., *et al.*: A predictive study of coronary heart disease. *JAMA*, **189**:103–110, 1964.

ROSENOW, J. H., and WATKINS, R. W.: Attitude, stress, and disease. *Modern Medicine*, **35**:33–41, 1967.

RUBIN, VERA (ed.): Culture, society and medicine. *Ann NY Acad Sci*, Art. 17, **84**:783–1060, 1960.

SAUNDERS, LYLE: *Cultural Difference and Medical Care*. Russell Sage Foundation, New York, 1954.

SCHIMMEL, ELIHU M.: The hazards of hospitalization. *Ann Intern Med*, **60**:100, 1964.

SCHUSTER, DONALD: Prediction of follow-up driving accidents and violations. *Traffic Safety*, **12**:17–21, 1968.

Seidl, L. G., et al.: *Bull Hopkins Hosp.* **119**: 299–315, 1966.

Shapiro, Samuel, et al.: The H.I.P. study of incidence and prognosis of coronary heart disease. *J Chronic Dis*, **18**:527–58, 1965.

Shaw, Lynnette: The practical use of projective personality tests as accident predictors. *Traffic Safety*, **9**:34–72, 1965.

Smith, Jay W., et al.: Studies on the epidemiology of adverse drug reactions. *New Eng J Med*, **274**:998–1002, 1966.

Spain, David: Problems in the study of coronary atherosclerosis in population groups. *Ann NY Acad Sci*, Art. 17, **83**:816–34, 1960.

Stamler, J.: Epidemiology of atherosclerotic coronary heart disease. *Postgrad Med*, **25**:610, 1959.

—— et al.: Prevalence and incidence of coronary heart disease in strata of the labor force of a Chicago industrial population. *J Chronic Dis*, **11**:405–20, 1960.

Syme, Leonard S.: Cultural mobility and coronary heart disease in an urban area. *Amer J Epidem*, **82**:334–46, 1966.

Tillman, William A., and Hobbs, G. E.: The accident-prone automobile driver: A study of the psychiatric and social background. *Amer J Psychiat*, **106**:321–31.

—— et al.: Group therapy amongst persons involved in frequent automobile accidents. *Prevention of Highway Injury*, 63–69. Highway Research Institute, University of Michigan, Ann Arbor, Mich., 1967.

Tobachnik, N., and Litman, R. E.: Character and life circumstance in fatal accident. *Psychoanal Forum*, **1**:65–74, 1966.

Tracy, Richard E.: Sex difference in coronary disease: Two opposing views. *J Chronic Dis*, **19**:1245–51, 1966.

United Nations: *Population and Vital Statistics*. Statistical Papers, Ser. A, Vol. XX, no. 2, New York, 1968.

U.S. Department of Transportation: *Alcohol and Highway Safety*. A Report to the Congress from the Secretary of Transportation. August 1968.

U.S. Public Health Service: Chronic respiratory disease control program. Report of the task force on chronic bronchitis and emphysema. *National Tuberculosis Assoc Bull (Mount Morris)*, **53**:1–23, 1967.

——: *The Health Consequences of Smoking*. 1696, 1967.

——: *Smoking and Health:* Report of the Advisory Committee to the Surgeon General of the Public Health Service. 1964.

——, National Center for Health Statistics: *Coronary Heart Disease in Adults— U.S., 1960–1962*. Pub. no. 1000, series 11, no. 10, 1965.

——, ——: *United States Life Tables by Causes of Death: 1959–1961*. Vol. 1, no. 6, Pub. no. 1252, Vol. 1, no. 6, 1968.

——, National Vital Statistics Division: *Mortality by Industry and Cause of Death Among Men 20–64 Years of Age*. Vital Statistics, Special Reports, Vol. 53, no. 4, 1963.

Van Itallie, Theodore B., and Felch, William C.: Reflections on the pathologic physiology of atherosclerosis. *New Eng J Med*, **263**:1179–84, 1960.

Wardwell, Walter I., et al.: Social and psychological factors in coronary heart disease. *J Health Hum Behav*, **4**:154–65, 1963.

Wellin, Edward: Implications of local culture for public health. *Applied Anthro*, **16**:16–18, 1958.

White, Neil K., et al.: The relationship of the degree of coronary atherosclerosis with age in men. *Circulation*, **1**:645–54, 1950.

Winkelstein, W., et al.: The relationship of air pollution and economic status to total mortality and selected respiratory system mortality in men. *Arch Environ Health (Chicago)*, **14**:162, 1967.

Wintrobe, Maxwell: *Clinical Hematology*, 6th ed., 643 pp., Lea and Febiger, 1967.

WOLF, S., *et al.*: Changes in serum lipids in relation to emotional stress during rigid control of diet and exercise. *Circulation,* **26**:379, 1962.

WORLD HEALTH ORGANIZATION: *Epidemiological and Vital Statistics Report: Ten Leading Causes of Death for Selected Countries in Africa, South and Central America and Asia,* no. 2, 1967.

————: *Epidemiological and Vital Statistics Report: Ten Leading Causes of Death for Selected Countries in North America, Europe and Oceania,* no. 1, 1967.

————: *1954 Expert Committee on Alcohol, First Report. WHO Techn Rep Ser,* no. 84. Geneva, no. 14.

————: *Morbidity Statistics—12th Report of the WHO Expert Committee on Health Statistics. WHO Tech Rep Ser,* no. 389.

————: *Third Report on the World Health Situation, 1961–1964.* Official Records of the World Health Organization, no. 155, Geneva, 1967.

————: *World Health Statistics Annual,* Vol. 1. *Vital Statistics and Causes of Death,* 1967.

————: *World Health Statistics Annual,* Vol. 2. *Infectious Diseases,* 1968.

WYNDER, E. L., *et al.*: Epidemiology of persistent cough. *Am Rev Resp Dis,* **91**:679–700, 1965.

ZWI, S., *et al.*: Cigarette smoking and pulmonary function in healthy young adults. *Amer Rev Resp Dis,* **89**:73–81, 1964.

PART THREE

The Administration of Health Services

13

The Administration of Public Health

Alonzo S. Yerby

INTRODUCTION

Public health administration may be defined as those managerial activities necessary for the organized promotion and protection of the health of a community. When public health administration is a governmental function, it may be considered to be a specialized branch of public administration. Health administration may be defined as those activities necessary to carry out a health function through the medium of an organization created for this purpose. By this definition public health administration is a categorical branch of health administration. The question is whether the "public" or the "health" characteristic is dominant.

From the standpoint of its evolution, public health administration has been more closely related to health professionals and matters affecting health than it has been related to public administration. Public involvement in health has taken place when events have given rise to major outbreaks of disease or to development of widespread discomfort or disability. When nineteenth-century reformers, armed with data relating high death rates to unsanitary living and working conditions, cried out for corrective action, they equated the public good with the protection of the health of the individual. Their language was forceful, their intent quite clear.

One of the primary prejudices . . . which sanitary reform has to encounter, is a vague apprehension of undue interference. All regulations for securing cleanliness and removing filth are apt to be considered as invasions of the privacy of the domestic health and the person, and amounting to an impertinent intermeddling, in matters concerning which it is insulting even to be inquisitive. But in reality the object of sanitary reform is to free the citizen from the vile fetters with which the acts of others have actually bound him, and to leave him free to pursue the natural tendency towards civilization and refinement, rather than to assume any arbitrary contest over his actions. We believe it to be quite true that it

363

always injures the individual to do for him what he ought, and is able, to do for himself. But the operative workman must live in the city, or starve; and if selfish wealth has made the city such that he cannot find a cell in it which is not a living tomb, saturated with corruption,—then he is not left to the freedom of his own actions, but is subject to an abominable bondage caused by the conduct of others. The strength and skill of Hercules could not enable the city artisan of Glasgow to live in purity, and if legislation cleanses the Augean stable, it is not doing for him what he should have been left to do for himself, but only saving him from suffering by the selfishness of third parties beyond his reach."

(*Edinburgh Review*, January 1850, p. 213, as quoted in Shattuck, L.: *Report of the Sanitary Commission of Massachusetts*, Boston, 1850.)

However, the zeal of the reformer did not always motivate the early sanitary commissions and boards of health that were appointed as an outcome of the demand for sanitary reform. Often unable to marshall the facts and unwilling to take action, their effectiveness was minimal.

Continuing public demand the involvement of physicians and other health professionals gradually led to the establishment of health departments capable of taking effective action. Laws were passed calling for the reporting of births and deaths and the causes of death and for the reporting of certain communicable diseases. Environmental sanitation was improved, particularly through the provision of community water supplies and sewerage disposal systems.

Discoveries of the nature of contagion and the mode of spread of disease producing microorganisms led to efforts to protect water supplies, food, and milk from contamination. With the discovery of immunizing agents came organized programs for the immunization of susceptible populations.

Some early public health agencies, notably the New York City Health Department, pioneered in the field of child health. Nurses were employed to teach child care to mothers living in poor neighborhoods, and low-cost pasteurized milk was distributed to families with small children. The milk stations that were established for this purpose soon became well-baby clinics. Advice and guidance on child care was given to the mother, and the babies were examined for abnormalities of growth and development and were immunized against smallpox and other infectious diseases.

The passage of federal legislation in 1912 establishing the Children's Bureau and the enactment of the Sheppard-Towner Act in 1921 provided the framework and financial aid needed to encourage the states to promote and extend child health services. The Social Security Act of 1935 and its Title V authorized the Children's Bureau to make annual grants to the states to assist in the extension and improvement of maternal and child health services. During World War II, the Children's Bureau was called upon to administer the Emergency Maternity and Infant Care Program for the wives of servicemen.

The willingness of the Congress to enact laws and appropriate funds for personal health services for mothers and children represented a significant and new role for public health in the United States. Prior to this development the care of individuals had been accepted as a public concern when such care had been considered necessary to protect other members of the community. This had been the justification for the establishment at public expense of institutions for the mentally ill and for persons suffering from tuberculosis and other communicable diseases.

Medical care of individuals as provided for in the Crippled Children's Program and the Wartime EMIC Program established one other important precedent. These programs were the first in the United States under public health auspices to establish standards affecting the quality of the care provided. The Children's Bureau required that each state participating in the programs, with the help of expert professional committees, establish standards governing the qualifications of physicians and the adequacy of maternity, newborn, and orthopedic services in hospitals providing services under the Crippled Children's and EMIC Programs.

The addition of personal health services as a function of public health departments strengthened the role of physicians and other health professionals in these agencies. Schools of Public Health came into being and began to attract physicians who wished to pursue careers as health officers. In time, graduation from a school of public health became a prerequisite for the directors of most public health departments throughout the United States.

The transition from sanitary reform to a health service agency established the primacy of the physician administrator in the field of public health. However, there were other factors related to or growing out of this development. As a professional, the physician viewed this role as apolitical. He encouraged and often insisted upon arrangements to insulate him from politics. He preferred to be appointed by and answer to a board of health (usually dominated by physicians) rather than be appointed by a mayor or governor. When appointed for a specific term the board and the incumbent health officer favored a term of office not coterminous with that of the chief executive. In some states laws were enacted that limited membership on boards of health to practising physicians or to members of the state medical society. The physician chosen as health officer under these circumstances often considered his first loyalty to be to his professional colleagues and their interests.

This emphasis on professionalism tended to weaken the concept of the health officer as a public servant and explains in part the lack of identification of public health with public administration. Although preoccupation with the professional role may have protected health departments from some of the harmful effects of political patronage and from political intervention on behalf of certain special interests groups, it was not an unmixed blessing. Chief executives unable to control health departments as they controlled other branches of government sometimes reacted with indifference to health department requests for more adequate support. Health officers eschewing a political role failed to act politically to accomplish desirable ends. The insulation against political interests was bought at the price of becoming beholden to the (also) special interests of the health establishment.

Schools of public health, somewhat unwittingly, perpetuated this state of affairs. Frequently key professors were recruited from the ranks of well-known health commissioners. The curricula of such schools tended to emphasize professional constraints rather than public responsibility and public need. By a curious bit of reverse logic the public aspect of public health administration became a limiting factor in the further evolution of the field. Public health came to mean only those things that were not considered the preserve of voluntary, proprietary, and other private interests in the health field. The traditional American distrust of government, the individualism of most physicians, and the fear of economic competition served to restrict public health to those activities that the private sector was unwilling or unable to undertake. The development and spread of compulsory health insurance programs in Europe was viewed by many Americans as a great evil and something to be avoided at all costs. The phrase "socialized medicine" became a rallying cry for those who opposed any expansion of governmental effort in care or in the prevention of illness. Medical societies and other groups took upon themselves a watchdog function to prevent governmental health agencies from extending their functions into provision of personal health services.

Health departments were restricted to a secondary or residual role in contrast to the private sector. Voluntary nonprofit agencies with funds derived from philanthropic sources or public subscription became the innovators of the public health field. Inherently more flexible than government and free to select the problems they would attack, their accomplishments and contributions to the field of public health were great indeed.

A major factor in the development of public health administration in the United States was the establishment of schools of public health in the first half of the twentieth century (see also Chapter 5). Aided and stimulated by health-oriented philanthropic agencies such as the Rockefeller Foundation and the Commonwealth Fund, schools of public health were established in a number of major universities including California, Columbia, Harvard, the state universities of Michigan, Minnesota, and North Carolina, also Tulane, Yale, and the Medical Faculty of Zagreb, Yugoslavia. The development of schools of public health in close association with or as part of schools of medicine served to strengthen the scientific and professional base of the public health administration. The proper emphasis on health, however, tended to obscure the need to be concerned with administration. Little contact was made with other university programs concerned with administration. The social sciences, public administration, and business administration were thought not to be relevant to the teaching of health administration by the physician administrators turned teachers. Students were required to take descriptive courses that catalogued health agencies and organizations. Administrative functions, such as planning, budget preparation, and evaluation, were taught as technical, almost mechanical, activities without a conceptual base. There was no theory, there were no hypotheses to be tested, only anecdotes and experiences presented as principles.

Physicians completed such training and took jobs as public health administrators only to learn that the principles were often not applicable, and they then learned by trial and error or they failed. In a field dominated by specialization, the public health administrator with one year of postgraduate training was neither a specialist in health nor a specialist in administration.

CHANGING ROLE OF THE PUBLIC HEALTH AGENCY

Over the past decade the role and function of the public health agency has undergone significant change. There has been an alteration of activities in the field of environmental health and a growth in activities related to the provision of personal health services.

The change in environmental health activities has been a reflection of the change in the nature and source of environmental health hazards. Public health agencies have had a traditional concern for the problems associated with substandard housing, unsafe disposal of human waste, poor food hygiene, and the contamination of drinking water. Although substandard housing remains as a significant problem, substantial gains have been made in the protection of water supplies, in the provision of sanitary sewerage systems, and the hygenic production and serving of foods.

Offsetting these gains have been the enormous growth in atmospheric pollution, and the disposal of industrial wastes in streams, rivers, and oceans, and the growing military, industrial, and medical use of radioactive substances. Frequently, the sources of pollutants and contaminants of air and water are located at great distances from the affected areas. Carried by the winds or the flow of waters, pollutants travel across geographic and political boundaries. Corrective action by local or even state health agencies acting alone is not feasible under these circumstances.

For this and other reasons, separate agencies concerned with air pollution, the protection of water resources, and the control of the use and disposal of radioactive substances have been established. These agencies are often organized on a regional or interstate basis. They may involve appropriate health officials in an advisory capacity but they tend to be under the direction of engineers rather than public health physicians.

The increase in the involvement of public health agencies with personal health services has been caused by the growing importance of chronic degenerative diseases and the passage of a number of federal laws that have had the effect of extending the responsibility of state and local public health agencies.

Chronic illness has replaced infectious disease as the primary cause of death and morbidity in industrialized nations. In the United States only one type of infectious disease (influenza and pneumonia) now ranks among the 15 leading causes of death (Table 13-1).

In general, the major causes of death, heart disease and cancer and vascular lesions affecting the central nervous system, are conditions for which specific preventive measures are not available. Many of the diseases in this grouping, however, respond quite well to adequate therapy. Often the institution of treatment during the early stages of the disease retards its progress and prevents the development of disabling sequelae. For this reason early detection of many chronic degenerative diseases is considered a necessary public health activity. Multiphasic screening programs have been instituted by health departments to improve the over-all rate of early disease detection at the community level (see Chapter 8). These programs are organized efforts to detect abnormal variations in body function that have been shown to be associated with certain disease conditions. In general, persons who have positive findings on the basis of screening examinations are referred to their personal physicians for diagnosis and treatment. Because many people do not have a personal physician public health agencies have found it necessary to arrange for medical care in many instances. In some jurisdictions, health departments operate hospitals for the care of chronically ill patients as well as conduct detection and educational programs concerned with specific chronic diseases.

TABLE 13-1
Mortality from 15 Leading Causes of Death: United States, 1963 *
[Ranked on the basis of the List of 60 Selected Causes of Death. Numbers after
causes of death are category numbers of the Seventh Revision of the
International Lists, 1955]

Rank Order	Cause of Death		Rates per 100,000 Population	Per Cent of Total Deaths
	All causes		961.9	100.0
1.	Diseases of heart	400–402, 410–443	375.4	39.0
2.	Malignant neoplasms, including neoplasms of lymphatic and hematopoietic tissues	140–205	151.4	15.7
3.	Vascular lesions affecting central nervous system	330–334	106.7	11.1
4.	Accidents	E800–E962	53.4	5.6
...	Motor vehicle accidents	E810–E835	23.1	2.4
...	Other accidents	E800–E802, E840–E962	30.3	3.1
5.	Influenza and pneumonia, except pneumonia of newborn	480–493	37.5	3.9
6.	Certain diseases of early infancy	760–776	33.3	3.5
7.	General arteriosclerosis	450	19.9	2.1
8.	Diabetes mellitus	260	17.2	1.8
9.	Other diseases of circulatory system	451–468	12.9	1.3
10.	Other bronchopulmonic diseases	525–527	12.3	1.3
11.	Cirrhosis of liver	581	11.9	1.2
12.	Suicide	E963, E970–E979	11.0	1.1
13.	Congenital malformations	750–759	11.0	1.1
14.	Other hypertensive disease	444–447	6.7	0.7
15.	Ulcer of stomach and duodenum	540, 541	6.5	0.7
...	All other causes	Residual	94.8	9.9

* Mortality Trends in the United States, 1954–1963. National Center for Health Statistics, Series 20, no. 2, U.S. Dep. of Health, Education, and Welfare.

In addition to the impact of chronic illness on the programs of health departments, there have been enacted by the United States Congress a number of measures designed to improve the availability of medical care to certain high-risk population groups. These laws have provided funds to the states to permit them to provide or purchase medical care for the indigent, the medically indigent, children, and pregnant women, and to supplement the care available to aged persons covered under compulsory and voluntary health insurance.

For the most part, the basic responsibility for these programs has been placed in departments of public welfare, but health departments are called upon to develop and to administer standards and conditions that must be met by participating health institutions and practitioners. In some states health departments have been made responsible for the administration of all phases of these medical-care programs except the determination of financial eligibility.

The inadequacy of health resources and their poor distribution has led to the enactment of additional legislation giving a central role to state public health agencies in the planning of health services for the entire population.

The changing role of the public health agency is to be seen in the report *Educational Qualifications of Physician-Directors of Official Health Agencies* by the American

Public Health Association. The Association statement described the three major areas of responsibility of public health agencies as

1. Promotion of personal and community health;
2. Maintenance of a healthful environment; and
3. An aggressive attack on disease and disability.

The report goes on to state that the official health agency should furnish primary leadership in assuring that all community health needs are met. The report adds, however, the somewhat gratuitous qualification that this goal is to be accomplished either through direct provision of services or indirectly through other official and voluntary agencies and the private sector. Because public health agencies lack both the legal mandate and the resources to meet *all* community health needs, their efforts must complement and supplement the activities of a wide variety of agencies and individual practitioners.

Turning to the matter of priorities and methodology, the APHA report states:

> The emphasis is on physical and mental health with primary prevention of disease where possible; or if not, then with secondary prevention through battling the progress of illness; prevention or treatment of the complications of sequelae; and rehabilitation. This is achieved through analysis and improvement of (1) the systems which provide for the delivery of health services, (2) the quality of health care which these systems provide, and (3) the adequacy of facilities and manpower in these systems for giving quality health care to the entire community.

Here we note that in addition to its role as a provider of services the public health agency is called upon to monitor the services provided by others and to improve them. For services it finds wanting, the report indicates that they are to be improved by (1) comprehensive health planning, (2) coordination, and (3) encouragement of community action and of research. There is no mention of the conflicts that are inherent in the complex role of monitor, supervisor, catalyst, and provider of services.

THE NEED FOR A THEORY OF PUBLIC HEALTH ADMINISTRATION

The complexity of the role of the public health administrator is a reason in itself why health administration deserves study and research. If health administration is to become a discipline in its own right, or even a specialized branch of public administration, it must evolve a body of theory. Gordon McLachlan, commenting on current research in medical care, described as universal and perplexing questions the deployment of skills and money and the establishment of policies concerned with the rate and direction of the development of health services in totally different kinds of areas (MacLachlan, 1964). He concludes that indeed it is all too evident that we are suffering from the lack of a theory of administration of health services. This deceptively simple observation is one of the core problems in the organization and delivery of health services. We lack a body of theory that is applicable and holds true in a variety of situations. We lack predictive tools to help lessen, if not avoid, the continuing reliance on trial and error.

Theory must grow out of testable and tested hypotheses; health administrators, however, have not taken the time to develop them. Research in health services, a long-neglected area, recently has begun to reach respectable proportions. Investigators in the United States, Canada, Latin America, Scandinavia, and the United Kingdom are publishing the results of their studies dealing with such matters as health organizations, the need for and utilization of health services, the measurement of health service effectiveness, the design of health facilities, and the evolving role of the social sciences in health administration.

Another explanation for the lack of theory in health administration is the fact that for many years schools of public health taught "public health practice" without reference to the social sciences. Little or no recognition was given to those aspects of social science theory that are highly relevant to the activities of the health administrator. Fortunately, the situation has changed. Schools of public health are broadening the teaching of public health practice to encompass the administration of all forms and types of health services. Cooperative research and teaching efforts are developing between schools of public health and schools of government, business administration, and law. Departments of health administration have drawn upon the faculties in departments of economics and political science, and sociologists, social anthropologists, and social psychologists have been invited to participate in the teaching of health administration. One university department of health services administration now has twelve different fields represented on its faculty.* A recent text on health administration devotes the first four of its thirteen chapters to general administration theory, an introduction to the social sciences, behavioral sciences, and organization and economic analysis. In its introduction the authors underscore the vastness of the field, the great variety of activities involved in administration, and the recent development of systematic thinking about the administrative process. They cite the work of Cole who has suggested that three phases in the evolution of administration can be distinguished: the empirical, the rational, and the cognitive. Empirical or traditional administration is the pragmatic rule-of-thumb approach. Rational administration began to develop about the turn of the century with the rise of "scientific management." It is concerned with techniques such as budgeting, work study, planning, and market research. Cognitive administration, the third and current phase, is a blending of sophisticated techniques and an appreciation of the interrelationship between the administrative unit and highly dynamic environment. It stresses adaptability to change as a requisite for organizational efficiency and survival.

The growth and development of computer technology has not only made possible the storage and instant retrieval of vast amounts of data; it has facilitated the development of a systems approach to the analysis of a wide variety of functions and operations. Systems analysis, operations research, and mathematical simulation have provided valuable tools and techniques for making quantitative measures of effectiveness and efficiency in functional and in economic terms. The application of these

* The Harvard School of Public Health's Department of Health Services Administration includes among its faculty persons from the fields of public health, hospital, medical care, and business administration, law, nursing, health education, political science, social anthropology, biostatistics, systems analysis, and operations research, and economics.

quantitative methods to the health field has added a much needed scientific dimension to health administration (see Chapter 9 for a fuller discussion).

Health administration must be acutely aware of the implication of scientific, technological, and social change. Lacking the constraints of a competitive market, it must rely heavily on effective administration to promote efficiency of operation. Because the product it seeks to produce is better health for communities of men through the judicious marshaling of the capabilities of healing professionals, it is a calling of high purpose that demands the very best of its practitioners.

HEALTH ORGANIZATIONS

By definition, the health administrator is concerned with health organizations. The organization is his natural and necessary environment. Unlike the physician or nurse, the administrator working alone is impotent. He is like a musician without an instrument or perhaps more like a conductor without an orchestra. He must work within and through the structure of an organization.

In general, public health organizations have developed out of *ad hoc* arrangements created to deal with specific problems. Early health departments came into being and grew by accretion as problems were identified that were susceptible to collective action. There were programs for the control of certain environmental health hazards, which in time were subdivided into separate programs for the protection of water, milk, food, housing sanitation, and so on. There were programs for the control of communicable diseases and often separate programs for the control of tuberculosis.

At the same time it became necessary to organize some programs on the basis of clientele. The programs for infants and pregnant women were followed by separate clientele-based programs for school children and preschool children.

Because health problems were rarely spread evenly over a community, it became necessary to organize programs on a geographic basis concentrating resources in areas of greatest need. The work of the early settlement houses and the success of child health stations, both located in poor neighborhoods much in need of services, led to the establishment of district health centers in Boston, New York, and other cities. These centers became a decentralized focus for the attack on prevalent health problems of the poorer sections of the city. As cities grew in size and complexity, health districts were delineated. Because these tended to be based on some arbitrarily chosen unit size of population their location reflected population density, which was in itself a direct correlation of the magnitude of health problems.

As public health agencies grew in size and in variety of functions they found it necessary to organize certain functions on the basis of process. Budget preparation and fiscal control, record keeping and reporting, and personnel administration became separate units although sometimes they were located in loosely organized bureaus or divisions of administration.

Thus, as Schaefer (1968) has noted, although administrative theory suggests the structuring of organizations according to program, clientele, area, or process, public health agencies found it necessary to employ all four of these patterns. The need for the organization to be based on different and somewhat conflicting models led inevitably to high levels of internal tension, conflict, and struggle for power and control.

Often unaware of the body of administrative theory that would have permitted the forecasting of some of the conflicts, health administrators tried various *ad hoc* arrangements of function in an effort to reduce the organizational tensions to tolerable levels. Those arrangements that seemed to work, at least for a while, became organizational principles. Apparently successful agencies came to be viewed as models of organization, which could be copied or at least adapted to other areas or other problems. The inherent unsoundness in this approach led to frequent reorganizations of health agencies in which new foci of tensions were substituted for, or sometimes erected upon existing ones.

International Health Organizations

Health organizations exist in a profusion of forms and sizes, and their functions vary from those that may limit their concerns to a single disease affecting a small discrete population to an organization whose concern is the health of the entire world. We begin our discussion with international organizations and we will trace their evolution from those with limited purposes to the global concern for world health.

The forerunners of today's international health organizations were International Sanitary Conferences. The first such conference was convened in Paris in 1851 to consider maritime quarantine requirements to control the spread of cholera and thereby render "important services to the trade and shipping of the Mediterranean, while at the same time safeguarding the public health" (WHO, 1958). The reference of trade before health was perhaps symbolic, because only three of the twelve participating nations ratified the convention. By 1865 these three nations, France, Portugal, and Sardinia, withdrew from the convention. Between 1851 and 1897 ten International Sanitary Conferences were held but not one was effective.

In 1902 the First International Sanitary Convention of the American Republics met in Washington, D.C. By this time medical science had made significant progress in determining the cause and methods for control of such dread diseases as plague, cholera, typhoid, smallpox, malaria, and yellow fever and nations were willing to cooperate in mutual efforts of health protection. The discovery of the mode of transmission of yellow fever and the subsequent eradication campaign in Havana shortly before the Convention also contributed to its success, which culminated in the establishment of the Pan American Sanitary Bureau, the first international health agency. Although the Pan American Sanitary Bureau was a regional organization, it exchanged epidemiologic intelligence with the Egyptian Sanitary, Maritime, and Quarantine Board and later developed cooperative relations with the Health Organization of the League of Nations.

In 1903 the eleventh International Sanitary Conference was held in Paris. This Conference revised the work of four previous conventions and consolidated them into the International Sanitary Convention of 1903. Perhaps more important was the initiation of efforts to establish an international health office. Four years later, in 1907, delegates from Belgium, Brazil, Egypt, France, Great Britain, Italy, Netherlands, Portugal, Russia, Spain, Switzerland, and the United States met in Rome and signed an agreement for the creation in Paris of *L'Office International d'Hygiene Publique*. *L'Office* concerned itself with the problems of control of yellow fever, plague, cholera, malaria, tuberculosis, typhoid, hookworm infestation, meningitis, and sleeping sickness. It also gave consideration to the hygiene of schools, places of work, and of food and to the construction and administration of hospitals. Although *L'Office* did not engage in field work, it served as an international information bureau and as a forum for the discussion and subsequent development of recommendations for the solution of public health problems, which were common to several nations. It called attention to the need for international agreements on the standardization of sera and vaccines and recommended compulsory notification of contagious forms of tuberculosis and tuberculosis deaths and of cases of leprosy. It recommended that central government should be party to the control by local governments of the purity of drinking water and sanitary disposal of human waste.

The next major development in international health organization was the creation of the Health Organization of the League of Nations in 1923. Article XXIII of the Covenant of the League of Nations provided that member nations should take steps in matters of international concern for the prevention and control of disease. Article XXIV established the principle that all international bureaus and existing general treaties shall be placed under the direction of the nations who were party to these endeavors.

These provisions of the Covenant, together with outbreaks of epidemic disease in several war-ravaged countries of Europe, set the stage for an international health agency within the framework of the League of Nations. In keeping with the provision of Article XXIV efforts were made to bring *L'Office International d'Hygiene Publique* under the jurisdiction of the League. These efforts failed largely because the United States, in refusing to join the League of Nations, also refused to consent to any international organization of which it was a member being combined with the League. As a result *L'Office* and the Health Organization of the League existed as an autonomous international health organization (WHO, 1958) for 30 years. A workable but not clear-cut division of responsibility developed between *L'Office* and the Health Organization. *L'Office* continued to supervise and work for improvement of international quarantine measures. It also concerned itself, however, with the international standardization of diphtheria antiserum and with the control of narcotic drugs. The Health Organization was first engaged in emergency programs to assist eastern European nations in their efforts to control major epidemics of typhus. An epidemiological intelligence service was established for the purpose of collecting and publishing data on the worldwide status of epidemic disease.

In 1923 the League established a malaria commission, which indicated a new approach in international efforts to control communicable diseases. Prior to that time emphasis had been placed on preventing the spread of infectious diseases between countries. The mission of the Malaria Commission was to study and to advise on the most effective methods of control of malaria anywhere in the world and irrespective of the probability of its spread to other countries.

Other pioneering efforts of the League included the establishment of a Cancer Commission and the subsequent publication of a series of annual reports on the results of radiotherapy of cancer of the uterus.

Technical commissions were established on such varied subjects as biological standardization, housing, physical fitness, typhus, leprosy, medical and public health training, rural hygiene, the unification of pharmacopoeias, and nutrition. The work of the technical commission on nutrition and its report on the physiological basis of nutrition is considered to be one of the most outstanding efforts of the Health Organization of the League.

Goodman (1965) has concluded:

"The seeds of both success and failure were planted in the Health Organization of the League almost from its foundation. Success, because it began with the then enormous prestige of the League behind it and because it was created at a time when the needs of international medicine had expanded and could not be met by the previously existing bodies and thus it had a really useful technical job to do. Failure, because the decline of the League as an instrument of world government—or even of world opinion— inevitably reacted on all its work and because of the existence of two independent bodies, the *Office* and the Health Organization, was a constant irritant, sometimes beneficial, but on the whole harmful. . . . The proof of the value of the Health Organization's work is that what it created has not been abandoned, but taken over by newcomers and extended, very largely on the original foundations."

Interim International Health Organizations

During World War II the Health Organization was isolated in neutral Switzerland with both work and staff greatly curtailed. *L'Office* in German-occupied Paris was unable to function as an international health agency. The disruption and destruction caused by the war created millions of homeless people, many of whom were unable or unwilling to return to their countries of origin. To deal with the enormous problem of war refugees, President Franklin D. Roosevelt suggested that the Allied Nations establish an international agency. UNRRA—the United Nations Relief and Rehabilitation Administration—came into being in 1943. UNRRA was given the responsibility of: assisting governments in the rehabilitation of their health services, the health protection of 13 million persons displaced by war until they could be repatriated, and the provision of medical care for the 3 million persons who could not be repatriated or resettled. In 1945, UNRRA also took over the quarantine and epidemic intelligence services of *L'Office*. In spite of its natural preoccupation with war refugees UNRRA was able to develop and secure ratification of two new conventions on the control of yellow fever.

UNRRA was phased out in 1947 when its international health activities were transferred to the Interim Commission of the World Health Organization, and its responsibility for medical care for displaced persons given over to the newly formed International Refugee Organization with which the author served in 1948 and 1949. IRO continued the provision of preventive and therapeutic medical services to a dwindling group of displaced persons in camps in the French, British, and United States Zones of Germany and in Italy. In 1949 IRO instituted a program of rehabilitation for seriously disabled persons to bring them to the point that they might be resettled.

The World Health Organization

At the end of World War II there were four international health organizations in existence: (1) the Pan American Sanitary Organization, (2) *L'Office International d'Hygiene Publique*, (3) The Health Organization of the League of Nations, and (4) the Health Division of the United Nations Relief and Rehabilitation Administration. PASO was a regional organization with its activities limited to Latin America and the United States. *L'Office*, under the pressures of war and the German occupation of Paris, had relinquished its concern for international quarantine matters to UNRRA, a temporary agency concerned primarily with the many problems of resettlement or repatriation of the refugees and displaced persons created by the war. Not one of the existing agencies was in a position to assume responsibilities for international health on a world-wide scale.

The United Nations Conference on International Organization met in San Francisco in 1945 to adopt and sign the charter of the United Nations. The original draft failed to mention health, but delegates from Brazil and China, who were physicians, succeeded in obtaining the adoption of a declaration recommending that a general conference be convened for the purpose of establishing an international health organization. This farsighted declaration went on to recommend that the plan for an international health organization give full consideration to the question of the relationship of such an organization and to methods of associating it with existing and future national and international health organizations.

The Economic and Social Council, which has been created by the General Assembly of the United Nations in January of 1946, adopted a resolution calling for an "international conference to consider the scope of, and the appropriate machinery for, international action in the field of public health and proposals for the establishment of a single international health organization of the United Nations" (WHO, 1939). The resolution provided for the establishment of a Technical Preparatory Committee to prepare a draft agenda and proposal for consideration by the conference.

The Technical Preparatory Committee met in Paris in March and April of 1946 under the chairmanship of Professor René Sand of Belgium. It prepared the conference of agenda and a draft constitution for the proposed health organization. The International Health Conference was convened at New York on June 19, 1946. It had the distinction of being the first international conference held under the auspices of the United Nations. Health, at first an afterthought, had moved to the forefront of consideration by the international body. Dr. Thomas Parran, Surgeon General of the United States Public Health Services, was elected President of the Conference and with minor changes the draft constitution was adopted as the Constitution of the World Health Organization.

The Conference also established an Interim Commission of the World Health Organization and initiated steps leading to the assumption by WHO of the duties and function of *L'Office International d'Hygiene Publique* and the eventual integration of the Pan American Sanitary Organization and the Pan Arab Regional Health Bureau, which had been recently established at Alexandria by the Arab League.

The Constitution of the World Health Organization is considered a landmark in the development of the concepts of public health and social medicine. In the 20 years of its existence there has been but one amendment in 1960, i.e., to change the membership of the Executive Board from eighteen to twenty-four.

The preamble to the Constitution and its first two articles are reproduced below:

THE STATES parties to this Constitution declare, in conformity with the Charter of the United Nations, that the following principles are basic to the happiness, harmonious relations, and security of all people:

Health is a state of complete physical, mental and social well-being and not merely the absence of disease or infirmity.

The enjoyment of the highest attainable standard of health is one of the fundamental rights of every human being without distinction of race, religion, political belief, economic or social condition.

The health of all peoples is fundamental to the attainment of peace and security and is dependent upon the fullest co-operation of individuals and States.

The achievement of any State in the promotion and protection of health is of value to all.

Unequal development in different countries in the promotion of health and control of disease, especially communicable disease, is a common danger.

Healthy development of the child is of basic importance; the ability to live harmoniously in a changing total environment is essential to such development.

The extension to all peoples of the benefits of medical, psychological and related knowledge is essential to the fullest attainment of health.

Informed opinion and active co-operation on the part of the public are of the utmost importance in the improvement of the people.

Governments have a responsibility for the health of their peoples which can be fulfilled only by the provision of adequate health and social measures.

ACCEPTING THESE PRINCIPLES, and for the purpose of co-operation among themselves and with others to promote and protect the health of all peoples, the contracting parties agree to the present Constitution and hereby establish the World Health Organization as a specialized agency within the terms of Article 57 of The Charter of the United Nations.

OBJECTIVE

Article 1

The objective of the World Health Organization (hereinafter called the Organization shall be the attainment by all peoples of the highest possible level of health.

FUNCTIONS

Article 2

In order to achieve its objective, the functions of the Organization shall be:

(a) to act as the directing and co-ordinating authority on international health work;

(b) to establish and maintain effective collaboration with the United Nations, specialized agencies, governmental health administrations, professional groups, and such other organizations as may be deemed appropriate;

(c) to assist governments, upon request, in strengthening health services;

(d) to furnish appropriate technical assistance and, in emergencies, necessary aid upon the request or acceptance of governments;

(e) to provide or assist in providing, upon the request of the United Nations, health services and facilities to special groups, such as the peoples of trust territories;

(f) to establish and maintain such administrative and technical services as may be required, including epidemiological and statistical services;

(g) to stimulate and advance work to eradicate epidemic, endemic and other diseases;

(h) to promote, in co-operation with other specialized agencies where necessary, the prevention of accidental injuries;

(i) to promote, in co-operation with other specialized agencies where necessary, the improvement of nutrition, housing, sanitation, recreation, economic or working conditions and other aspects of environmental hygiene;

(j) to promote co-operation among scientific and professional groups which contribute to the advancement of health;

(k) to propose conventions, agreements and regulations, and make recommendations with respect to international health matters and to perform such duties as may be assigned thereby to the Organization and are consistent with its objective;

(l) to promote maternal and child health and welfare and to foster the ability to live harmoniously in a changing total environment;

(m) to foster activities in the field of mental health, especially those affecting the harmony of human relations;

(n) to promote and conduct research in the field of health;

(o) to promote improved standards of teaching and training in the health, medical and related professions;

(p) to study and report on, in co-operation with other specialized agencies where necessary, administrative and social techniques affecting public health and medical care from preventive and curative points of view, including hospital services and social security;

(q) to provide information, counsel and assistance in the field of health;

(r) to assist in developing an informed public opinion among all peoples on matters of health;

(s) to establish and revise as necessary international nomenclatures of diseases, of causes of death and of public health practices;

(t) to standardize diagnostic procedures as necessary;

(u) to develop, establish and promote international standards in respect of food, biological, pharmaceutical and similar products;

(v) generally to take all necessary action to attain the objective of the Organization.

The remaining articles define the membership, and structure of the organization. Membership is open to all states including nonmembers of the United Nations, and territories not responsible for the conduct of their international relations are permitted to join as Associate Members if nominated by the nation having such authority.

The structure of the organization consists of a World Health Assembly, an Executive Board, and a Secretariat. The Assembly is an annual congress of member nations to which each member may send three delegates. Its functions include the establishment of policy, review and approval of the budget, and the appointment of the Director-General.

The Executive Board consists of twenty-four persons elected by the Assembly on the nomination of member nations. Board members serve for three terms and eight members are elected annually. The Executive Board prepares the agenda and the budget for the Assembly and is responsible for the execution of adopted policies.

The Secretariat consists of the Director-General and technical and administrative staff. Article 37 of the Constitution defines the international civil-servant status of each member of the staff and calls on individual staff members and the member nations to respect this condition. The Constitution also confers on the Director-General the sole authority for the appointment of staff subject to staff regulations approved by the Health Assembly. The Constitution states that the primary consideration in the employment of the staff shall be to assure efficiency, integrity, and maintenance of the internationally representative character of the Secretariat. In practice it appears that at times efficiency and integrity have given way to international representation. On the whole, however, the Director-Generals have been able to assemble and retain a remarkably competent staff. Some member nations have weakened the concept of the international civil servant by insisting on periodic replacement of its nationals who are members of the Secretariat without reference to their productivity or value to the organization.

As of June, 1966, WHO had 126 member nations including three associate members. On the decision of the First World Health Assembly the city of Geneva, Switzerland, was chosen as the organization's headquarters.

The major activities of WHO are shown in Figure 13-1.

WHO Relations with Nongovernmental Organizations. Article 71 of the Constitution of WHO authorizes the development of suitable arrangements for consultation and cooperation with nongovernmental organizations. The Third World Health Assembly (1950) established criteria for admitting nongovernmental organizations into an official relationship with WHO. Such organizations must be concerned with matters falling within the competence of WHO and must pursue their aims and purposes in conformity with the spirit and purposes of the WHO Constitution. In addition, nongovernmental organizations must be of recognized standing, must represent a substantial proportion of persons organized for participation in the particular fields in which they operate, and must have a directing body and authority to speak for their members through authorized representatives. More than forty nongovernmental organizations have established a formal relationship with WHO; among these are the International Association for the Prevention of Blindness, the International Council

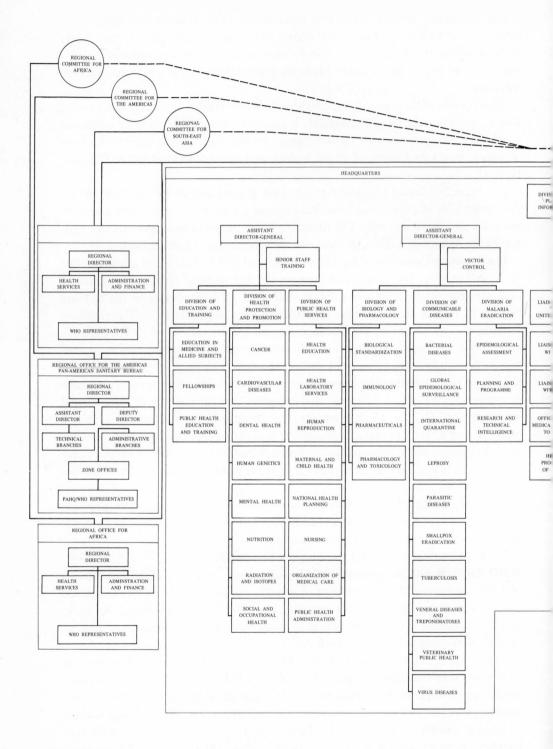

REGIONAL COMMITTEE FOR AFRICA

REGIONAL COMMITTEE FOR THE AMERICAS

REGIONAL COMMITTEE FOR SOUTH-EAST ASIA

HEADQUARTERS

DIVIS...
\ PL...
INFOR...

REGIONAL DIRECTOR

HEALTH SERVICES

ADMINISTRATION AND FINANCE

WHO REPRESENTATIVES

REGIONAL OFFICE FOR THE AMERICAS
PAN-AMERICAN SANITARY BUREAU

REGIONAL DIRECTOR

ASSISTANT DIRECTOR

DEPUTY DIRECTOR

TECHNICAL BRANCHES

ADMINISTRATIVE BRANCHES

ZONE OFFICES

PAHQ/WHO REPRESENTATIVES

REGIONAL OFFICE FOR AFRICA

REGIONAL DIRECTOR

HEALTH SERVICES

ADMINSTRATION AND FINANCE

WHO REPRESENTATIVES

ASSISTANT DIRECTOR-GENERAL

SENIOR STAFF TRAINING

ASSISTANT DIRECTOR-GENERAL

VECTOR CONTROL

DIVISION OF EDUCATION AND TRAINING

DIVISION OF HEALTH PROTECTION AND PROMOTION

DIVISION OF PUBLIC HEALTH SERVICES

DIVISION OF BIOLOGY AND PHARMACOLOGY

DIVISION OF COMMUNICABLE DISEASES

DIVISION OF MALARIA ERADICATION

LIAIS...
UNITE...

EDUCATION IN MEDICINE AND ALLIED SUBJECTS

CANCER

HEALTH EDUCATION

BIOLOGICAL STANDARDIZATION

BACTERIAL DISEASES

EPIDEMOLOGICAL ASSESSMENT

LIAIS...
WI...

FELLOWSHIPS

CARDIOVASCULAR DISEASES

HEALTH LABORATORY SERVICES

IMMUNOLOGY

GLOBAL EPIDEMOLOGICAL SURVEILLANCE

PLANNING AND PROGRAMME

LIAIS...
WI...

PUBLIC HEALTH EDUCATION AND TRAINING

DENTAL HEALTH

HUMAN REPRODUCTION

PHARMACEUTICALS

INTERNATIONAL QUARANTINE

RESEARCH AND TECHNICAL INTELLIGENCE

OFFIC...
MEDICA...
TO...

HUMAN GENETICS

MATERNAL AND CHILD HEALTH

PHARMACOLOGY AND TOXICOLOGY

LEPROSY

HE...
PRO...
OF...

MENTAL HEALTH

NATIONAL HEALTH PLANNING

PARASITIC DISEASES

NUTRITION

NURSING

SMALLPOX ERADICATION

RADIATION AND ISOTOPES

ORGANIZATION OF MEDICAL CARE

TUBERCULOSIS

SOCIAL AND OCCUPATIONAL HEALTH

PUBLIC HEALTH ADMINISTRATION

VENERAL DISEASES AND TREPONEMATOSES

VETERINARY PUBLIC HEALTH

VIRUS DISEASES

378

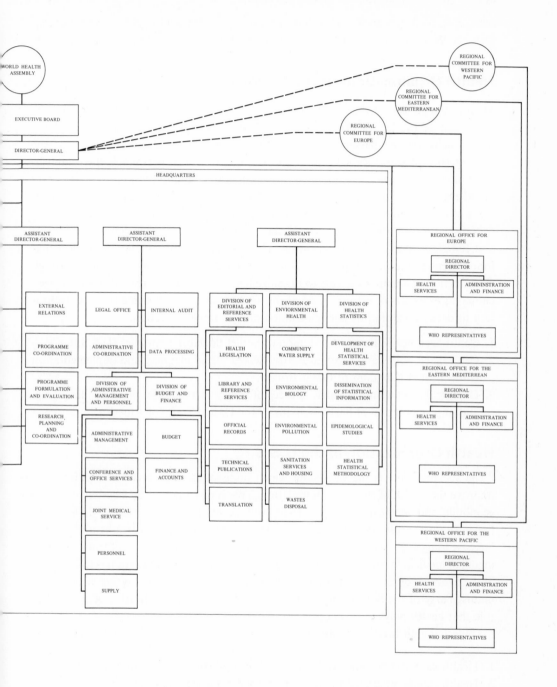

FIGURE 13-1. Organization of the World Health Organization.

of Nurses, the International Hospital Federation, the International Pediatric Association, the World Federation for Mental Health, and the World Medical Association.

Health Organizations at the National Level

Most of the nations of the world have given a high priority to the promotion and the protection of the health of their citizens. National health efforts have taken many forms including the passage of laws regulating activities related to health or the prevention of disease; the education and training of health personnel; the establishment of clinics, hospitals, and related institutions; the direct provision of medical care or the provision of subsidy or insurance against the costs of illness; and the establishment of an organizational structure to implement national health policies.

National health organizations established by government vary widely in their forms and functions, and many classification schemes are possible. In the discussion that follows centralization of authority has been selected as a means of establishing a rough classification of a nation's efforts to organize health activities. Three nations have been chosen as examples of extremes and of the median on a scale running from centralization to decentralization of policy formulation and implementation.

1. Centralized health authority—Union of Soviet Socialist Republics (U.S.S.R.).
2. Centralized policy and fiscal authority, decentralized planning and implementation —the United Kingdom of Great Britain.
3. Decentralized and multicentric sources of policy formulation, planning, financing, and implementation of health activities—the United States of America.

Health Organization in the U.S.S.R.

"The socialist state is the only state which undertakes to protect and continuously improve the health of the whole population. This is provided for by a system of socioeconomic and medical measures. There will be an extensive program designed to prevent and sharply reduce diseases, wipe out mass infectious diseases and further increase longevity. The needs of the urban and rural population in all forms of highly qualified medical services will be met in full." This ambitious declaration is to be found in the *Program of the Communist Party* as adopted by the 22nd Congress of the Communist Party of the Soviet Union on October 31, 1961. It is indicative of the central role that health plays in Soviet policy.

Underlying all health activities in the Soviet Union are the following principles.

1. Health care services are available and free to all through a state-run system.
2. Health care is integrated through centralized planning and direction.
3. The primary objective of the health care system is the prevention of illness and the promotion of health.
4. The state provides for the education of all health personnel.

A brief description of the political organization of the U.S.S.R. is necessary for the understanding of the organization of the health care system.

The Union of the Soviet Socialist Republics consists of 15 republics, each named for the predominating ethnic or national group. Within the 15 Union Republics there are 20 Autonomous Republics representative of smaller national groups, and eight Autonomous Regions. This complex of republics is divided into 112 administration districts called oblasts, which in turn are divided into 2,638 subdistricts called *rayons*. The smallest administrative unit, the uchastok, or microrayon, has a population of about 4,000 persons. There are about 10 uchastoks to a rayon, which has an average population of about 40,000 persons. In the Ukranian Republic, with a population of 45,000,000, there are 475 rayons and 26 oblasts.

The Union Republics, Autonomous Republics, and Autonomous Regions each elect a Soviet of Workers Deputy, who appoints a chief executive and heads of the departments or ministries. The appointed ministers form an administrative body called the Council of Ministers. The highest legislative body is the Supreme Soviet of the U.S.S.R., which is elected by popular vote on the basis of one representative (Deputy) for each 300,000 people. The Supreme Soviet appoints the highest executive and administrative body, the Council of Ministers. Article 68 of the constitution defines the function of the Council of Ministers as one of coordination and direction of the ministries of the U.S.S.R. Article 49 of the constitution gives to the Presidium (essentially an executive committee) of the Supreme Soviet the right to annul decisions and orders of Soviet ministers and republican ministers if they do not conform to law. Authority to suspend questionable orders or directives of national and republican ministries is delegated to the Council of Ministers. The Council of Ministers consists of a Chairman, First Deputy Chairman, a number of vice-chairmen, the ministers of the U.S.S.R., and the chairmen of a few state committees. The Constitution of the U.S.S.R. and the Constitution of the Union and Autonomous Republics provide for the protection and improvement of the health of the people. The most important health organization in the Soviet Union is the Ministry of Health.

The Ministry of Health plans the total health program including the provision of manpower, facilities, and supplies. It is responsible for the planning and coordination of medical research, the provision of environmental health services, the development and supervision of the pharmaceutical and medical equipment industries, the supervision of the Ministries of Health of the Republics, the conduct of international health relations, and the establishment of norms which form the basis of national health planning. Field has described the ministry as a large service bureaucracy, pyramidal in shape and hierarchical in nature, composed of a series of departments or administrations, each one concerned with one phase of medical services and dependent for its financial and other logistic sustenance on allocations from the state budget.

The Ministry is divided into the following departments.

1. Department of Preventive and Curative Medicine.
   Responsible for prophylactic and therapeutic services for adults including hospitals and related institutions and research institutes.
2. Department of Medical Care and Prophylaxis for Mothers and Children.
   Responsible for prophylactic, obstetric, and therapeutic services for mothers and prophylactic, therapeutic, and custodial care of children.
3. Central Sanitary-Epidemiologic Department.
   Responsible for environmental health services, including control of hazards of radiation and the prevention and control of communicable disease.
4. Department of Planning and Finance.
   Responsible for standards, planning, and financing of hospitals.
5. Department of Medical Personnel.
   Responsible for graduate and postgraduate training of physicians and the training of paramedical personnel.
6. Department of Pharmaceuticals.
   Responsible for production and the quality of all drugs including antibiotics.
7. Department of Biological Products.
   Responsible for production of vaccine, sera, and other biologics.
8. Department of Medical Equipment and Technical Apparatus.
   Responsible for design and production of medical equipment.

9. Department of Supplies.
   Responsible for supplying equipment, drugs, and supplies to all hospital, polyclinic and related facilities.
10. Department of Foreign Affairs.
    Responsible for international health matters.

According to Field (1967) the Departments of Pharmaceuticals, Biologics, and Medical Equipment are combined in one department.

The Ministry of Health also contains the Academy of Medical Sciences and a number of research and postgraduate institutes. The Academy of Medical Sciences is considered the most important medical institution in the U.S.S.R. Membership in the Academy is considered to be a great honor. The Academy is charged with the responsibility of furthering scientific research in medicine and in establishing priorities and an over-all plan for medical research throughout the Soviet Union.

Other institutes that are part of the Ministry of Health include the Central Institute for Advanced Medical Studies. Founded in 1930, the Central Institute is responsible for the promotion and scientific development of medical specialization, the training of research workers and teachers to staff other institutions, and the training of clinical specialists. On the direction of the Ministry of Health the Central Institute develops model curricula and teaching methods to be employed in the training of medical specialists in other postgraduate institutes throughout the U.S.S.R. The research activities of the Institute are related to its educational responsibilities and must have the approval of the Scientific Council of the Academy of Medical Sciences. This approval assures conformity with the Five-Year Medical Research Plan of the U.S.S.R. as promulgated by the Academy of Medical Sciences and authorized by the Ministry of Health.

The Central Institute contains four faculties: Surgery, Therapy (Medicine), Biomedical Sciences, and Sanitation and Hygiene. The Faculty of Sanitation and Hygiene bears a close resemblance to a graduate school of public health in the United States. It is divided into seven specialized departments: (1) Public Health Organization, (2) Communal Hygiene, (3) Industrial Hygiene, (4) Nutrition, (5) Hygiene of Children and Adolescents, (6) Radiation Hygiene, and (7) Epidemiology. In addition there are three general departments which serve the entire Institute: (1) Marxism-Leninism, (2) History of Medicine, and (3) Foreign Languages. Biostatistics is included in the Department of Public Health Organization.

Students are admitted to study in the Faculty of Sanitation and Hygiene on the recommendation of the Ministry of Health of the U.S.S.R. or of a republican ministry of health. Priority is given to persons serving as Health Ministers, Deputy Health Ministers, Directors of Sanitary-Epidemiologic at the Republic or oblast level.

Another institute within the Ministry of Health is the Semashko Institute of Public Health Administration. Named for Dr. N. S. Semashko, the First Health Commissar of the Soviet Union, this institute is concerned with the collection of data and the conduct of research in respect to the organization and supervision of health services, health planning and health economics, and the scientific organization of health personnel. Statistical data on morbidity, mortality, utilization of health services, costs and health personnel are collected and analyzed. These data are used to determine the health status of the country and to develop norms for services, staffing norms, and work load norms for health personnel. These norms play a vital role in the planning of health services and the location and staffing of health facilities. Every health facility throughout the U.S.S.R. is expected to conform to the staff and work load norms established for that class of institution.

Other institutes within the Ministry include the Central Institute for Tuberculosis, which is responsible for the development of methods of control, diagnosis and treatment of tuberculosis; and the Institute for Design of Medical Establishments which, as its name implies, is concerned with the development of standards for health facilities and for design research.

From the above description of the Ministry of Health and its related institutes it should be noted that there is significant centralization of research, training of health personnel, and planning and development of health facilities. Five-year research plans are developed in Moscow according to priorities determined by the Ministry. All health research must be consonant with the national plan for health research.

Similarly the content of curricula and the methodology of teaching at both graduate and undergraduate professional and para professional schools must conform to centrally developed schema. The uniformity of the appearance and the functional aspects of Soviet hospitals, polyclinics, sanatoria, and so on, reflect the development of prototype plans at the national level. Similar uniformity exists in the staffing, work loads of personnel, and to a significant degree the actual care of patients is standardized.

National Ministries in the U.S.S.R. are of two types. All-union ministries and union-republic ministries. All-union ministries are those with direct responsibility for administration of all the activities under their jurisdiction. This would be comparable to the Departments of Commerce, Labor, or Agriculture in the United States. Union-republican ministries are those which share administrative functions with counterpart ministries at the republic level. This would be roughly comparable to the U.S. Department of Health, Education, and Welfare, which exercises many of its functions through counterpart agencies at the state level. The Ministry of Health of the U.S.S.R. is an example of the union-republican type. The Ministry of Health of the U.S.S.R. provides national direction to all health activities and has responsibility for planning, supervision, and financing of all health programs and services including the production of health manpower. The ministry of health of a republic is responsible for health planning for the area under its jurisdiction and for the operation of its health resources. Unlike the relationships between the health agencies of the U.S. Department of Health, Education, and Welfare and state health departments, the ministry of health of a Soviet republic's plans must conform to detailed normals established in Moscow and to the national health plan. Moreover, the operations of the republic's health resources are supervised by the Ministry of Health of the U.S.S.R. through review and analysis of statistical and other reports and by direct supervisory and inspectional visits by personnel from the Ministry or ministerial institutes. Standardization of health functions and activities is expected and enforced.

A Republican Ministry of Health.   As an example of a republican ministry of health, we shall consider the Ministry of Health of the Ukrainian Republic. The Ukrainian Republic, located in the southwestern corner of the Soviet Union, has a population of 45 million persons. The population is about evenly divided between those employed in industrial or agricultural pursuits. The republic is divided into 25 oblasts (regions) and 475 rayons (subregions). The population of a rayon varies from 30,000 to 100,000 persons.

The Minister of Health is appointed by the Minister of the Republic on the recommendation of the Minister of Health of the U.S.S.R. Figure 13-2 is the organizational chart of the Ukrainian Ministry of Health.

It should be noted that no sharp distinction is made between mental health and physical health in the Soviet Union. Facilities and services for the mentally ill include psychoneurological clinics (some with in-patient beds), psychiatric services as part of general polyclinics, therapeutic workshops, day hospitals, psychiatric hospitals, and psychiatric colonies, which are for persons with serious but stable psychiatric disabilities. These services are administered as an integral part of the division or bureau of medical services.

At the oblast level there is a regional health department, which consists of an executive office, a medical advisory committee, administrative and fiscal staff, an environmental health and epidemic control unit, a unit for medical and preventive services for adults, and a unit for medical and preventive services for women and children.

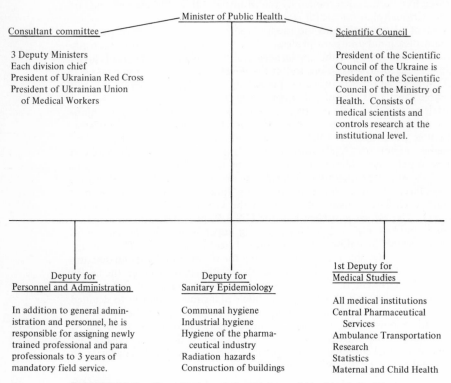

Minister of Public Health

Consultant committee

3 Deputy Ministers
Each division chief
President of Ukrainian Red Cross
President of Ukrainian Union
   of Medical Workers

Scientific Council

President of the Scientific
Council of the Ukraine is
President of the Scientific
Council of the Ministry of
Health. Consists of
medical scientists and
controls research at the
institutional level.

Deputy for
Personnel and Administration

In addition to general administration and personnel, he is
responsible for assigning newly
trained professional and para
professionals to 3 years of
mandatory field service.

Deputy for
Sanitary Epidemiology

Communal hygiene
Industrial hygiene
Hygiene of the pharma-
   ceutical industry
Radiation hazards
Construction of buildings

1st Deputy for
Medical Studies

All medical institutions
Central Pharmaceutical
   Services
Ambulance Transportation
Research
Statistics
Maternal and Child Health

FIGURE 13-2. Organization of the Ministry of Health of the Ukraine.

At the municipal level there is a city health department consisting of an executive officer, administrative and fiscal officers, a medical statistician, a director (inspector) of adult medical and preventive services, a director for women and children's medical and preventive services, and a sanitary-epidemic control officer, who also serves as the republic sanitary inspector for the town.

At the rayon, or district, level the district hospital serves as the unit of administrative authority. In districts that do not contain a hospital, the polyclinics, which are divisions of the hospital serving the district, become basic administrative units.

Throughout the hierarchial network there is a system of supervision that extends from the Ministry of Health of U.S.S.R. through every administrative and service level to individual posts (*feldscher*) in rural areas. Hospital performance is reviewed at the republic level, polyclinic performance is supervised by hospital physicians. Rayon physicians are supervised by polyclinic physicians. Feldschers are supervised by rayon physicians. Supervision involves review and evaluation of performance and the grading of subordinates. Physicians are awarded grades I through V. The higher the grade, the higher the salary and the greater the opportunity for advancement (Field, 1967).

It is difficult to assess the effects of the degree of centralization of authority and control of health services. It has resulted in a high degree of uniformity and rigidity. Innovation is not encouraged nor is change likely to occur except as determined and initiated at the top of the pyramid, the Ministry of Health of the U.S.S.R. The prevailing, or perhaps official, point of view of Russian health leaders is that the Soviet Union has created the ideal health service system model and that innovation and change in the structure are irrelevant. Soviet health officials view their objective as the full implementation of the goal set by the Programme of the Communist Party "to protect and continuously improve the health of the whole population." They see no need to look for or test other models of a health service system.

It is fair to say that the Soviet centrality of planning and resource allocation has assured the availability of health services throughout the territorial limits of one of the largest nations on earth.

A discussion of the policy and goal-setting role of the Communist Party does not fall within the scope of this paper. Suffice it to say that the over-all goals and policies of the Ministry of Health of the U.S.S.R. are determined by, or at the least must be consonant with, the goals of the Communist Party of the U.S.S.R. The essential questions are (1) to what extent are goals determined by a political party that claims membership of a small proportion of the population, representative of and in the best interests of the Soviet people; and (2) how effective is the Russian health service system in meeting the needs of the citizenry of the U.S.S.R. Objective studies of these questions would be most valuable.

Health Organization in the United Kingdom

Health organization in the United Kingdom would place approximately at the mid-point on a scale denoting centralization of authority. The centralization of health authority in the Soviet Union might represent one extreme of central control, and the United States would represent an extreme of decentralized control. A paradox in this observation is the fact that both the Soviet Union and the United States are structurally federal forms of government with sharing (in widely divergent ways) of authority with the national and state or republic governments. The United Kingdom on the other hand has only a national government. There are no British equivalents of states or republics and hence no state or republican governmental structure between the national and local levels. Although local government does indeed exist in Britain, it is subject to the national authority of Parliament, operates under the supervision of national ministries, and derives more than half its funds from national appropriations (Time, Inc., 1961). Nonetheless, there is more decentralization of authority for health services than in the U.S.S.R., though considerably less than in the United States.

At the request of the Crown, and on recommendation to the Prime Minister, the Government is formed by appointing Ministers who are in charge of various ministries (departments) of government. A Minister may or may not be a member of the Cabinet. (The present Minister of Health is not a Cabinet member.) The Minister is assisted by Parliamentary Secretaries and Under-Secretaries, who are selected from the House of Lords or the House of Commons. The chief administrative officer of a ministry is the Permanent Secretary, who is a career civil service officer with tenure, having advanced up the ladder of administrative grades from Assistant Principal to Principal, to Assistant Secretary, to Under-Secretary, to Permanent Secretary. The Permanent

Secretary is an administrator and not a professional or specialist in the area of concern of the ministry. In the Ministry of Health there is a Chief Medical Officer, who is a physician appointed by the Permanent Secretary. Although the Chief Medical Officer is responsible to the Permanent Secretary, he has the right of access to the Minister. The nonmedical members of the Ministry carry out the executive functions, and the Chief Medical Officer and his subordinate health professionals serve as advisers.

The present structure of health organization and administration in the United Kingdom is based largely upon the National Health Services Act of 1946. Section One of the Act states

It shall be the duty of the Minister of Health to promote the establishment in England and Wales of a comprehensive health service designed to secure improvement in the physical and mental health of the people of England and Wales and the prevention, diagnosis and treatment of illness. . . .

Not all health and health-related services come under the jurisdiction of the Ministry of Health. The Department of Education and Science is responsible for school health services and the care and education of handicapped children. The Home Office is responsible for the implementation of the Dangerous Drug Acts. The Ministry of Agriculture, Fisheries, and Food is responsible for the purity and sanitation of food. The Ministry of Housing and Local Government is responsible for the supervision of water supplies and sewage disposal.

The National Health Service. Early in the planning of the National Health Service it was recognized that a high degree of administrative autonomy was desirable to avoid political or fiscal domination or unwarranted governmental invasion into areas of professional concern. However, having decided that the major source of support would have to come from general tax revenue, the control of Parliament and the Treasury over appropriations was inevitable. There were proposals that the National Health Service be administered by an autonomous public corporation. This was unacceptable inasmuch as public corporations are generally self-financing, and the National Health Service would be almost wholly dependent on appropriations of tax funds. It was decided to place the National Health Service within the Ministry of Health, but to have Parliament cast one vote for the entire National Health Service appropriation. The Treasury retained authority to redistribute funds between major divisions, such as hospital services, whereas the Minister of Health may redistribute funds within a major division. In this manner, appropriate fiscal accountability has been retained without serious sacrifice of autonomy.

Decentralization of Administration. Although the over-all responsibility rests with the Ministry of Health, local administration is divided between three independent bodies. Hospitals and specialists' consultation services are the responsibility of 15 regional hospital boards; general practitioner, dental, pharmaceutical, and optical services are the responsibility of 138 local executive councils; and paramedical services (bedside nursing, midwifery, medical social work, physical therapy, homemakers, ambulance transportation, and so on), custodial care institutions, and conventional public health services are the responsibility of 148 local health authorities. In addition, in England and Wales, but not in Scotland, the 26 university teaching hospitals are responsible to

Boards of Governors, which by-pass the Regional Hospital Boards and answer directly to the Ministry of Health.*

Each of the boards, councils, and authorities receives an annual block grant to enable it to carry out its functions. The allocation of the National Health Service Budget among the component units is the responsibility of the Minister of Health.

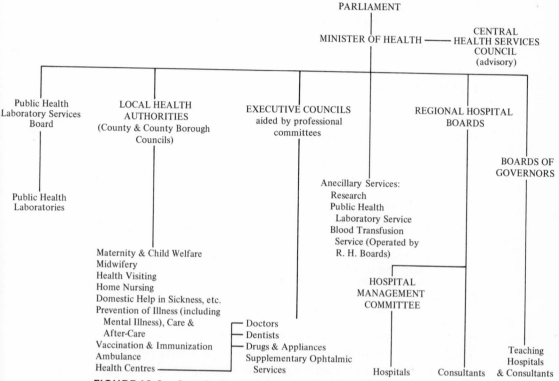

FIGURE 13-3. Organization of the National Health Service in England and Wales.

Administration of the National Health Service, England and Wales. The Minister of Health is responsible for the National Health Service (see Figure 13-3). He is advised by a twenty-three-member Central Health Services Council. Answering to the Minister are Executive Councils, Regional Hospital Boards, and Local Authority (Health) Services.

1. The Executive Councils are an outgrowth of the old Insurance Committees of the former National Health Insurance. The Executive Councils consist of 25 members, eight selected by the Local Health Authority, seven by the local medical committee, three by the local dental committee, two by the local pharmaceutical committee, and five by the Minister of Health. The Executive Councils are responsible for:

   a. General practitioner services.
   b. Dental services.
   c. Pharmaceutical services.
   d. Optical services.

* In Scotland, the University teaching hospitals are responsible to Medical Education Committees, which in turn are responsible to the Regional Hospital Boards, which, like the Local Health Authorities and the Executive Councils, are responsible to the Department of Health for Scotland, which comes under the Secretary of State for Scotland. Ambulance services in Scotland are operated by voluntary associations.

General practitioners and dentists having rejected the roles of civil servants or officials of local government accepted a contractual arrangement with the Executive Councils. The Councils receive and disburse the capitation funds, handle the records of physicians' panels, investigate complaints, and enforce regulations.

2. Regional Hospital Boards. There is a Regional Hospital Board for each of the 15 hospital regions. Each region contains at least one university teaching hospital. These hospitals are responsible through their Boards of Governors to the Minister of Health. The Regional Hospital Boards are appointed by the Minister of Health with physicians constituting not more than one quarter of the membership. The Regional Hospital Boards are responsible for the organization, administration and planning of:

   a. General hospitals.
   b. Special hospitals including mental hospitals.
   c. Specialists' services.

   Day-to-day administration of individual hospitals is the responsibility of hospital management committees appointed by the Regional Hospital Boards. The Regional Hospital Boards also appoint the consultants and senior medical and dental staff of the hospitals.

3. Local Health Authority Services. The Local Health Authority Services are responsible for:

   a. Ambulance transportation.
   b. Health visiting (public health nursing).
   c. Home nursing.
   d. Homemaker services.
   e. Custodial care institutions.
   f. Public health services and the operation of health centers, which may provide space for the offices of general practitioners.
   g. Midwifery services.
   h. Supervision of mentally ill persons living at home.*

Scope of Medical Care Under the National Health Service.   Everyone in Great Britain, including visitors, is entitled to unlimited care without waiting periods. Exceptions are persons who come to the United Kingdom for the purpose of obtaining medical care. Care is inclusive and consists of

1. General practitioner family doctor care.

2. Specialist care.

3. Hospital care including psychiatric, emergency, and rehabilitation services.

4. Dental care.

5. Drugs and appliances.

6. Ophthalmic services.

7. Maternity care.

8. Home nursing.

9. Ambulance transportation.

10. Homemaker services.

Charges are made for the following

1. Two shillings and sixpence for each item prescribed by the doctor or dentist (except as noted below).

* Treatment of ambulatory mentally ill persons is provided in mental health clinics attached to hospitals.

2. £2 10s. for dental treatment and half cost of dentures up to a maximum of £5. Students, children under 16, expectant mothers, or mothers who have had a child in the last 12 months, and Old Age Pensioners are not charged for dental care.
3. £1 10s. average for eyeglasses.

Other Functions of the Ministry of Health. In 1959 the Public Health Laboratory Service was transferred from the jurisdiction of the Medical Research Council and placed under the control of the Minister of Health. The Public Health Laboratory Service operates a network of Public Health Laboratories throughout England and Wales. A Public Health Laboratory Services Board advises the Minister on matters pertaining to the operation of public health laboratories.

Statutory Health Bodies that Exist Outside the Ministry of Health. Parliament has established a number of national bodies with important health functions that are independent of the Ministry of Health. These include

1. Medical Research Council.
2. General Medical Council.
3. General nursing councils.
4. Midwives boards.
5. General Dental Council.
6. Council for the Professions Supplementary to Medicine.

THE MEDICAL RESEARCH COUNCIL. The Medical Research Council is charged with the responsibility of promoting and supporting research in the biomedical sciences. The Council is composed of twelve members. Its chairman is a layman, and the Chief Medical Officers of the Ministry of Health of the United Kingdom and of the Departments of Health of Scotland and Ireland attend the meetings of the Council. The Council is responsible to the Crown through a Committee of the Privy Council.*

The Council operates the National Institute for Medical Research, which is located in London, and administers a program of grants to support research in special institutes, hospitals, universities, and laboratories.

In recognition of the importance of clinical research, the Council has appointed a Clinical Research Board to promote research in this field.

THE GENERAL MEDICAL COUNCIL. The General Medical Council is responsible for safeguarding the professional standards and conduct of physicians. Its functions include registration of physicians; the setting of standards of medical education, professional ethics, and discipline; and the publication of the British Pharmacopeia. The General Medical Council is responsible to the Crown through the Privy Council. The 47 members of the Council are selected in the following manner 8 (5 physicians and 3 laymen) are appointed by the Crown, 18 are chosen by universities, ten are chosen by the Royal Medical College, and 11 are elected by registered medical practitioners resident in the United Kingdom.

GENERAL NURSING COUNCILS. General nursing councils were established in England and Scotland to establish standards for nurse registration and to develop the content of nurse education in hospitals. The general nursing councils are responsible to the Crown

---

* A body of distinguished citizens appointed by the Crown to oversee certain governmental functions.

through the Privy Council. The General Nursing Council for Scotland has 26 members of whom 13 are elected by the nursing profession, 2 are appointed by the Privy Council to represent universities, and 11 are appointed by the Secretary of State.

THE CENTRAL MIDWIVES BOARDS. The central midwives boards were established to set standards of training and discipline for midwives. The boards must contain persons interested in maternity services. Some members are elected by midwives and others are appointed by the Minister of Health to represent the universities, the royal colleges, local health authorities, medical officers of health, and the Queen's Institute of District Nursing.

THE GENERAL DENTAL COUNCIL. The General Dental Council performs for the dental profession the same functions that are carried out by the General Medical Council for the medical profession. Its membership is similarly composed and chosen.

THE COUNCIL OF PROFESSIONS SUPPLEMENTARY TO MEDICINE. The Council of Professions Supplementary to Medicine is responsible for registration, educational standards, examination, and discipline of chiropractors, dietitians, medical laboratory technicians, occupational therapists, physical therapists, x-ray technicians, and remedial gymnasts. Each professional or technical group has a separate board. The council is responsible to the Crown through the Privy Council and consists of 21 members, 7 of whom are physicians.

The Role of Local Government in the Provision of Health Services in the United Kingdom. The National Health Services Act places the responsibility for a variety of services on local health authorities. These authorities are parts of county boroughs, administrative counties, urban districts, rural districts, and boroughs within metropolitan London. There are 174 major local health authorities in England and Wales and 30 other authorities with delegated health functions. Local health authorities are responsible to the Minister of Health for supportive health services provided for under the National Health Service and mental health services provided for under the Mental Health Acts. In addition, local health authorities are responsible for a number of health services that come under the jurisdiction of other departments of national government including the Ministry of Housing and Local Government; the Department of Education and Science; the Ministry of Agriculture, Fisheries, and Food; the Ministry of Labor; the Home Office and the Medical Research Council. These services include the following

1. Environmental health services.
    a. Communicable disease control.
    b. Seaport hygiene and quarantine.
    c. Housing sanitation.
    d. Water sanitation.
    e. Sewerage sanitation.
2. School health services.
3. Occupational health services.
4. Food and drug administration.
5. Public health laboratory services.
6. Research.

The local authorities are composed of three representatives elected from each ward within the county areas or boroughs. The elected councilors form a council and are required to appoint a number of committees including a Health Committee. The council also is required to appoint a Medical Officer of Health and a Sanitary Inspector. The Medical Officer of Health serves as secretary to the Health Committee and is advisory to the council. He is expected to inform himself in respect to all matters affecting the public health within his district, to determine, to the extent feasible, the causes of diseases and other health problems, and to develop means for the prevention or control of health hazards.

In carrying out his various responsibilities, the Medical Officer of Health may be assisted by several Assistant Medical Officers of Health and a staff of health visitors (public health nurses), district nurses (registered nurses who provide bedside care of the sick), district midwives, social workers, mental welfare workers (persons with some social work training), sanitary inspectors, and home help (homemakers).

Authority and Control in the British Health Service System. Britain has achieved a remarkable degree of unity of purpose and approach in respect of health goals and, through a number of laws enacted by Parliament, has created a mechanism for organizing and financing health services including research and the production of health manpower. Parliament, which in Britain exercises supreme power, has employed a number of instruments and organizational patterns that have retained central control at the national level although providing a certain amount of autonomy in the administration of health services at the community level and in the regulation of the professions. Opportunities have been provided through elected and appointed councils and boards for professional and lay participation in planning, standard setting, and administration.

Parliament has made certain councils, such as statutory councils, responsible not to itself but to the Crown through the device of having Queen's Privy Council exercise supervisory oversight. Of course, Parliament retains the right to alter or even abolish the Councils if it deems appropriate. Moreover, Parliament permits the council members to be chosen jointly by the Crown and the profession to be regulated.

The executive councils that govern the provision of general practitioner, dental, and pharmaceutical services answer to the Minister of Health and thus to Parliament. Their membership, however, is determined by the professional groups involved and by the Local Health Authority, which is in turn a part of elected local government.

Regional hospital boards, which govern the provision of hospital and specialists' services, are appointed by the Minister of Health after consultation with universities, local health authorities, bodies representing the medical profession, voluntary associations, employers, and trade unions. Thus Parliament through the Minister retains ultimate authority, yet the requirement of consultation in respect to appointments provides an opportunity for the professions, agencies, and groups effected, and the general public, to have a voice in the selection of board members. In the case of the teaching hospitals, the Board of Governors is appointed by the Minister of Health but three fifths of the members are nominated in equal numbers by the university, the teaching staff, and the Regional Hospital Board for the area in which the hospital is situated. Similarly, the hospital management committees, which are responsible for the administration of individual hospitals, are appointed by regional hospital boards in consultation with local health authorities, executive councils, and the senior physicians and dentists working in the hospitals.

Thus, we see that although Parliament exercises both legislative and executive power numerous provisions are made for citizen (lay and professional) participation in administration, including management and planning of health services.

Finally, the prestigious royal colleges and the medical and dental associations exert influence in matters relating to hospital appointments and the conditions of participation of physicians and dentists in the National Health Service.

It may be concluded that Britain has provided ample checks and balances to safeguard the interests of the people, the professions, and the Treasury in its effort to protect the mental and physical health of the people of England, Scotland, and Wales.

Health Organization in the United States

There are three salient characteristics of health organization in the United States (1) pluralism, (2) multicentric sources of goal setting and decision making, and (3) fragmentation of effort. Pluralism is exemplified by the fact that most personal health services are provided by the private sector, most preventive health services (personal and environmental) are provided by the public sector. Moreover, there are numerous examples in which the lines of demarcation between public and private domain in the health field are blurred or even reversed. In an open society founded on a deep distrust for centralized governmental authority, it is perhaps inevitable that there would develop numerous foci in and out of government where health goals are determined and health programs sponsored. These two factors, pluralism and multicentricity, have led inexorably to fragmentation of effort. With no agency or body, even at the highest level of government, constituted in a manner to permit the determination of national health policy or the establishment of national health goals, it becomes a game in which anyone may play (Cohen, 1968). The multiplicity of participants assures on the one hand a multiplicity of goals, and on the other hand that goals so set are at best fragmentary and at worst irrelevant or self-serving.

Historically, health programs and organizations have come into being as the answer to a specific problem. The oldest federal health agency, the Public Health Service, began in 1798 as the Marine Hospital Service. Its sole purpose was to provide medical and hospital care to merchant seamen. Over the years it was granted a piecemeal collection of functions whenever Congress was convinced that a health problem of sufficient magnitude required action at the federal level.

A major consideration underlying this state of affairs is the fact that the Constitution does not specifically delegate any public health powers or responsibility to the federal government. When the Congress has enacted laws pertaining to the health of the public it has done so under the general provisions of the Constitution relating to (1) the regulation of foreign and interstate commerce, (2) the promotion of the general welfare, (3) the levying of taxes, and (4) the authority of the President (with the consent of the Senate) to enter into treaties with foreign nations.

Under the federal system of government the state is sovereign. The states have reserved the right to regulate matters affecting health within their borders. This right has been exercised in the passage of laws requiring the registration or licensure of health professionals, the supervision and inspection of health institutions, the control of communicable diseases, the control of environmental health hazards, the involuntary confinement of mentally ill persons, the regulation of the production and sale of drugs and biologics, and the collection of vital statistics.

Federal law in these areas must be limited to federal territories unless the matter relates to interstate or foreign commerce. Hence, there are no federal laws that are generally applicable in respect to the licensure of health professionals or facilities, or the confinement of the mentally ill. Federal laws exist in reference to the interstate nature of many environmental health hazards, particularly the contamination of air and water and the safety of food and drugs produced for interstate commerce. Even the collection of vital statistics is based on the voluntary cooperation of the states.

Perhaps equally important in understanding the patterns and configurations of health organizations and programs in the United States is the tradition of voluntarism in health matters. This tradition can be traced to voluntary efforts that flourished in England in the seventeenth and eighteenth centuries and led to the establishment of hospitals, medical schools, and societies for the improvement of the medical profession. Moreover, there was the still earlier tradition of the church in providing care to the sick and the destitute (often made so by illness or death of the breadwinner).

In addition to the establishment of voluntary hospitals, medical schools, dispensaries, and convalescent homes, there developed in the United States at the beginning of the twentieth century that peculiarly American institution, the voluntary health agency, which grew out of the health concerns of interested citizens. It is, in general, an organization designed to focus public attention and stimulate action in respect to a specific health problem, such as tuberculosis, or the health problems of a particular group, e.g., mothers and children, or the poor. Many of the early voluntary agencies began by developing a nursing service or a clinic and almost all of them have devoted some of their resources to financing health services. In recent years they have tended to concentrate their efforts in the fields of research and health education of the public, leaving service more and more to government.

Still another factor in the pluralism of the American health effort has been the dominant role played by organizations of health professionals, particularly physicians. Organized medicine, as it is called in the United States, has carried out the traditional functions of professional societies, self-improvement and self-regulation. Since the early nineteen-twenties, however, organized medicine has played a vigorous role of militant opposition to government involvement in the provision or the financing of personal health services. This pattern of opposition has taken many forms. It has included such activities as the support of state legislation restricting membership on state boards of health to practising physicians, or legislation requiring a majority of physician members on the governing boards of nonprofit health-insurance plans. It has been notable for large and costly campaigns to defeat federal legislation related to the provision or financing of medical care and has even included opposition to disability pensions and federal aid to medical education. Campaigns have been conducted to defeat candidates for election to Congressional or state legislatures who are considered to be sympathetic to a larger or expanded role of government in the health field.

The influence of organized medicine and other health organizations on the Congress is such that protective caveats are often written in Federal legislation. Public Law 89–97, the law providing health insurance for the aged, contains the following provision in Title XVIII, Section 1801:

"Nothing in this title shall be construed to authorize any Federal officer or employee to exercise any supervision or control over the practice of medicine or the manner in which medical services are provided . . . or to exercise any supervision or control over the administration or operation of any such institution (providing health services)."

And in Section 2(a) of Public Law 89–749, the Comprehensive Health Planning and Public Health Services Amendments of 1966 there is the statement that:

"Federal assistance must be directed to support the marshaling of all health resources —national, state, and local—to assure comprehensive health services of high quality for every person, but without interference with existing patterns of private professional practice of medicine, dentistry, and related arts."

A question may well be raised as to whether the assurance of high quality of health services for every person can in fact be realized without interfering with existing patterns of private professional practice of medicine, dentistry, and related arts.

These and many other factors underlie the pluralistic, multicentric, and fragmentary state of health organization of health services in the United States.

Health Organization at the Federal Level.   Fragmentation of health responsibility at the federal level is perhaps best seen in the fact that the following major federal agencies administer health programs

1. Department of Agriculture.
2. Civil Service Commission.
3. Department of Defense.
4. Department of Health, Education, and Welfare.
5. Department of Housing and Urban Development.
6. Department of the Interior.
7. Department of Justice.
8. Department of Labor.
9. National Aeronautics and Space Administration.
10. Office of Economic Opportunity.
11. Small Business Administration.
12. Department of State.
13. Veterans Administration

(Committee on Interstate and Foreign Commerce, 1966)

As an indication of the magnitude of involvement of some of the above agencies, the amount of funds budgeted for medical and health-related programs is revealing. For the fiscal year 1965, a total of 5.16 billion dollars was budgeted. Of this amount the Department of Health, Education, and Welfare accounted for 2.21 billion, the Veterans Administration 1.26 billion, and the Department of Defense 1.06 billion. For the fiscal year 1969, it is estimated that the total for budgeted funds for medical and health-related activities will amount to 9.78 billion dollars. Of this amount DHEW will account for 5.07 billion, the Department of Defense 1.85 billion, and the

Veterans Administration 1.53 billion. In addition to budgeted funds, it is estimated that 5.78 billion dollars will be spent for medical care from the Trust Fund of the Social Security Administration.

The Department of Health, Education, and Welfare. The Department of Health, Education, and Welfare can trace its antecedents to the establishment of the Marine Hospital Service in 1798. Its present form as an umbrella organization for federal agencies concerned with the general welfare of the people of the United States can be traced to the establishment in 1939 of the Federal Security Agency at a subcabinet level. In his message to Congress accompanying the Reorganization Plan No. 1 of 1939, President Franklin D. Roosevelt stated—

I find it necessary and desirable to group in a Federal Security Agency those agencies of Government, the major purpose of which is to promote social and economic security, educational opportunity, and the health of the citizens of the Nation.
(*Congressional Record*, 76th Congress, 1st Session)

The agencies brought together in the Federal Security Agency were the Social Security Board, then an independent agency; the U.S. Employment Service, then in the Department of Labor; the Office of Education, then in the Department of Interior; the Public Health Service, then in the Treasury Department; the National Youth Administration, then part of the Works Progress Administration; and the Civilian Conservation Corps, an independent agency. In 1940 the Food and Drug Administration was transferred from the Department of Agriculture, and in 1946 the Children's Bureau was transferred from the Department of Labor to the Federal Security Administration.

In 1953, under President Dwight D. Eisenhower, a cabinet level Department of Health, Education, and Welfare was established and had assigned to it all of the agencies and functions of the Federal Security Agency. DHEW, like its predecessor, the Federal Security Agency, has been plagued by a lack of administrative unity and common purpose. Many of its agencies have strong traditions and most of them predate the establishment of the Department. Not only do they serve varying constituencies, they relate to different committees of the Congress. Astute agency heads have found it possible to utilize public support for their mission to influence Congress to support their program budgets at levels in excess of the amounts approved by the Secretary and the President.

The disparate nature and size and importance of the component agencies of DHEW have challenged successive Secretaries to develop a cohesive department with mutual goals.

By the time John W. Gardner became the fifth Secretary to head DHEW it had "grown like Topsy into a giant composed of nearly 100,000 employees, working for eight major agencies and more than 200 subagencies and divisions with a fiscal 1966 budget of $7.7 billion and for fiscal 1968, $12.2 billion. Many of the agencies had become little baronies whose long-time employees jealously guarded their domains against all attempts at innovation." (DHEW, 1968.)

Secretary Gardner undertook a major reorganization of DHEW, which was carried forward by Secretary Wilbur Cohen, who succeeded him in the spring of 1968. The current organization of DHEW is shown in Figure 13-4.

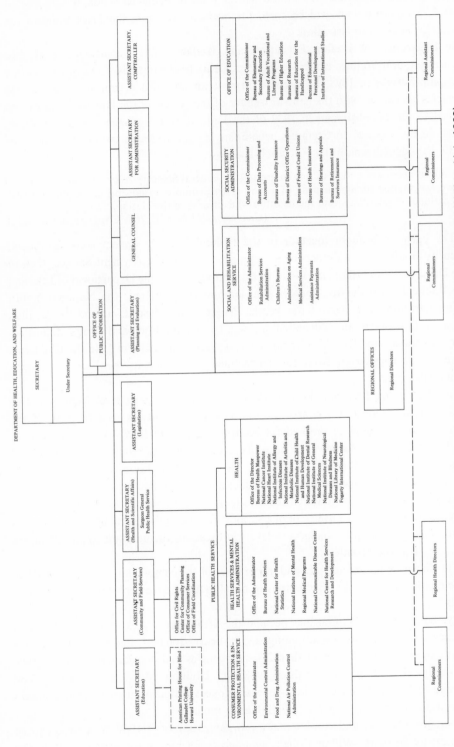

DEPARTMENT OF HEALTH, EDUCATION, AND WELFARE

SECRETARY

Under Secretary

OFFICE OF PUBLIC INFORMATION

ASSISTANT SECRETARY (Education)

American Printing House for Blind
Gallaudet College
Howard University

ASSISTANT SECRETARY (Community and Field Services)

Office for Civil Rights
Center for Community Planning
Office of Consumer Services
Office of Field Coordination

ASSISTANT SECRETARY (Health and Scientific Affairs)

Surgeon General
Public Health Service

ASSISTANT SECRETARY (Legislation)

ASSISTANT SECRETARY (Planning and Evaluation)

GENERAL COUNSEL

ASSISTANT SECRETARY FOR ADMINISTRATION

ASSISTANT SECRETARY, COMPTROLLER

PUBLIC HEALTH SERVICE

CONSUMER PROTECTION & EN-VIRONMENTAL HEALTH SERVICE

Office of the Administrator
Environmental Control Administration
Food and Drug Administration
National Air Pollution Control Administration

HEALTH SERVICES & MENTAL HEALTH ADMINISTRATION

Office of the Administrator
Bureau of Health Services
National Center for Health Statistics
National Institute of Mental Health
Regional Medical Programs
National Communicable Disease Center
National Center for Health Services Research and Development

HEALTH

Office of the Director
Bureau of Health Manpower
National Cancer Institute
National Heart Institute
National Institute of Allergy and Infectious Diseases
National Institute of Arthritis and Metabolic Diseases
National Institute of Child Health and Human Development
National Institute of Dental Research
National Institute of General Medical Sciences
National Institute of Neurological Diseases and Blindness
National Library of Medicine
Fogarty International Center

SOCIAL AND REHABILITATION SERVICE

Office of the Administrator
Rehabilitation Services Administration
Children's Bureau
Administration on Aging
Medical Services Administration
Assistance Payments Administration

SOCIAL SECURITY ADMINISTRATION

Office of the Commissioner
Bureau of Data Processing and Accounts
Bureau of Disability Insurance
Bureau of District Office Operations
Bureau of Federal Credit Unions
Bureau of Health Insurance
Bureau of Hearings and Appeals
Bureau of Retirement and Survivors Insurance

OFFICE OF EDUCATION

Office of the Commissioner
Bureau of Elementary and Secondary Education
Bureau of Adult Vocational and Library Programs
Bureau of Higher Education
Bureau of Research
Bureau of Education for the Handicapped
Bureau of Educational Personnel Development
Institute of International Studies

REGIONAL OFFICES

Regional Directors

Regional Commissioners

Regional Health Directors

Regional Commissioners

Regional Commissioners

Regional Commissioners

Regional Assistant Commissioners

FIGURE 13–4. Organization of United States Department of Health, Education and Welfare (July 1968).

396

That this latest reorganization does not go far enough in resolving the problems of coordination may be seen in the recommendation of the Subcommittee on Investigation of DHEW of the Committee on Interstate and Foreign Commerce of the House of Representatives—that there is a need to establish a single organizational focus of federal health authority and responsibility by establishing a separate Department of Health. The Subcommittee in considering the health activities of other federal departments made the distinction between agencies whose health programs are a means to the fulfillment of another administrative mission and those for which health programs are a primary concern. It recommended inclusion of only the latter type of activity in a Department of Health.

In addition to the reorganization of DHEW in 1968, Secretary Cohen addressed himself to the problem of coordination of the health activities of other federal departments and agencies. Secretary Cohen recommended to President Lyndon Johnson that the Secretary of HEW be made responsible for coordinating all federal health policies and programs and be authorized to establish a Federal Interdepartmental Policy Council composed of ranking representatives of each department and agency having a substantial role in discharging the federal responsibility for the promotion of health among the general population and among segments of the population such as military personnel, veterans, and other beneficiaries of federal health services. The proposed council would report through the Secretary to the President.

Another approach to the problem of the formulation of national health policy was taken by the National Advisory Commission on Health Manpower, which was appointed by President Johnson in 1966. This commission stated that the national government needed continuing advice from a source that concerns itself with the entire spectrum of governmental and nongovernmental health activities. The commission recommended the establishment of a Council of Health Advisers composed of nongovernment experts reporting to the public and the President through the Secretary of HEW.

The Organization of Health Services at the State Level.   It is perhaps not surprising that like the federal government, states have not been able to avoid fragmentation of authority and effort in the health field. "A partial listing of state agencies that have health responsibilities would include the following departments of health, welfare, agriculture, education, and vocational rehabilitation; mental health and separate mental retardation authorities; hospital construction authorities; special boards and commissions, such as those concerned with industrial accidents, alcoholism, narcotics, and drugs; river and water authorities; public works agencies; and housing and planning organizations" (U.S. Depart. of HEW, 1966).

Like the federal government some states have attempted coordination through the establishment of umbrella agencies combining health and welfare activities. Although states are sovereign, their sovereignty in health and welfare matters has been eroded by their necessary dependence on the federal government for financial support for vital programs. Increasingly since the nineteen-thirties, states have been forced to look for federal grants-in-aid support for a multitude of public services for which states are responsible. In the health field, DHEW makes financial aid available to state health agencies through 158 separate grant-in-aid programs. These grants provide support for research, training of health personnel, construction of health facilities, and the provision of health services. The grants are of two kinds, formula and project grants. Formula grants are allotted to states on the basis of formulae related to population, per capita income, and prevalence of the health problem; and states are required to match the federal contribution by providing a mandatory percentage of the cost of the program. Project grants may be awarded to state agencies or any appropriate public or private nonprofit agency. Project-grant aid is of limited duration and may or may not require the recipient agency to supply matching funds.

Formula grants often contain the stipulation that states designate "single state agencies" to receive and administer grant funds. This requirement began in the nineteen-thirties when Congress felt that it had to prod the states into establishing appropriate administrative units that could carry out the intent of the federal program and be held accountable for the proper use of federal aid. This requirement, however, has tended to cause the proliferation of state agencies and has hampered the adoption of flexible policies governing the use of federal aid by the states.

STATE HEALTH DEPARTMENTS.   Each of the fifty states has a health department headed by a physician typically appointed by the Governor on the recommendation of the State Board of Health. It is the function of the department to carry out certain health functions that are usually defined in law or in the policies and regulations adopted by the board. These include environmental sanitation, the prevention and control of disease, the collection of vital statistics, and the provision of hospital care for persons with tuberculosis or other chronic diseases. Where there is not a separate department of mental health, the state health department usually is responsible for the operation of hospitals and other facilities and services for the mentally ill and the mentally retarded. State health departments usually are responsible for the supervision and licensure of health facilities. This function has been strengthened by the federal requirements in Public Law 89–97 pertaining to the supervision of health facilities participating in the care of the aged. The licensure and registration of health professionals often are functions of separate boards or of state departments of education.

With few exceptions, state health departments administer the federal-state program for handicapped children originally called the Crippled Children's Program. In some states the operation of this program is decentralized by delegation to local health departments. The state health department maintains administrative control usually by retaining the authority for approval of eligibility and the treatment program for each child accepted.

Other than the handicapped children's program and the provision of certain hospital services, state health departments usually do not provide preventive medical and dental services to groups such as mothers and children nor do they inspect local food establishments or housing. These functions, and often many more, are delegated to local health departments, and the state agency performs a supervisory role and reviews the performance of its local counterpart.

Local Health Departments.   Local health departments are to be found in all major cities and in many towns and counties. A considerable number of people, however, particularly in rural areas, are not served by local health departments. Local health departments are headed by an executive officer who is usually, but not always, a physician. He is appointed by the mayor or chief executive of the city, usually on the advice of the local board of health. Local health departments exercise certain legislative functions delegated to them by states and may adopt health codes that must be consistent with state health laws. Local health departments are primarily concerned with matters that directly affect the health of the residents of the local community, including the sanitation of food, water, housing, and the control and prevention of communicable and other diseases, and the provision of direct care to certain high-risk groups such as pregnant women, children, the aged, and the poor. In respect to the poor there is a dichotomy of function in that welfare departments are generally responsible for medical care for persons receiving financial aid for other necessities of life. Recently with the expansion of federal aid to the states for the provision of medical care to certain categories of indigent and medically indigent persons, local and state health departments have become involved in varying degrees in arranging for or providing health services for the poor and for persons who are self-supporting but are unable to pay for medical care.

Voluntary Health Agencies. Voluntary health agencies exist at national, state, and local levels. They play an important role in the identification of health problems and in devising approaches designed to solve them. Voluntary health agencies have concerned themselves with such varied functions as the support of the education of health professionals; the support of research pertaining to the causes, prevention, and cure of specific diseases; the direct provision of health care to special groups or to individuals with specific diseases; the provision of rehabilitation services to the handicapped; the provision of institutional care of the aged and infirm; health care, meals, and house-keeping services to disabled, chronically ill, or aged persons living in their own homes; health care of mothers and children; and the promotion of standards of health care. Voluntary agencies are inherently more flexible in their operations than governmental agencies and they are often able to obtain the services of health professionals who would not work for government. On the other hand, they tend to concentrate on pieces of the mosaic of health problems reflecting the interests of their leaders or donors rather than the importance or magnitude of the health need.

By demonstrating concern and devising solutions, they have pioneered in many health fields pointing the way for the establishment of governmental responsibility. In recent years government, particularly at the national level, has seized the initiative for innovation. As voluntary agencies have begun to experience difficulties in raising funds by public subscription, and as the cost of services and research in the health field have sharply risen, voluntary agencies have assumed a new role—that of agent for the governmental agency. Voluntary agencies are assuming many service and research functions under contract to governmental agencies, employing their flexibility, know-how, and resourcefulness in a new form of partnership to serve the health of the people.

CONCLUSIONS

The pluralism and the decentralization of authority for planning and research, and for the development of manpower, facilities, and services, has permitted and encouraged innovation and the development of a wide variety of approaches in the health field. The opportunity for innovation and for the flexible use of various mechanisms and models has been bought at the cost of fragmentation, gaps in coverage, and duplication of effort. Centralized planning at national, regional, state, or local levels has been repugnant to many health professionals, professional societies, and health organizations. Although planning has come to be recognized as a necessity, the Congress has enacted a bewildering variety of federal laws each dealing separately with such matters as health care of children, mothers, Indians, the poor and the aged; health facilities; health manpower; mental illness; heart disease, cancer and stroke; rehabilitation of the disabled; and air and water pollution. In many instances these laws call for planning and action by separate and often competing or conflicting groups at regional, state, and local levels. Pluralism, so much a part of American life, will continue in the field of health. In the United States, and perhaps elsewhere, the health administrator must be a generalist, gifted and flexible, and dedicated to the high purpose of better health for people.

REFERENCES

COHEN, W.: *Health in America: The Role of the Federal Government in Bringing High Quality Health Care to All the American People*—A Report to the President by the Secretary of Health, Education, and Welfare. Washington, D.C., June 14, 1968.

COMMITTEE ON INTERSTATE AND FOREIGN COMMERCE, HOUSE OF REPRESENTATIVES: *Investigation of HEW*. Washington, D.C., Oct. 13, 1966.

Congressional Record, **84**, Part V, 4710, 76th Congress, 1st Sess.

Encyclopedia Britannica, **19**:729. Chicago, 1953.

FIELD, M. G.: How socialized medicine works in the Soviet Union. *The Progressive*, 44–47, March 1958.

———: *Soviet Socialized Medicine*. The Free Press, New York, 1967.

FORSYTH, G.: *Doctors and State Medicine*. Pitman Medical Publishing Co., London, 1966.

GOODMAN, N. M.: International health organizations. In Hobson, W. (ed.): *The Theory and Practice of Public Health*. Oxford University Press, London, 1965.

HER MAJESTY'S STATIONERY OFFICE: *Health Services in Britain*. London, 1960.

———: *National Health Services Act*. London, 1946.

MACHLAN, G. (ed.): *Problems and Progress in Medical Care*. Oxford University Press, London, 1964.

MEDICAL WORLD NEWS: Reorganizing "Health" in HEW. *Medical World News*, 58–64, 1968.

PAN AMERICAN HEALTH ORGANIZATION: *Task Force on Health at the Ministerial Level*. The Organization, Washington, D.C., 1964.

PETERS, R. J., and KINNARD, J. (eds.): *Health Services Administration*. E. & S. Livingstone Ltd., Edinburgh, 1965.

Programme of the Communist Party of the Soviet Union. Foreign Languages Publishing House, Moscow, 1951.

Report of the National Advisory Commission on Health and Manpower, **1**:76–77. U.S. Government Printing Office, Washington, D.C.

SCHAEFER, M.: Current issues in health organization. *Amer J Public Health*, **58**:1192–99, 1968.

TIME, INC.: *Britain*. Time, Inc., New York, 1961.

U.S. DEPARTMENT OF HEALTH, EDUCATION, AND WELFARE: *Advisory Committee on HEW Relationships with State Health Agencies*—Report to the Secretary. Washington, D.C.

U.S. PUBLIC HEALTH SERVICE: *Hospital Services in the U.S.S.R.*, Pub. no. 930-F-10. November 1968.

————, NATIONAL CENTER FOR HEALTH STATISTICS: *Mortality Trends in the United States, 1954–1963*.

WORLD HEALTH ORGANIZATION: *The First Ten Years of the World Health Organization.* The Organization, Geneva, 1958.

————: *World Health Organization Manual.* The Organization, Geneva, 1967.

YERBY, A. S.: Medical care in the Soviet Union. *Medical Care*, **6**: 280–85, 1968.

14

Community and Governmental Responsibility in Delivery of Medical Care to the Individual

George G. Reader

INTRODUCTION

Although in much of the world there has been a long history of governmental provision of health services to individuals, it has been a somewhat new development in the United States. This chapter will deal with the recent rapid growth of governmental responsibility and its implications for the future.

The common pattern in Colonial America was public subscription through voluntary contribution for needed health services. In the late eighteenth century, for example, dispensaries and hospitals were founded by leading citizens. The Pennsylvania Hospital was the first in the country in the modern meaning of the word and was organized by Dr. Thomas Bond and Benjamin Franklin. The New York Hospital similarly was founded by Dr. Samuel Bard and Sir Henry Moore, who was Governor of the New York colony and headed the assemblage attending the first graduation of medical students from King's College (Columbia). On that occasion Dr. Bard eloquently urged on the community the need for a general hospital, which appeal met with an immediate response. Both hospitals were granted some provincial funds, but the major support came from wealthy donors.

With the organization of the federal government the Marine Hospital Service was developed after a British model to provide medical care for merchant seamen. The act for the relief of sick and disabled seamen was passed by the Congress on July 16, 1798, and from this stemmed the first federal efforts in public health, as well as in direct service to patients.

Medical services had been provided to troops during the Revolution, of course, but a Navy Medical Corps was not organized until 1811 and the Army not until 1818. Since then the federal government has entered directly into the care of a number of groups, Indians, veterans, freed slaves, lepers, drug addicts, federal prisoners, interned Japanese during World War II, and migratory farm workers.

Local governmental responsibility for medical services in the community at large was slower to emerge. Physicians donated their services to indigent patients, and municipal funding of health facilities did not occur widely until the late nineteenth century.

SOCIAL RESPONSIBILITY FOR HEALTH SERVICES

With this strong tradition of free enterprise and private philanthropy in the United States, true social responsibility for health care has only reached a significant level of acceptance in recent years. The definition incorporated into the preamble to the constitution of the World Health Organization in 1946 stated:

The enjoyment of the highest attainable standard of health is one of the fundamental rights of every human being without distinction of race, religion, political belief, economic or social condition.

Its endorsement came as a shock to many persons in the United States. Although some in the medical profession felt that ratification of the WHO charter implied acceptance of socialized medicine, today most physicians are willing to accept the idea that health care is a right rather than a privilege. They quarrel over how the care should be provided; many feel that it is their personal philanthropic prerogative to minister to the sick poor. They resent being pre-empted by other agencies. Many businessmen and economists, on the other hand, believe that health care is a commodity and should be available only to those who can afford it. There is a consensus that no person should be allowed to die for lack of treatment, but medical services other than emergency care are subject to dispute.

There is of course some question as to whether medical care always improves health. At times a great many expensive services have been made available to a community without discernible alteration in the usual indices of health, such as neonatal mortality, morbidity statistics, and death rates. Other factors such as sanitation, food, housing, and employment may well be more important than medical treatment. In terms of improving the health of an individual, a distinction may eventually have to be made between those services that are essential and those that might be considered luxuries. Certainly a broken leg needs to be splinted, but the common cold may run its self-limited course without a visit to a physician or exhibition of drugs. Some preventive services are also open to question on the basis of their proved efficacy. Immunization against poliomyelitis will protect in most cases and will certainly reduce the incidence in a community. Primary prevention of coronary artery disease or of cancer, on the other hand, is still uncertain. Many medical services are mainly a source of comfort and support to the patient without any evidence that they have more than a placebo effect; witness the injection of vitamins to restore flagging energies. As the costs of health care rise, third parties including government may be expected to raise questions about what is necessary for patients and what is not. It is generally conceded today, however, that patients at all economic levels have a right to access to health services and that these must be paid for by society if the person is unable to meet the cost himself. The rest of this exposition will consider how government at all levels has met this obligation or failed to meet it, both directly and indirectly.

HEALTH CARE PROVIDED DIRECTLY BY GOVERNMENT

Because it is often confusing to understand how the responsibilities and authority of various levels of government interrelate, it is desirable first to consider what levels are involved generally in health care before going on to discuss examples of what each has done and is doing. Local government has concerned itself traditionally in the United States with protection of its own community from the threat of disease. As was noted previously, the first concern was with construction of health facilities and provision of services to prevent epidemics. Pesthouses came first and hospitals for the sick poor later. As the concept of public health began to take hold at the local level, however, more direct services were developed, such as child health clinics, venereal disease and tuberculosis treatment and control programs, and the management of narcotic and alcohol addiction. Except for child health, the element of service to the individual tended to be secondary to the motivation of protection of the community. In recent years, however, direct service to people has become a primary aim.

State government has always tried to deal with health problems that are larger than local communities can cope with or that cross the lines between one or more localities. Mental health long ago became too large an issue for municipalities, and most states found it necessary to move in and provide institutional facilities for the mentally disturbed. State governments have also served as channels for federal programs, finding this a convenient way to distribute tax funds equitably and still retain the concept of "states rights."

The federal government usually has provided direct health care to specific groups in the population, such as merchant seamen and migrant workers, who would not otherwise receive it. The federal government also acts in a stimulatory and advisory capacity with state and local health departments. More recently, however, there has been an inclination, and in some instances a mandate, to reach out directly to people in local communities where health services have previously been inadequate.

PERSONAL HEALTH SERVICES PROVIDED BY LOCAL COMMUNITIES

In most communities in the United States today local government attempts to discharge its responsibility for provision of health services to those who cannot afford private care by maintaining hospitals in the large centers or by contracting to pay for services in voluntary hospitals. Hospital bed care is thus available to all members of the community, and is usually supplemented by clinic care for those who cannot afford physicians' fees. In many areas of the United States, though, physicians still prefer to see indigent patients in their offices and charge a token fee or nothing. They may sometimes be reimbursed by the local welfare department.

The health department usually conducts clinics for venereal disease and tuberculosis as part of its control program, and often supports child health stations and dental clinics. These are often staffed by practicing physicians and dentists who are paid something for their participation. Dentistry rarely goes beyond filling and extracting teeth, and maternal and child health concentrates on prophylactic immunizations and health practices rather than on treatment. Family planning is often a part of this service. In New York and other large cities the health department may also extend its preventive activities to chronic illness because this has become numerically the most pressing urban health problem of the day (see Chapter 12). Diagnostic services are provided, as well as preventive health activities such as antismoking clinics, anti-coronary clubs, and cancer detection services. Because secondary prevention of complications in chronic illness is usually more successful than primary prevention, however, and requires careful study of patients and follow-up, there is a growing tendency for health departments to engage in long-term responsibility for management of the chronically ill. More recently the emphasis on provision of direct services, particularly to the deprived, has increased greatly so that many local health officers are now looking into ways to participate in delivery of services to people who would not otherwise have adequate health care. This is a shift from an older philanthropic attitude of providing comfort for the sick poor to a much more aggressive and constructive approach to raising the level of health of the whole community through improved health services. The neighborhood health center to be discussed in detail below is one such manifestation. Many feel that the future of the official public health agency in an industrialized society such as ours lies in organizing the provision of health services to maximize their effects rather than merely trying to reduce the level of threat from epidemics and environmental hazards. Modern public health in the United States encompasses both prevention and treatment.

STATE HEALTH SERVICES

As has been indicated, state governments tend to take on large-scale problems that are beyond the resources of local communities. In the smaller states this may mean actual direct general service in the local communities, and almost everywhere it includes provision of mental health care. Not uncommonly the mental health budget represents the largest segment of the state budget in that it supports the construction and maintenance of mental hospitals as well as payment for the care rendered therein. Since the development of psychotropic drugs, there has been greater emphasis on local ambulatory care for psychiatric patients, but the need for mental hospitals continues to increase beyond the resources of local jurisdictions.

In New York State the government supports treatment of narcotic addicts, too, through a system of shelters somewhat analogous to the mental hospital system. It also provides treatment for cancer patients as part of the research endeavor of the Roswell Park Institute, and supports a number of general hospitals in conjunction with education of health professionals under the auspices of the State University.

FEDERAL ACTIVITIES

The federal government gives health services to a number of special interest groups, as has been noted. It also has direct responsibility for members of the armed forces and their dependents and for veterans. In conjunction with the research activities of the National Institutes of Health it supports the Clinical Center, a large hospital that provides subjects and a setting for clinical investigation. As one example of its direct services and their effects, the Indian Health Program will be considered next.

The Indian Health Program.   The Indian Health Program is one of the best and most successful efforts in the federal government's role in providing direct health services and is worth considering in some detail. Until 1954, when Public Law 83–568 transferred the maintenance and operation of hospital and health facilities for Indians to the Public Health Service, Indian health had been the responsibility of the Department of the Interior. Earlier in the last century it had been under the United States Army. Prior to assignment to the Public Health Service, implementation of health services had been somewhat desultory. The Public Health Service, however, given a full mandate to improve the health of the Indians and Alaska natives, has made most remarkable strides since 1954. It is an indication of what can be done through application of modern public health principles, attending to sanitary facilities and housing as well as applying preventive and curative techniques. Within ten years neonatal deaths were reduced 44 per cent for Indian babies and 50 per cent for Alaska native babies. Tuberculosis death rates were reduced 56 per cent and 84 per cent respectively, and gastroenteric disease death rates 60 per cent. Tuberculosis was the leading cause of death in 1949 and dropped to ninth place by 1966. Gastroenteritis as a cause of death dropped from fifth place in 1951 to tenth place in 1964. Indians lived to an average age of 44 years in 1966, compared with an age of 38 eight years before, a gain of six years. The leading causes of death by 1963 were—

Indian	Alaska Native
Heart disease	Accidents
Accidents	Diseases of early infancy
Influenza and pneumonia	Influenza and pneumonia
Malignant neoplasms	Heart disease
Diseases of early infancy	Malignant neoplasms
Vascular lesions	Vascular lesions
Cirrhosis of liver	Cirrhosis of liver

This indicated a shift away from infectious disease and toward chronic illness. The high accident rate shows that the life remains rugged and hazardous.

Although life expectancy has been increased, it is still only 63.9 years for Indians compared with 70.2 for the general United States population. Death rates are much higher, too, for Indians than for the general population in many of the controllable diseases, indicating that there is more yet to be accomplished. In 1965, however, 381,000 persons were being cared for by 5,275 health personnel on a budget of about 63 million dollars. Nearly 60 per cent of the personnel today are of Indian descent, and training represents a significant part of the activities budgeted. This whole endeavor can in some ways be looked upon as a model of government medicine, both for developing countries and for the underprivileged in our own society. (U.S. Public Health Service, 1966.)

REGULATORY FUNCTIONS OF GOVERNMENT IN PERSONAL HEALTH SERVICES

At many levels and in a number of ways, government attempts to protect its citizens from poor health care. Licensure of health professionals has the longest history in this endeavor and has almost always been a function of state government. The aim of licensing examinations for physicians and other practitioners is to determine that they are qualified before they enter into practice. It is a safeguard only of the qualifications of new practitioners, however, because once a license is given, it becomes a right of the practitioner. He retains this right unless it can be shown that he has broken the law, and then it can be revoked only by due process. There are no repeat licensure examinations.

The Federal Government.   The United States federal government does not grant licences but it does set standards in many ways. The Food and Drug Administration (FDA) supervises the quality and efficacy of drugs and to a degree even influences prescribing practices indirectly by monitoring the directions and recommendations of manufacturers. Federal legislation providing health benefits also sets standards, such as those for the care of crippled children. It has also specified appropriate construction standards for health facilities under the Hill-Burton Act. Under the Medicare Act it specified the type of service to be provided within hospitals in extended care facilities and in home health services, including staffing patterns.

Many local jurisdictions have developed codes for hospital and nursing home staffs, requiring a specific level of training for chiefs of service and those identified as specialists. This is a trend that may be expected to continue. Under Title XIX of the Medicare Act, much of the determination of quality standards is left to the states, and many have developed quite detailed regulations governing providers of service to beneficiaries under this program. There is a growing tendency, in fact, to require quality controls of all health services paid for by public moneys.

Government has also taken a less direct interest in supervising the composition of boards of insurance companies, such as Blue Cross, and in the practices of insurance underwriters as they relate to reimbursement for personal health services.

Perhaps the most potentially pervasive influence, however, is Public Law 89–749, passed by the Congress in 1966 and amended by Public Law 90-174. These together are known as the Partnership in Health Act, or the Comprehensive Health Planning Law. This is a complicated piece of legislation, and only the sections that bear on personal health services will be discussed at this point. There are two features of considerable significance, one a grant program to encourage states to develop a single state-wide health-planning agency that will have the power to pass on development of health facilities and services within the state, and the other a project-grant section, which allows nonprofit community agencies to apply for funds for direct service to individuals. State planning-grant applications "must show that preventive, diagnostic, treatment and rehabilitative programs shall include special attention to the health needs of high risk population groups in terms of age, economic status, geographic location, or other relevant factors." Most states have hastened to designate such a planning agency and have begun to examine health services within the state. Such attention by an official agency is very likely to result in setting of standards to improve quality, although it is too soon as yet to determine the ultimate consequences nation-wide. Likewise it is too early to know how effective the project-grant system will be in improving health services in neighborhoods of large cities and in local communities. This may, however, be the beginning of a new form of governmental influence on health services stemming from the federal government but reaching down through the states to the local community level. The designation, *Partnership in Health*, is meant to imply just this kind of relationship, a part of the "creative federalism" that has been a hallmark of the Johnson Administration. (U.S. Office of Comprehensive Health Planning, 1967.)

INDIRECT SUPPORT OF HEALTH SERVICES

Today the government pays a large part of the bill for health services. A study by Nora Piore of the health budget of New York City for 1964–65 prior to implementation of Medicare, showed that one third of the total cost of personal health services rendered to families was borne by government and one half of the cost of care for hospitalization. Since Medicare the proportion has, of course, gone up considerably. Government is now deeply in the business of support of indirect health services as well as those direct services that have already been noted (Piore, 1965).

Workmen's Compensation

One of the oldest forms of indirect support and regulation of health services, one that goes back to the turn of the century in some states, is legislation requiring insured support of employees injured at work. Workmen's compensation is government-sponsored rather than government-funded, and the laws vary from state to state. All the states today have workmen's compensation programs, and all are paid for by employers although the terms of the benefits are set by state law. In most jurisdictions cash support benefits are emphasized rather than medical care. Although some states have attempted to regulate the quality of medical benefits offered, there is generally considered to be too little emphasis on modern concepts or rehabilitation in the various programs.

MEDICARE

With the economic depression of the 1930's came the first organized effort on a national scale to deal with medical indigency. The Social Security Act of 1935 established the Old Age, Survivors, and Disability programs of the federal government.

These are insurance programs providing retirement benefits and survivor's benefits for the spouse. Except for disability payments and support for vocational rehabilitation, these did little for a number of years to affect personal health services. It was not until 1965 that momentum built up to a point where the Congress was ready to provide support of personal health services for the aged. The election of 1964 had been a landslide for the Democratic Party and provided a mandate for passage of amendments allowing health insurance benefits. The Medicare Bill was introduced into the House of Representatives as HR I and into the Senate simultaneously as S I. It was taken up by the Ways and Means Committee of the House, and after much discussion and organized opposition from the American Medical Association in the form of an extensive advertising campaign, a revised version emerged from the Committee as HR 6675. This bill incorporated some of the concepts of insured physician payments proposed by the American Medical Association in another bill, which they had supported, called Eldercare, in addition to the original hospital insurance provisions of Medicare. And it added a section, Title XIX, which revised and greatly expanded the Medical Assistance to the Aged Act (Kerr-Mills). The House Ways and Means Committee report described the over-all purpose of the bill as follows:

First to provide a coordinated approach for health insurance and medical care for the aged under the Social Security Act by establishing—

(1) A basic plan providing protection against the costs of hospital and related care financed through a separate payroll tax and separate trust fund;
(2) A voluntary "supplementary" plan providing payments for physicians' and other medical and health services financed through small monthly premiums by individual participants matched equally by Federal Government revenue contributions; and
(3) A greatly expanded medical assistance program for the needy and medically needy which would combine all the vendor medical provisions for the aged, blind, disabled, and families with dependent children, now in five titles of the Social Security Act, under a uniform program and matching formula in a single new title.

Second, to expand the services for maternal and child health, crippled children, and the mentally retarded, and to establish a 5-year program of "special project grants" to provide comprehensive health care and services for needy children of school age or preschool age.

Third, to revise and improve the benefit and coverage provisions and the financing structure of the Federal old-age, survivors', and disability insurance system by—

(1) Increasing benefits by 7 per cent across the board with a $4 minimum increase for a worker retiring or who retired age 65 or older;
(2) Continuing benefits to age 22 for children attending school;
(3) Providing actuarially reduced benefits for widows at age 60;
(4) Liberalizing the definition and waiting period for disability insurance benefits;
(5) Paying benefits on a transitional basis to certain persons currently 72 or over who are now ineligible;
(6) Increasing the amount an individual is permitted to earn without losing benefits;
(7) Amending the coverage provisions by:
   (a) Including self-employed physicians;
   (b) Covering cash tips;
   (c) Liberalizing the income treatment for self-employed farmers;
   (d) Improving certain State and local coverage provisions;
   (e) Exempting certain religious groups opposed to insurance;
(8) Revising the tax schedule and the earnings base so as to fully finance the changes made; and
(9) Making other miscellaneous improvements.

Fourth, to improve and expand the public assistance programs by—

(1) Increasing the Federal matching share for cash payments for the needy aged, blind, disabled, and families with dependent children;
(2) Eliminating limitations on Federal participation in public assistance to aged individuals in tuberculosis and mental disease hospitals under certain conditions;
(3) Affording the States broader latitude in disregarding certain earnings in determining need for aged recipients of public assistance;
(4) Making other improvements in the public assistance titles of the Social Security Act.
(Committee on Ways and Means, House of Representatives, 1965)

This bill, HR 6675, was passed by the House and then by the Senate and became Public Law 89-97.

In 1967 Congress modified the law slightly. These current amendments to the Social Security Act can be summarized in somewhat simplified form as follows:

Benefits Under Title XVIII

The benefit period (originally called a spell of illness) ends as soon as a beneficiary has not been an in-patient of any hospital or extended care facility for 60 days in a row.
Part A Benefits. These include up to 90 hospital days in each benefit period, and may be extended by the lifetime reserve of 60 days.

Up to 100 extended-care-facility days in each benefit period if there have been three days in a hospital first.

Up to 100 home health visits for each benefit period Part A helps pay for in a hospital—

Semiprivate room (2–4 beds) and all meals, including special diets.
Operating room charges.
Regular nursing services (including intensive care nursing).
Drugs furnished by the hospital.
Laboratory tests.
X-ray and other radiology services.
Medical supplies such as splints and casts.
Use of appliances and equipment furnished by the hospital.
Medical social services.

In an extended care facility—

Semiprivate room (2–4 beds) and all meals, including special diets.
Regular nursing services.
Drugs furnished by the extended care facility.
Physical, occupational, and speech therapy.
Medical supplies such as splints and casts.
Use of appliances and equipment furnished by the facility.
Medical social services.

Part A helps pay through a home health agency for—

Part-time nursing care.
Physical, occupational, or speech therapy.
Part-time services of home health aides.
Medical social services.
Medical supplies furnished by the agency.
Use of medical appliances.

Part B Benefits.   Part B benefits are obtained by paying a monthly premium and the first $50 for covered services in each calendar year. Part B pays 80 per cent of the reasonable charges for all additional covered services. Part B helps pay for Physician Services—

Medical and surgical services by a doctor of medicine or osteopathy. (Part B cannot make payment for services performed outside the United States.)

Certain medical and surgical services by a doctor of dental medicine or a doctor of dental surgery.

Certain services by a podiatrist within the limits authorized by the State in which he practices.

Other services that are ordinarily furnished in the physician's office and included in his bill. These include

Diagnostic tests and procedures.
Medical supplies.
Services of his office nurse.
Drugs and biologicals that cannot be self-administered.

Part B helps pay for Hospital Outpatient Benefits—

Laboratory and other diagnostic services.
X-ray and other radiology services.
Emergency room services.
Medical supplies.

For Home Health Benefits—

Part-time nursing care.
Physical, occupational, and speech therapy.
Part-time services of home health aides.
Medical supplies furnished by the agency.
Use of medical appliances.

For Other Medical Services and Supplies—

Diagnostic procedures, such as laboratory tests and x-ray services, furnished by participating facilities or approved independent laboratories.*

Radiation therapy.*

Surgical dressings, splints, casts, and similar devices.*

Devices (other than dental) to replace all or part of an internal body organ. This includes corrective lenses after a cataract operation.*

Rental or purchase of durable medical equipment prescribed by a physician to be used in the patient's home.

Certain ambulance services.

Certain portable diagnostic x-ray services.

Drugs and biologicals that cannot be self-administered.†

Title XIX

The amendment of the Medical Assistance Act (Kerr-Mills) was "for the purpose of enabling each State to furnish (1) medical assistance in behalf of families with dependent children and of aged, blind, or permanently and totally disabled individuals, whose

---

* If a patient is in a hospital or extended care facility and, for some reason, hospital insurance cannot pay for these services (for example, because he has used up his benefit days), medical insurance can help pay for them.

† Summarized from *Medicare: A Reference Guide for Physicians*, U.S. Social Security Administration, 1968.

income and resources are insufficient to meet the costs of necessary medical services, and (2) rehabilitation and other services to help such families and individuals attain or retain capability for independence or self-care." It was intended to improve the deficiencies of Kerr-Mills and to complement Title XVIII. Under it each state to obtain federal funds must submit a plan to be approved by the Secretary of Health, Education, and Welfare. The state programs have been called by various names, MediCal in California and Medicaid in New York, for example. New York State was one of the first to submit a plan and it set the eligibility level at $6,000 for a family of four. Within a few months considerable public opposition developed to such liberality. Congress also feared that high eligibility levels under Title XIX might prove too much of a drain on the national budget and amended it to set national limits on eligibility. New York immediately lowered its eligibility limits and cut benefits, not wanting to assume the additional costs of the program itself. Most other states have been more cautious about offering benefits in the plans they have submitted.

It is somewhat early to tell the impact of the state plans on health services because all of them have not been fully implemented. As with Title XVIII, however, states will set standards for the health care that is to be reimbursed, and the scrutiny of both federal and state government will be upon the distribution, cost, and quality of personal health services to a degree never found in the past. Where public funds flow, public interest inevitably follows.

An Era of Change

The impact of the Social Security Amendments of 1965, even though not yet fully developed, may be considered revolutionary in terms of their scope and in the fundamental changes that will result in American health practices. Most importantly, a precedent has been established for use of government funds for the health care of a large segment of the population, all those over 65, using the insurance principle and without a means test. It is likely that these benefits will gradually be extended to other groups, such as widows under 65 and the disabled.

Although many predicted that hospitals would be flooded by applicants, this has not occurred. The elderly seem no more eager to be hospitalized unnecessarily than they were before. Utilization of service has gone up, and expenditures have been somewhat higher than expected. Utilization has been largely related to need, but expense has risen because of the rising costs of health services. Reimbursement for hospitalization under Medicare is based on true costs, and that basis has provided an impetus to hospital personnel, who have traditionally been underpaid, to demand and get higher wages.

Aside from increases in utilization and costs, two of the most significant changes the legislation has wrought in practice to date have been its effect on hospital accounting practices and on the development of utilization review procedures. Medicare has caused hospitals all over the country to put in uniform accounting systems and to analyze their cost structure to determine their real costs in billing the Social Security Administration. These changes have brought a new and more businesslike outlook to hospitals, as well as providing comparable data for large numbers of hospitals. In the long run it is likely to make more rational an industry that has traditionally viewed itself as a charitable enterprise. Eventually, in fact, it may be possible to apply cost-benefit effectiveness techniques with consequences that may be profound.

Utilization review was required by Medicare with the hope that it would cut down on overuse of hospital beds. Each hospital and extended care facility, in order to qualify as a provider of services under the Act, is required to have a utilization review committee with at least two physician members. Composition and function of the committee are monitored by the state and by the Medicare intermediary. There are two functions to be served, the first is educational through review of a random sample of admissions; the second is a review of all long-stay cases to confirm the patient's need for continuation of the level of care he is receiving. Utilization review has had the effect of introducing peer supervision of physicians' performance into the hospitals and nursing homes of the country. It has raised the level of visibility of physician activity and made the analysis of patient management in many institutions a routine. Although utilization review is not yet pursued conscientiously everywhere, it cannot help but have important consequences for the quality of health services throughout the United States.

REGIONAL MEDICAL PROGRAMS

Another indirect way that the federal government is seeking to support and influence the distribution of personal health services is through Public Law 89-239, which established the Regional Medical Program "to make available the best possible patient care for heart disease, cancer, stroke, and related diseases." It is in a sense a companion piece of legislation to the Partnership in Health Act and seeks somewhat similar ends through another channel.

Following World War II, the federal government began supporting biomedical research on a large scale. In 1947 the national expenditure for research totaled $87 million and by 1967 had reached $2.257 billion; much of this was tax money channeled through the National Institutes of Health to the universities, medical schools, and teaching hospitals of the country. Because there had been some feeling on the part of President Johnson and his advisers that research findings from this massive effort were not being applied rapidly and effectively enough, the President appointed a Commission on Heart Disease, Cancer, and Stroke, the three leading causes of death. The report of that commission, issued in December 1964, focused attention on the delivery of health services to combat these diseases. It recommended a network of regional centers based on medical schools and suggested a grant mechanism to implement it analogous to the extramural grant program of the National Institutes of Health. The Congress, however, after listening to a number of spokesmen for the health interests of the country, particularly representatives of practicing physicians and community hospitals, passed The Regional Programs Act, incorporating a different concept, that of regional cooperative arrangements among existing health resources. The emphasis was on a "grass roots" initiative with advisory committees in each region composed of representatives of practicing health professionals as well as of the medical schools. A planning grant for a region is sought first to be followed by regional and subregional operating project grants. Most of the 50 regions of the country have planning grants, and operational grants are now beginning to be funded. The Division of Regional Medical Programs was first placed under the National Institutes of Health, but with the reorganization of the Department of Health, Education, and Welfare it has subsequently been moved to the Health Services and Mental Health Administration (1968).

It is too early to tell whether the Regional Medical Programs will be effective in "speeding research knowledge to the patient's bedside," but it is likely to be a considerable impetus to the already developing accretion of service networks around medical centers. There will be competition for Congressional appropriations with the Partnership in Health Act in promoting regionalism, and whichever is able to show the better results will probably get the bulk of the money in the future.

PROBLEMS AND PROSPECTS FOR THE FUTURE

In summarizing this chapter it is appropriate to indicate some of the future trends. There is clear evidence from the activities now receiving priority in the federal government of a desire to relate more directly to the local community, spurred by the need to combat poverty, particularly in the cities. Local government, too, has shown growing concern for improving health care as a community measure, whereas state government has become much more deeply involved in planning, standard-setting, and quality control.

Much of the recent legislation, reports of governmental committees, and trends of implementation have stressed comprehensiveness of care. This final section will deal, therefore, with a definition of comprehensive care, one of its manifestations, the neighborhood health center, and the organizational attempts that have been made or are necessary on the part of the government to carry out this concept.

Comprehensive Care

The term "comprehensive care" is undoubtedly an old one, but can be most usefully traced back to the 1949 *Annual Report of the Commonwealth Fund.* In that report Geddes Smith made a distinction between the older scientific revolution in medicine and the need for new dimensions in the second half of the twentieth century. In addition to scientific medicine the report suggested that preventive, constructive, social, and comprehensive aspects of medicine should be stressed. "Comprehensive" was described as the type of medicine in which "doctors deal with patients whole instead of in parts." The term came to stand for all the new dimensions, however, and to imply prevention, rehabilitation, and social medicine as well as physician responsibility alone. Mainly as a result of the effort and inspiration of Dr. Lester Evans of the Commonwealth Fund, it came to be incorporated formally into the teaching programs of a number of medical schools. A major experiment in teaching comprehensive medicine, which was supported by the Commonwealth Fund, was that at Cornell University Medical College. In the Cornell Comprehensive Care and Teaching Program comprehensive care was defined as "coordinated, continuous, complete, family-oriented, compassionate care of patients through each episode of their illnesses" (Reader and Goss, 1967).

At the level of the individual this type of care requires an active planning and administrative role for the physician to bring all the necessary services, as well as fellow health professionals, into play in the service of the patient. When comprehensive care is extended to the community level, it requires a service system that coordinates the health facilities and levels of care for the inhabitants of a region to provide both a complete range of services and the most efficient use of them. The Medicare Act implicitly recognized the principles of comprehensive care in its reimbursement for care in hospital, doctor's office, home, and extended care facility, and in providing for utilization review to move people through the system to less expensive and yet effective levels of care. What is still seriously lacking is an effective coordinating role for government in this activity in most jurisdictions.

The Neighborhood Health Center

One of the experimental approaches to provision of comprehensive care for people living in slum areas has been the neighborhood health centers first sponsored by the Office of Economic Opportunity. There are a number scattered about the major cities of the United States, each somewhat different from the others, and some cities such as New York have begun to fund them themselves. Some will be funded under the project grants of the Partnership in Health Act. Many consider them to be the best answer to the problem of provision of comprehensive care to people, particularly the medically indigent, at the local level. In general they are group practice clinics for ambulatory care, with a back-up hospital that supplies major hospital services and admits the patients when hospitalization is required. They serve defined geographic areas, however, and take complete responsibility for all the medically needy in their district. In most of them there has been some conflict with the community over control of operations, and there is a growing tendency to believe community representatives should have a considerable share in the nonprofessional decisions relating to their operation. Thus far most have all the unfortunate aspects of crowded, unattractive municipal hospital clinics; but they are far more accessible and are providing much in the way of health services not hitherto utilized. They must still be looked upon as somewhat experimental until they have had longer trial and further variations, and until innovations have been attempted. They are already sufficiently institutionalized, however, so that one regional planning organization, the Health and Hospital Review and Planning Council of Greater New York, has developed guidelines that must be followed under the authority delegated to planning councils by New York State's Folsom Act (Health and Hospital Review and Planning Council of New York, 1967).

Government Efforts at Coordination

In an effort to rationalize health services in a number of jurisdictions and to make administration more efficient, government has attempted to respond by fostering the merger of health and welfare departments. In a number of communities, too, hospitals, ambulatory services, and public health have been brought together under one authority. In New York City, for example, the Lindsay administration has developed a Health Services Administration encompassing the former departments of Hospitals, Health, Mental Health, and the Medical Examiner's office. The aim is to make the whole system of municipal health services work together. This attempt has so far not been successful, and another approach, the formation of a nonprofit Health Services Corporation, has been recommended. Problems of cost and public accountability under the authority system have not been resolved, however, and it has not as yet proved acceptable as a solution. But as health planning grows in momentum as a governmental function, and as governmental responsibility for delivery and reimbursement for health services grows, more effective administrative mechanisms than those presently available may be expected to emerge at each level of government. (Commission on the Delivery of Personal Health Services, 1967.)

REFERENCES

COMMISSION ON THE DELIVERY OF PERSONAL HEALTH SERVICES: *Comprehensive Community Health Services for New York City*. Report dated 1967.

COMMITTEE ON WAYS AND MEANS OF THE HOUSE OF REPRESENTATIVES: *Social Security Amendments of 1965*. U.S. Government Printing Office, Washington, D.C., 1965.

CONANT, RALPH W.: *The Politics of Community Health*. Public Affairs Press, Washington, D.C., 1968.

HEALTH AND HOSPITAL REVIEW AND PLANNING COUNCIL OF NEW YORK: *Guidelines for Evaluating Neighborhood Clinics and Health Centers*. Mimeo. Report dated Apr. 24, 1967,

LYNCH, MATHEW J. G., and RAPHAEL, STANLEY S.: *Medicine and the State*. Thomas, Springfield, Ill., 1963.

MARSTON, ROBERT Q.: To meet the nation's health needs. *New Eng J Med*, **279**:10, 520–24 September 1968.

NATIONAL COMMISSION ON COMMUNITY HEALTH SERVICES: *Action—Planning for Community Health Services*. Public Affairs Press, Washington, D.C., 1967.

PIORE, NORA: Metropolitan medical economics. *Sci Amer*, 212:19, 1965.

READER, GEORGE G., and GOSS, MARY E. W. (eds.): *Comprehensive Medical Care and Teaching*. Cornell University Press, Ithaca, N.Y., 1967.

SHRYOCK, RICHARD HARRISON: *Medicine and Society in America: 1660–1860*. Cornell University Press, Ithaca, N.Y., 1962.

SOCIETY OF THE NEW YORK HOSPITAL: *Society of the New York Hospital: Commemorative Exercises, One Hundred and Fiftieth Anniversary, 1771–1921*. The Society, New York. 1921.

STRAUS, ROBERT: *Changing Environmental Hazards: Challenges to Community Health*. Public Affairs Press, Washington, D.C.

———: *Financing Community Health Services and Facilities*. Public Affairs Press, Washington, D.C., 1967.

———: *Health Administration and Organization in the Decade Ahead*. Public Affairs Press, Washington, D.C., 1967.

———: *Health Care Facilities: The Community Bridge to Effective Health Services*. Public Affairs Press, Washington, D.C., 1967.

———: *Health Is a Community Affair*. Harvard University Press, Cambridge, Mass., 1967.

———: *Health Manpower: Action to Meet Community Needs*. Public Affairs Press, Washington, D.C.

STRAUS, ROBERT: *Medical Care for Seamen:* The origin of Public Medical Service in the United States. Yale University Press, New Haven, 1950.

U.S. HEALTH SERVICES AND MENTAL HEALTH ADMINISTRATION: *Guidelines: Regional Medical Programs, Revised May 1968.*

U.S. OFFICE OF COMPREHENSIVE HEALTH PLANNING: *Information and Policies on Grants for Health Services Development.* Mimeo., July 20, 1967.

————: *Information and Policies on Grants to States for Public Health Services.* Mimeo., June 15, 1967.

U.S. PUBLIC HEALTH SERVICE: *Indian Health Highlights.* U.S. Government Printing Office, Washington, D.C., 1966.

————: *The Indian Health Program of the U.S. Public Health Service.* U.S. Government Printing Office, Washington, D.C., 1966.

————, INDIAN HEALTH PROGRAM: *To the First Americans.* Second Annual Report.

U.S. SOCIAL SECURITY ADMINISTRATION: *Medicare: A Reference Guide for Physicians.* U.S. Government Printing Office, Washington, D.C.

WILSON, ROBERT N.: *Community Structure and Health Action:* A Report on Process Analysis. Public Affairs Press, Washington, D.C., 1968.

15

Preventive Medicine in Individual Practice

Jeremiah A. Barondess

INTRODUCTION

The role of the individual practitioner of medicine in relation to the prevention of disease has been changing in recent years, as have a number of other aspects of the delivery of health care.

Preventive medicine and public health have not, in the past, been areas that have attracted substantial interest or major creative effort from medical practitioners; there have been several reasons for this. First, those attracted to the practice of medicine in the classical sense have, by and large, been primarily engaged by an interest in the diagnosis, and more especially, the treatment, of established disease in individuals. Second, medical school curricula, although providing some acquaintance with concepts and techniques relating to public health and preventive medicine as applied to population groups, have generally given the student an inadequate appreciation of the opportunities and responsibilities in these areas that devolve upon the physician seeing individual patients on a one-to-one basis. Rather, this information has come to the medical student largely as a by-product of clinical instruction, spread through the clinical clerkship, time spent in the out-patient department, and postgraduate internship and residency training. Third, and most important, has been the classical impotence of the individual practitioner in relation to disease prevention (see Chapter 1). Thus, it is clear that the enhancement of life expectancy in medically sophisticated countries in the last 50 to 100 years has been due primarily to the adoption of such public health measures as the purification of water supplies, the proper handling and disposal of sewage, the control of insect vectors of disease, massive immunization procedures directed against specific infections, and other measures, rather than to the availability and application of effective preventive and therapeutic measures by the individual physician to the individual patient.

418

The impact of the physician on disease prevention and control is, however, changing, and will, no doubt, continue to do so. This change derives primarily from the advent of scientific investigation in medicine and from the insights it has provided into the pathogenesis and natural history of disease, as well as from the availability, for the first time, of large numbers of potent, and often specific, therapeutic agents. Application of these insights and treatment measures to the cohorts of individuals that constitute medical practices now provides the practitioner with opportunities and widespread responsibilities for effective action in relation to disease control and prevention. When one considers that over 90 per cent of American medical graduates ultimately choose individual practice for their professional lives, the potential leverage to be exerted in this area by practicing physicians can be visualized.

Concurrent with these changes has come an increasing awareness on the part of the public of much that goes on in the medical world. Newspapers and other media of communication have made millions of people conversant with procedures as complex as organ transplantation and hyperbaric therapy, and aware of such terms as *kwashiorkor* and *marasmus*. The proceedings of major medical meetings are reported in the press, and televised explanations of medical advances are commonplace. The resultant increasing medical sophistication of the population, together with social changes that have developed a demand for good medical care, in the broadest sense, as a basic right, serve to fuel further the alteration of the practitioner's role from an almost exclusively therapeutic one to a broader, more sophisticated and more effective involvement in the entire spectrum of health care activities, and to underscore the expansion of his interest from the treatment of established disease to a concern with the maintenance, as well as with the restoration, of good health, when and where possible.

In a real sense, all diagnostic and therapeutic activity has a preventive component, in that it seeks to forestall or interdict deterioration of the patient's health. Thus, the role of the modern practitioner is threefold; namely, the prevention of disease, the mitigation of established disease, and the eradication, when feasible, of established disease. In each instance the focus of the physician's attention is the individual, although the implications of the interactions of the individual with the community are also to be considered.

In connection with the physician's role in the area of disease prevention as applied to individuals, it is worthy of emphasis that the pressure of these responsibilities should be felt, and in fact sought, by those in every clinical specialty; not only by internists, pediatricians, and general practitioners, but by general surgeons, obstetricians, otorhinolaryngologists, and all others who render clinical care. Every medical contact, regardless of the precipitating event or presenting complaint, can and should be used by the physician as an opportunity to discover abnormalities that, if not identified and interfered with, might lead to the development of significant disease; such abnormalities may appear as lesions, biochemical aberrations (e.g., hypercholesterolemia), or habits (e.g., cigarette smoking), and are often of greater long-range importance to the patient's health than the immediate difficulty that has caused him to seek medical advice.

Some of the opportunities for the identification of these overt and latent threats to the patient's health will be considered in the ensuing sections of this chapter. Our ability to alter such lesions or trends varies widely, and the beneficial effect of such alteration, even when feasible, is not well established in many instances, though probable in others, and clear-cut in some. In each instance the physician must proceed on the basis of the best scientific information available at the time, and with appropriate care that his preventive and therapeutic measures do not, by virtue of being themselves potentially harmful, substitute one danger for another.

The following section, although not meant to be all-inclusive, indicates the scope of the physician's opportunities to identify trends and established disease, correction of which may enhance the patient's health outlook.

SCREENING OPPORTUNITIES IN PHYSICIAN-PATIENT CONTACTS

Skin

Cutaneous lesions of particular interest from the point of view of this chapter fall into two groups, namely those that are potentially premalignant and those that may reflect the presence of visceral or systemic disease.

In the first group are included solar keratosis, arsenical keratosis, Bowen's disease, and a few others.

Solar keratosis occurs primarily after middle age in fair-skinned individuals in areas of the body exposed to sunlight. Squamous cell carcinoma appears in a small number of these lesions, usually after a latent period of years. The keratotic lesion itself appears as an adherent, rough, brown, or yellowish scale, which may become thick and horny. Similar changes may appear in those exposed to ionizing radiation, radiant heat, and in workers exposed to pitch and other products of coal distillation.

Arsenical keratosis is a rare lesion that may also result in squamous cell carcinoma. The lesions appear chiefly on the palms and soles as small hyperkeratotic areas resembling corns. Bowen's disease and multiple basal cell carcinomas, chiefly on the trunk, may be associated.

Bowen's disease, characterized by a small, red, slightly scaly area occurring anywhere on the skin or mucosal surfaces, is an intraepidermal carcinoma, which may become invasive, with squamous cell characteristics. Many cases are thought to reflect exposure to trivalent arsenicals, either in medications or through industrial processes. In addition to the development of skin cancer, Bowen's disease is followed by systemic malignancy in about 25 per cent of cases (Graham and Helwig, 1964). This is most commonly in the respiratory, gastrointestinal, or genitourinary systems, and is noted, on the average, about five and a half years after the onset of the Bowen's disease.

Erythroplasia of Queyrat is probably Bowen's disease of the penis occurring in the uncircumcised, but lacks the association with visceral malignancy seen with Bowen's disease.

Cutaneous horn is a keratotic protuberance most common on the exposed areas, especially the upper face and the ears; it may undergo transition to squamous cell carcinoma.

Nevi are universally present in adults and rarely undergo malignant change. It is to be noted, however, that most melanomas arise from nevi. Current practice is to advise removal of nevi from areas in which they are subjected to chronic mechanical trauma, such as the beltline, the collar line, the feet, and areas under shoulder straps. Elevated, hair-bearing nevi appear less likely to undergo malignant change. Unevenness of pigmentation within a nevus and fuzziness of the pigmented margins are signs suggesting junctional activity and call for excision and histologic examination. Nevi should be excised surgically when they are removed, because malignant transformation has followed attempts to destroy them by local measures, such as electrodessication.

Certain skin lesions should alert the clinician to the possibility of systemic or visceral disease, especially malignancy. Among these are to be included acanthosis nigricans, which features primarily a brownish or black discoloration of the skin in flexural or in intertriginous areas associated with a soft, velvety appearance of the involved skin. Warty or pedunculated lesions may appear in the involved area. Acanthosis nigricans in adults is associated with abdominal or pelvic malignancy, chiefly adenocarcinoma, in over 90 per cent of cases, though other tumors, including lymphomata, have been seen. In perhaps 20 per cent of cases the cutaneous lesions antedate other clinical evidence of the neoplasm.

Erythema multiforme, erythema nodosum, diffuse exfoliative dermatitis, and various vesicular or bullous dermatoses may be seen in association with almost any type of internal malignancy as well as with drug hypersensitivity and various infections. The varied skin lesions of dermatomyositis should call to mind the association of this condition with internal malignancy, especially carcinoma.

Other conditions of a systemic nature that may be associated with skin lesions of varying degrees of specificity or suggestiveness include such diverse disorders as disseminated lupus erythematosus, scleroderma, sarcoidosis, hyperlipemia, hemochromatosis, Cushing's syndrome, the purpuras, leukemia, gout, diabetes mellitus, neurofibromatosis, cirrhosis of the liver, Ehlers-Danlos syndrome, and carotenemia in myxedema. The physician must be alert to the possibilities of early diagnosis and therapy presented by the galaxy of cutaneous changes that may be seen, and should view every skin lesion as a potential suspicion-arouser of possibly remediable or preventable disease.

Eye, Ear, Throat, Oral Cavity

In relation to eye disease per se, the chief condition to which attention has been directed in an effort to prevent visual loss is glaucoma. It should be noted that there is a lack of scientifically acceptable evidence that treating the patient with an established glaucomatous field defect does him good in the sense of preventing further loss of visual field (Graham, 1966). Nevertheless, sophisticated ophthalmologic opinion believes that it does; hence, considerable effort has been expended to locate presymptomatic glaucomatous individuals. Although measurement of intraocular pressure by tonometry has been used very widely for this purpose, recent evaluations raise serious questions about the validity of tonometry as a case-finding procedure, particularly as applied to the general population (Graham, 1966; Cochrane, 1967). Present evidence suggests that visual field examinations are more reliable, and that case-finding techniques should be applied especially to first-degree relatives of established cases of chronic glaucoma, in whom the incidence of the disease may be between 8 and 10 per cent.

Funduscopic examination of the eye may provide evidence suggesting a number of systemic disorders, treatment of which may exert some protective effect on the patient's health. Among these may be noted hypertensive disease, diabetes mellitus, hyper-lipemia, arterial disease, blood dyscrasias of various types, and increased intracranial pressure owing to brain tumor, subdural hematoma, or a variety of other causes. The discovery of funduscopic evidence of these or other major systemic conditions should be followed by appropriate investigations so that evidence of established disease, either symptomatic or presymptomatic, can be identified and approached thera-peutically, in the hope of some long-term benefit to the patient.

Aspects of ear disease that have been the object of preventive medical interest have chiefly revolved around hearing loss. Widespread screening examinations have sug-gested that up to 39 per cent of the general population have reduced auditory acuity (Oliver, 1967). Although much of this loss is irremediable in any fundamental sense by present techniques, some individuals may be benefited, or the rate of deterioration of hearing slowed, by attention to local disease of the ear, avoidance of acoustic trauma, discontinuation of potentially ototoxic drugs, and perhaps treatment measures directed against systemic conditions that may be associated with hearing loss, such as myxedema.

Examination of the oral cavity may reveal evidence of the glossitis of pernicious anemia; the dental abnormalities of congenital syphilis; early carcinomas of the lips, tongue, buccal mucosa, or pharynx; or flat, grayish patches of leukoplakia, a pre-malignant lesion often related to smoking or to chronic mechanical trauma from jagged teeth, ill-fitting dentures, cheek-biting, and so on. Discovery of any of these abnor-malities provides an opportunity for the prevention or reduction of morbidity in the individual.

Cardiovascular System

The potential prevention of morbidity in cardiovascular disease relates to a number of entities, primarily arteriosclerotic cardiovascular disease, hypertensive cardiovascular disease, rheumatic fever, and bacterial endocarditis.

Arteriosclerotic Cardiovascular Disease.   The most important mode of clinical expres-sion of arteriosclerotic cardiovascular disease is ischemic heart disease, which is based anatomically on coronary artery atheroma in almost all cases. A variety of factors have been shown to influence the risk of development of ischemic heart disease, and a number of others are suspected of playing a role. Some of these predisposing factors are potentially alterable by means of medical manipulation and others are not; even in relation to those that are manipulatable, long-term studies establishing a beneficial effect on the course of ischemic heart disease and/or on life expectancy as a result of medical management are lacking, in most instances. Thus, in this area perhaps more than in most others, the physician, even while attempting to protect his patient as far as possible from the risk of developing ischemic heart disease, must maintain an awareness of the distinction between measures of scientifically proved efficacy and those that seem likely to help but are not yet of established usefulness; he must be ready to modify, add to, or abandon those in the latter group as new evidence accumulates.

The risk factors that, to this point, appear operative in ischemic heart disease are family incidence, arterial hypertension, hyperlipidemia, obesity, cigarette smoking, presence of diabetes mellitus, physical inactivity, and perhaps socioeconomic status and unusually stressful occupations or life situations (see Chapter 12).

Although a history of ischemic heart disease in a patient's family is clearly not remediable, the effect of a strong family history, especially in the patient's parents or siblings, is worthy of note, as it is associated with an increased risk of the disease in the patient.

The presence of arterial hypertension is associated with an increased incidence of ischemic heart disease expressed as angina pectoris and acute myocardial infarction (Kannel *et al.*, 1965; Oliver, 1966). Angina pectoris may sometimes be relieved, but long-term studies establishing a reduction in the risk of acute myocardial infarction as a consequence of control by treatment of arterial hypertension are lacking, though this is not to say that such a relationship may not ultimately be established. Both in relation to the increased risk of ischemic heart disease and of other complications of arterial hypertension, attempts should be made to reduce blood pressure levels to normal, insofar as possible, when such patients are encountered.

Chronic elevation of levels of serum lipids appears clearly to be associated in some cases with an increased risk of symptomatic arteriosclerotic cardiovascular disease, including ischemic heart disease. Considerable confusion has long existed in the literature concerned with this area, some of which has been illuminated by recent studies on serum lipid fractionation (Fredrickson and Lees, 1965; Ahrens *et al.*, 1961). These studies have delineated several types of hyperlipemia.

In essential hypercholesterolemia serum cholesterol concentrations are elevated, whereas levels of triglycerides are normal or nearly so. There is a striking familial incidence of the disorder, which is associated with severe and premature atherosclerosis, frequently expressed as ischemic heart disease. Atheromatous disease of the aortic valve with resultant aortic stenosis may also be seen. Tendon xanthomata are common, as is corneal arcus. Myocardial infarction at early ages is common. The vascular disease in these patients is severe and often fulminating. Dietary treatment with replacement, as far as possible, of saturated by polyunsaturated fatty acids (avoidance of mammalian fats; substitution of fish and fowl as protein sources; use of corn oil in cooking) results in reduction of serum cholesterol concentrations and in mobilization of at least some tissue deposits of lipid-rich material, as exemplified by reduction in xanthomata. Whether similar reduction of lipid deposits in arterial walls can be accomplished, either by dietary means or new chemical agents, such as clofibrate, is not yet clear. Nevertheless, the usual course of the disease justifies efforts to interfere therapeutically with the abnormalities that have been identified.

Conditions characterized by elevation of serum triglyceride concentrations have also been defined. In some patients such hyperglyceridemia follows fat ingestion; the lipoproteins found in the blood of these patients appear to be, in effect, chylomicrons derived from post-prandial intestinal lymph. This disorder, which may be related to a deficiency of plasma lipoprotein lipase, is also familial. Hypercholesterolemia is not a feature, nor is accelerated vascular disease. This type of hyperglyceridemia appears to be uncommon.

In contrast, hyperglyceridemia following carbohydrate ingestion is more common. In one study of 286 patients with clinical atherosclerosis and hyperlipidemia, more than 90 per cent were found to have this type of abnormality (Kuo, 1967). These patients may or may not have associated hypercholesterolemia. A family history of diabetes mellitus is common, and carbohydrate intolerance can be demonstrated frequently; indeed, these patients may represent instances of latent diabetes, perhaps of a specific type. Serum triglyceride levels increase when the diet is rich in carbohydrate and fall when the fat intake is increased at the expense of carbohydrate. Clinical evidence of generalized atherosclerosis and ischemic heart disease is commonly noted in these patients. The serum lipid abnormalities can be reversed to a large extent by dietary alterations consisting of restriction of sugar intake and a carbohydrate allowance of 125 to 150 gm, supplied as starches. Again, the potential effect on atheromatous lesions and on the course of atherosclerotic disease of long-term alteration of serum lipid patterns by such measures remains to be defined.

The association of obesity and ischemic heart disease is well established (Kannel *et al.*, 1965). Coronary artery atheroma in the obese may be at least partially an expression of the hypertension and diabetes mellitus frequently seen in these patients; striking mitigation of these two disorders can often be accomplished by weight reduction in the obese. Although no studies are available bearing on the effects of long-term weight control on atheromatous lesions in the obese, significant amelioration of angina pectoris and improvement in the survival rates of obese patients who have sustained myocardial infarctions can be accomplished by such weight reduction (Mayer, 1966).

Further, the risk of developing clinical ischemic heart disease appears to be related to adiposity even in the absence of gross obesity (Reid *et al.*, 1967). Although reduction in this risk as a result of weight control over long periods has yet to be demonstrated, the physician is justified in attempting to reduce this long-term risk to his patients by encouraging leanness as a permanent state of affairs. In this connection it should be noted that there is no evidence that reducing diets of special composition (e.g., high-carbohydrate, high-fat, rice, and so on) have any advantage over general caloric restriction with a "normal" distribution of fat, carbohydrate, and protein calories. Indeed, as Mayer has pointed out (1966), some of these are potentially harmful; thus, the so-called "drinking man's diet," high in fat, with ad libitum consumption of calories and alcohol, not only tends to make the patient fat (and inebriated) but also may be highly atherogenic.

Cigarette smoking is associated with excess development of myocardial infarction in both men and women (Kannel *et al.*, 1965; Truett *et al.*, 1967). Sudden death, as an additional expression of ischemic heart disease, has also been associated statistically with cigarette smoking; the data in relation to angina pectoris are less striking, though some studies have shown an association. Other studies have indicated a relationship between cigarette smoking and stroke (Kannel *et al.*, 1965), and a great weight of clinical experience suggests that smoking exerts an adverse effect on atherosclerotic disease of peripheral arteries as expressed by intermittent claudication and gangrene. Although duration of cigarette smoking does not appear to bear a statistical relationship to clinical ischemic heart disease (in contrast to the data relating to lung cancer), the quantity of cigarettes smoked per day does relate to the death rates from coronary heart disease and to the incidence of acute myocardial infarction. Further, these risks appear to be reduced when cigarette smoking is abandoned (Boyle *et al.*, 1964). These facts appear to provide an opportunity for major prevention of morbidity and mortality in ischemic heart disease. The incidence of this disorder in the United States adds pressure to the physician's responsibility to do what he can, not only to discourage the use of cigarettes in those who already smoke, but to prevent adoption of the habit by the young. The importance of parental example has been suggested by a number of studies showing that the adoption of the cigarette habit by a child may be in part a function of whether or not his parents smoke.

Level of physical activity and existence of unusual types or levels of stress have been suggested as additional factors associated with the risk of developing ischemic heart disease; long-term studies will be required to clarify these issues. Thus, in relation to the question of stress, one unsettled problem is whether the stressful environment per se is responsible for the increased incidence of coronary heart disease that has been observed, or whether more or less specific personality types are prone to appear in stressful situations *and* to develop coronary heart disease, without a direct causal relationship necessarily being operative. Studies to this point have suggested that individuals characterized by excessive drive, aggressiveness, ambition, competitiveness, and a sense of time urgency are more likely to develop coronary heart disease than men without these traits. Other studies (Thomas and Ross, 1968) support the inference that some aspects of the psychological and social functioning of the individual may be correlated with the risk of developing ischemic heart disease. These issues must be developed and clarified before their usefulness in preventing coronary heart disease is clear.

Rheumatic Fever.   Preventive effort in relation to acute rheumatic fever and rheumatic heart disease has met with significant success. This effort revolves about two major areas, namely the prompt identification and adequate therapy of infections caused by Group A beta hemolytic streptococcal infections, and antimicrobial prophylaxis against recurrence of such infections in individuals with a history of acute rheumatic fever in any of its clinical forms. In relation to the former, a high index of suspicion for beta hemolytic streptococcal etiology of acute pharyngitis is essential. Throat cultures should be used widely, as the clinical characteristics of such infections are not reliable enough to prevent missing the diagnosis in a significant proportion of cases. Such infections, when present, should be treated promptly, preferably with penicillin in adequate doses for not less than ten days. Those allergic to penicillin may be treated with erythromycin for a similar period. Throat cultures should be obtained from contacts of these patients in an effort to identify and treat those who have been colonized by the organism. The success of such treatment of streptococcal infections in reducing the incidence of subsequent rheumatic fever has been well established. A related gradual reduction in the frequency of chronic rheumatic heart disease may be anticipated; clinical experience indicates that this may be occurring.

The prevention of recurrence of rheumatic fever in individuals with a past history of the disease revolves about the prevention of Group A beta hemolytic streptoccal infections. Continuous antimicrobial prophylaxis has been shown to be highly effective in this regard, and should be applied to all those with such a history; the proper duration of such prophylaxis has been debated, but among those with established rheumatic heart disease it should probably be lifelong; patients with a history of rheumatic fever but without heart disease should probably be carried on prophylaxis at least through early adult life. Prophylaxis may be carried out with daily oral penicillin or sulfonamides or with monthly intramuscular injections of benzathine penicillin G.

Bacterial Endocarditis.   Prevention of bacterial endocarditis is thought to be feasible under certain circumstances, and it seems highly likely that some cases of the disease can be prevented. Efforts in this direction are based on the predilection of the disease for previously damaged valves and congenital cardiac defects and on the not infrequent appearance of the disease after dental or urologic procedures, as these are often followed by bacteremia. Accordingly, patients with valvular or congenital heart disease should be given a brief course of antimicrobial therapy at the time of dental extractions, extensive periodontal work, or instrumentation of the urinary tract. For dental procedures penicillin is usually used, because the oral organisms most often responsible for bacterial endocarditis are usually highly sensitive to this agent. For urologic procedures tetracycline is ordinarily used. Therapy may begin a few hours to a day prior to the procedure, and should continue for 48 to 72 hours.

Hypertension.   Hypertension has been considered briefly in connection with its impact on the course of ischemic heart disease. Aside from this relationship, the reduction of high blood pressure can significantly increase survival in hypertensive patients. This is well established as regards malignant hypertension. In relation to patients with other grades of hypertension, those in whom blood pressure elevations are moderate to severe appear to be protected to a significant degree from the excess mortality associated with hypertension, especially that portion associated with renal failure and early stroke (Leishman, 1963). An additional aspect of the effort to return elevation of the arterial pressure to normal revolves about the early identification and proper treatment of patients with potentially remediable underlying causes for their hypertension. These causes include pheochromocytoma, coarctation of the aorta, aldosterone-secreting tumors of the adrenal cortex, Cushing's syndrome, unilateral kidney disease, and unilateral or bilateral renal artery stenosis. Such causes should be looked for in every patient with diastolic hypertension before chronic medical therapy is undertaken, in the hope that permanent cure or amelioration of the blood pressure elevation can be accomplished by appropriate therapy of the underlying process.

Genitourinary System

The major disorders of the genitourinary system in relation to which there are important preventive efforts to be made are diseases of the kidneys. A number of renal disorders present with or are based on fairly readily identifiable acute episodes, which often subside, with or without treatment, and may then be followed by long periods of continued pathologic change in the kidney in the absence of symptomatology; during this interval, which may last for years, it is difficult to identify the process in the kidney. Even in those few patients in whom it is characterized, therapeutic efforts are usually ineffective, because the factors responsible for continued activity of the lesion are poorly understood. The process proceeds, terminating, in many patients, in the clinical picture of renal insufficiency, based on extensive destruction of kidney parenchyma. The physician's most productive opportunity to interfere with this chain of events lies in prevention or mitigation of the initial insult.

Acute glomerulonephritis is one disorder that affords this opportunity. Recent studies indicate that most cases are caused by prior infection with group A beta hemolytic streptococci, with some strains (types 4, 12, 18, 25, 41, and the Red Lake strain) particularly involved. Although the details of the pathogenetic mechanism are unclear, the epidemiologic evidence is strong; not only has it resulted in the incrimination of the strains noted above, but it has defined seasonal fluctuations in the incidence of acute glomerulonephritis that parallel those of beta hemolytic streptococcal infections in general, and it has afforded some understanding of the epidemics of acute nephritis that are sometimes seen. The prevention of this disease is certainly its best management. Prevention is best accomplished with penicillin administered to those exposed during outbreaks of streptococcal disease due to nephritogenic strains, particularly in institutions, such as military installations, schools, and camps. Family contacts of cases of acute post-streptococcal glomerulonephritis should be subjected to throat cultures and given eradicative courses of penicillin if beta hemolytic streptococci are identified.

Although penicillin treatment of established streptococcal infection is of course indicated, it does not appear to lessen the risk of subsequent acute glomerulonephritis, unlike the experience in relation to acute rheumatic fever. Again unlike acute rheumatic fever, continuous antistreptococcal prophylaxis following a documented episode of acute glomerulonephritis has not found widespread use, because second attacks of the disease are uncommon. Some physicians give such patients daily oral penicillin during the seasons of relative prevalence of streptococcal infections; in addition, such prophylaxis should be undertaken when outbreaks of streptococcal disease are present in the community.

Pyelonephritis is a common renal lesion, one which has also been subjected to intensive study in recent years. Although the relationship between the acute and chronic forms of the disease is in several respects unclear, a significant proportion of patients with chronic pyelonephritis give a clear history of antecedent acute attacks. Because clear evidence is lacking that the pathologic process in the kidney in chronic pyelonephritis can be halted by presently available treatment methods, the reduction of morbidity and mortality from this disease is at present dependent upon successful attack on the acute form. A number of factors that predispose to acute pyelonephritis have been identified, and they should be sought in such patients in an effort to promote eradication of the infection and to reduce the risk of relapse or recurrence. Urinary tract obstruction, instrumentation (including catheterization) of the urinary tract, vesicoureteral reflux during micturition, and the presence of diabetes mellitus are among such predisposing lesions. Avoidance of catheterization, and especially of the use of indwelling catheters, except when absolutely necessary, should be practiced by all physicians. Relief of obstruction due to calculi, prostatic enlargement, and other causes may be required for the eradication of urinary tract infections. Prompt and adequate antimicrobial therapy of acute pyelonephritis is also important, in order that the degree of destruction of renal parenchyma in the affected area may be minimized. Similarly, effective therapy of infections of the lower urinary tract is important in reducing the risk of subsequent acute pyelonephritis. The object of such therapy should be sterilization of the urine, as demonstrated by appropriate bacteriologic techniques. Antimicrobial drugs should be selected on the basis of *in vitro* sensitivity tests of the offending organism, usually one of the enteric bacteria. Where possible, bactericidal, rather than bacteriostatic agents, should be employed.

That significant renal disease may be produced by drugs has been known for years. Thus, various antimicrobial agents, such as sulfonamides, kanamycin, the polymyxins, streptomycin, and colistin, have all been associated with greater or lesser degrees of renal toxicity, even when used in proper doses and with appropriate precautions. Most such instances of renal injury have been acute, rather than productive of chronic renal disease. Outdated, degraded tetracycline has been associated with an acquired type of Fanconi syndrome, usually reversible, but productive of substantial illness. Of perhaps greater concern, because of the widespread use of the drugs without medical control, is nephrotoxicity due to analgesic abuse. Formulations containing phenacetin have been incriminated. In general, although the pathogenesis of the interstitial nephritis seen in these patients is poorly understood, cumulative dosage of phenacetin ingested has exceeded 1 kg (Schreiner, 1962).

Other diagnostic and therapeutic measures that have been associated with renal injury include oral cholecystography with bunamiodyl (Orabilex), abdominal aortography using iodides, retrograde pyelography, ionizing radiation, and exposure to a variety of metals. Responsibility for recognition or avoidance in these instances rests with the physician.

The prevention of acute renal failure, chiefly by prompt recognition and effective treatment of shock, by avoidance of mismatched transfusions, by adequate management of acute infections, and by relief of acute obstruction of the urinary tract, presents additional opportunities for the avoidance of some instances of renal injury. Similarly, the recognition of lower urinary tract obstruction of longer standing may permit relief of otherwise intractable and advancing uremia.

A longer-term issue in the potential prevention of disease of the urinary tract has to do with the increased incidence of carcinoma of the bladder in cigarette smokers. This association, although not the foremost suggesting cigarette smoking as a cause of human disease, is an additional aspect of the problem that demands the physician's attention.

Respiratory System

The primary areas of attention in relation to prevention of pulmonary disease at present have to do with carcinoma of the lung and chronic obstructive pulmonary disease and their relation to cigarette smoking. Carcinoma of the lung is increasing rapidly in incidence in this country, and may be considered to be an epidemic disease at this time. Not only has the over-all frequency of the disease increased, but the attack rate among women, formerly a low-incidence group, has also risen sharply. Although the disease is unquestionably diagnosed now with more facility than it was twenty-five years ago, and although the population at risk has increased as more people have lived to relatively advanced ages, there seems little reason to doubt that the actual frequency of the disease has increased rapidly. In addition, salvage in lung cancer with present therapy is poor, with 5-year survival rates of 5 to 8 per cent in most centers. Although it is possible that intensive screening of large populations with resultant earlier diagnosis may improve this figure somewhat, Lilienfeld *et al.* (1966) present information suggesting strongly that a major reduction in morbidity and mortality in the disease can be accomplished only by prevention, at least until major advances in knowledge of the biology of cancer and in cancer therapy are forthcoming. Further, the evidence available at this time suggests that lung cancer may be largely a preventable disease. Cigarette smoking has been implicated as a cause of lung cancer, especially squamous cell carcinoma, not only by large retrospective studies, but by prospective ones as well (DHEW, 1964; PHS Rev., 1968 Suppl.). Though other factors, including air pollution in urban settings, inhalation of foreign materials such as asbestos, and individual propensity, are also likely involved in some cases, the weight of present information indicates strongly that cigarette smoking is the most important contributing factor in the genesis of lung cancer.

The issues in relation to chronic bronchitis and emphysema are also complex. Because of the common association of these two conditions and the difficulties involved in separating them clinically, they are now usually considered jointly as the usual basis of chronic obstructive pulmonary disease. This disorder, which is a common cause of respiratory disability and death, has been found to occur more commonly in cigarette smokers than in nonsmokers, and to be related to both the number of cigarettes smoked per day and the duration of smoking (Burrows *et al.*, 1965; *Health Consequences of Smoking*, 1968). Arrest or regression of chronic bronchitis and emphysema by presently available treatment modalities is probably not feasible, though acute infectious exacerbations can be controlled. Thus, attempts to reduce morbidity and mortality from chronic obstructive pulmonary disease must rely at present on efforts at prevention, of which discontinuation or avoidance of cigarette smoking appears to be the most important.

Cigarette smoking in the United States is an extremely widespread habit, presently indulged in, for example, by 52 per cent of adult males (Abelson, 1968). Although efforts to reduce this incidence must rely in part on governmental efforts to control cigarette advertising and distribution, and on positions taken by major medical organizations, the responsibility of the individual physician in acquainting his patients with the evidence and in encouraging them to make a conscious decision whether to smoke or not to smoke, is of key importance. The widespread publicity given to the adverse effects of smoking on health in recent years has apparently resulted in a leveling off, and perhaps a drop, in per capita cigarette consumption in the United States, and, probably of greater importance, has resulted in a widespread conviction among teenagers that smoking is injurious to health. Recent surveys have indicated that 80 per cent of this group expect that they will not or probably will not become smokers. This trend should be encouraged by every physician as a major aspect of his commitment to prevention of important aspects of bronchopulmonary and cardiovascular disease.

Other diseases of the lung with important preventive aspects include recurrent pulmonary embolization and the pneumoconioses. Lung injury from drugs (e.g., hexamethonium and hydralazine), although a well-established entity, is rare. Prevention of pulmonary embolization and infarction is attempted chiefly by early ambulation of postoperative and *post partum* patients, the use of elastic stockings or bandages in immobilized patients, and the administration of anticoagulant drugs to patients at risk of developing phlebothrombosis or mural thrombosis in the heart. The prevention of pneumoconiosis has revolved primarily about efforts at dust suppression, effective ventilation, and the use of protective masks in industries in which the risk is significant.

Gastrointestinal System

Preventive efforts in relation to gastrointestinal disease have chiefly to do with some aspects of cancer prophylaxis and with prevention of certain types of liver injury. Cancer prevention in the gastrointestinal tract has focused on the enhanced risk of carcinoma of the stomach in patients with pernicious anemia and on premalignant lesions of the colon. The increased frequency of gastric carcinoma in pernicious anemia is well established. Patients with the latter disorder should be evaluated recurrently with this association in mind; symptoms suggesting gastric dysfunction, or the appearance of guaiac-positive stools are indications for upper gastrointestinal x-ray studies; some feel that such x-rays should be done at intervals up to every six months in all patients with pernicious anemia, whether symptomatic or not.

Premalignant lesions of the colon include familial polyposis coli (but not the gastrointestinal polyposis of the Peutz-Jehger syndrome), villous adenomata, and chronic idiopathic ulcerative colitis. Familial polyposis coli is a rare disease transmitted as a Mendelian dominant trait, associated with a very striking tendency to the development of colon cancer. Prophylactic colectomy is the only known effective measure for the eradication of this risk. Relatives of patients with this disorder should be subjected to barium enema x-rays with air contrast to identify presymptomatic cases. Villous adenoma of the colon is a relatively uncommon lesion, usually occurring in the rectum or sigmoid, and associated with potential for malignant behavior. The lesion is usually polypoid and presents with rectal bleeding and the passage of large quantities of mucus, sometimes with associated hypokalemia. Adequate excision should be carried out when these lesions are found. In many cases this can be accomplished through the sigmoidoscope. As with any polypoid lesion of the large bowel, careful histologic examination of the excised tissue should be performed. The association of chronic idiopathic ulcerative colitis and carcinoma of the colon is well established. In general, carcinoma has developed in those patients with long-standing ulcerative colitis, particularly when the disease has been severe and unremitting. The impact of modern medical therapy of ulcerative colitis on the risk of carcinoma has not been established; hence a high index of suspicion must be maintained by the physician, and sigmoidoscopy and barium enema carried out whenever clinical events suggest superimposition of carcinoma as a possibility.

The common adenomatous polyp of the colon, once thought to possess significant potential for malignant transformation, now appears not to carry that risk (Castleman and Krickstein, 1962). It must be noted, however, that only proper histologic examination can distinguish definitely among the polypoid lesions of the colon (i.e., polypoid adenoma, villous adenoma and polypoid carcinoma) that may be encountered; this fact should be borne in mind, particularly in relation to small lesions removed at sigmoidoscopy.

Potentially preventable liver disease includes those lesions produced by the agents of viral hepatitis, by various drugs and anesthetic agents, and by alcohol. The type of viral hepatitis characterized by a relatively short incubation period and readily transmissible on person-to-person contact, i.e., so-called infectious hepatitis, is preventable in most cases, at least at the clinical level, through the intramuscular use of gamma globulin of human origin (Chapter 10). This material, even when prepared from plasma pools from donors with no history of the disease, apparently contains high titers of protective antibodies, and prevents overt hepatitis in exposed susceptibles in most cases; there is evidence that small doses, of the order of 0.01–0.02 ml per pound of body weight, permit subclinical infection in some instances, whereas larger doses, e.g., 0.1 ml or more per pound, are more likely to prevent infection from occurring. Which of these circumstances is preferable is unclear; thus, the former would presumably permit long-lasting active immunity to occur, though at the risk of at least a small incidence of chronic post-hepatitic liver disease. Because attack rates are high among family contacts of cases of infectious hepatitis, such individuals, along with other close contacts of cases, should receive gamma globulin. The material should also be administered to those traveling to hyperendemic areas. The use of this agent in patients who have received whole blood or plasma transfusions is unsettled at this time. Studies have shown that a significant proportion of cases of post-transfusion hepatitis occur after a relatively short incubation period. At least some of these undoubtedly represent instances of infectious hepatitis transmitted by transfusion, and would presumably be prevented or modified by the administration of moderate doses of gamma globulin (e.g., 0.02–0.06 ml per pound of body weight) after infusion of whole blood or plasma. It has also been suggested that long-incubation period hepatitis, so-called serum hepatitis, may be prevented to some extent by administration of 10 ml of gamma globulin after transfusion and again a month later. The evidence for this view is not at present solid. Until such time as it becomes so, it may be wisest to confine these large doses of gamma globulin to patients receiving large numbers of transfusions, with the attendant increased risk of hepatitis, and to those with pre-existent liver disease, who would presumably be more endangered than others by the superimposition of the viral disease. Finally, some proportion of the cases of post-transfusion hepatitis would be prevented if more rigorous indications for transfusion were insisted on, and if presently available preparations of human serum albumin were used more widely in place of blood and plasma in the treatment of situations requiring the expansion of plasma volume, since the use of albumin prepared by present techniques has not been associated with the transmission of viral hepatitis.

Drug-induced liver injury and some of the aspects of excessive use of alcohol are considered later in this chapter.

Neuromuscular System

Dysfunction of the neuromuscular system may reflect local disease confined to a single structure or a portion of the system (such as the peripheral nerves), or may be produced by a wide variety of diseases elsewhere in the body. Thus, preventive aspects of neuromuscular disease are concerned, on the one hand, with measures aimed at protecting against injury to the nervous system and/or skeletal muscles per se, and on the other, with evaluation of neuromuscular syndromes as expressions of established but possibly remediable or modifiable disease elsewhere.

In the first group are found specific opportunities for prevention of neurologic injury by infectious agents, such as immunization against poliomyelitis and chemoprophylaxis of meningococcal meningitis in contacts of cases (Chapter 10). Also in this group are situations in which recognition and appropriate therapy of systemic conditions may prevent specific neurologic syndromes, e.g., combined system disease in pernicious anemia. Also to be considered here are some aspects of cerebral vascular disease in relation to which anticoagulant therapy appears to be effective, either in terms of reducing the frequency of vascular insults to the brain, mitigation of the effects of such insults once under way, or both. Included in this group are cerebral embolization, so-called transient ischemic attacks, and the stroke-in-evolution. Attention to other conditions that may reduce the risk of cerebral infarction would include polycythemia and severe anemia, particularly in patients with established atheromatous disease of the cerebral vessels.

The neuromuscular syndromes that may be regarded as possible expressions of systemic or localized visceral disease are numerous. Confusion, delirium, and alterations of consciousness are among the most important of these, and may be caused by a wide variety of processes, including intoxications with drugs, heavy metals, or alcohol; metabolic disorders such as uremia, hepatic failure, hypoglycemia, various derangements of electrolyte metabolism and acid-base balance; hypoxia or widespread ischemia from any cause; endocrine disease, including hypothyroidism, adrenal cortical insufficiency, and parathyroid dysfunction, and a number of other disorders. Peripheral neuropathy and myopathy are also commonly seen as expressions of deep-seated disease, including carcinoma of a variety of types; in such instances evidence of peripheral neuropathy, myopathy, or both may antedate other clinical manifestations of the tumor by months. Thus, appearance of this neuromuscular syndrome without an apparent alternative cause requires a clinical, laboratory, and radiologic search for occult malignancy. Other causes of neuromyopathy, particularly peripheral neuropathy, include poisoning by various heavy metals and organic compounds, acute infections, notably diphtheria, alcoholism, diabetes mellitus, uremia, and collagen vascular disease. The occurrence of myasthenia gravis should bring to mind its association, in 15 to 20 per cent of cases, with thymic tumors.

Hematologic Disease

Disorders of the formed elements of the peripheral blood may reflect underlying disease of any organ system of the body, in addition to their evident relation to conditions that affect the blood-forming apparatus primarily. Prevention of primary insults to the hematopoietic tissues revolves at present chiefly around the careful use of drugs. A host of therapeutic agents have been incriminated as causes of bone marrow suppression with resultant anemia, leukopenia, and thrombocytopenia in various combinations, or with the induction of hemolysis. Others are less clearly related but any drug that the patient has been taking must be viewed as bearing a potential causative relationship to marrow suppression marked by diminution of any of the formed elements of the blood. Of the agents in current use those which are most commonly associated with marrow suppression are chloramphenicol, sulfonamides, and agents used in the chemotherapy of malignant disease (antimetabolites, folic acid antagonists, nitrogen mustards). Others include diphenylhydantoin (Dilantin), quinacrine (Atabrine), and perhaps certain antihistamines, antithyroid agents, phenylbutazone, procaineamide, and chlorpromazine. In addition, ionizing radiation, various organic solvents, hair dyes, and other antibiotics have been suspected or incriminated. The cautions to the physician in matching the risk of various therapeutic agents to the dangers of the disease to be treated are evident.

As in presenting syndromes relating to other organ systems, hematopoietic disorders may reflect the presence of underlying disease, recognition of which may aid in preventing morbidity and mortality. The most important of these is iron-deficiency anemia. Although this disorder is frequently due to the cumulative effects of menstrual blood loss in women in their menstrual years, it should always be regarded as a possible indication of chronic occult gastrointestinal bleeding, particularly in men or in postmenopausal women, and appropriate diagnostic studies should be carried out. A significant number of such individuals are ultimately shown to have presymptomatic gastrointestinal malignancy or peptic ulcer disease.

Other anemias may be found to be based on a large number of conditions, including vitamin B_{12} deficiency due to pernicious anemia, malabsorption from a variety of causes, or hypothyroidism; others may reflect the presence of lymphomatous disease, various hereditary and acquired hemolytic disorders, splenomegaly due to any cause, renal insufficiency, metastatic disease of the bone marrow, thymic tumors, and so on. Thrombocytopenia similarly may be a presenting manifestation of underlying disease, including bone marrow replacement or invasion, splenomegaly from any cause, a wide spectrum of acute infections, the collagen vascular diseases, and accelerated intravascular coagulation. Leukemoid reactions may be seen in a number of bacterial infections, malignant disease, especially with bone marrow metastases, sudden hemolysis or hemorrhage, severe burns, and in other conditions.

Endocrine System

The relation of certain endocrine disorders (pheochromocytoma, Cushing's syndrome, primary aldosteronism) to hypertensive disease has been considered. A number of other endocrinopathies present aspects germane to a discussion of preventive aspects of disease, but discussion here will be confined to two, namely the menopausal syndrome and osteoporosis. The question of replacement therapy in postmenopausal patients has been debated for years, and continues to be. Aside from treatment of the vasomotor instability and the local genitourinary complaints often seen in these patients, the relation of estrogen lack to the rate of progress of atherosclerosis has been an important issue in the discussion of replacement therapy.

An increased incidence of symptomatic coronary artery atherosclerosis in post-menopausal women and in patients castrated before the naturally occurring menopause has been established. Further, a change toward the male pattern in the serum lipoproteins has been noted in these patients, and has been reversible with estrogen therapy. Although direct biological connections between estrogen metabolism and the development of atheromatous lesions have not been established experimentally, many believe that the epidemiologic and biochemical observations noted above justify estrogen replacement more or less routinely in menopausal women in an effort to prevent to some degree the development of atherosclerotic cardiovascular disease. Initiation of such therapy must be with the realization that its usefulness for this purpose has not been clearly established.

Postmenopausal osteoporosis, demonstrable ultimately in most women who live a number of years beyond the menopause, appears to be related in part to estrogen lack, though calcium intake and level of physical activity also seem to be involved. It is to be noted that senile osteoporosis also occurs in men, though later in life than in women. In addition, a number of metabolic abnormalities have been noted in osteoporotic patients, the relative importance and interrelationships of which are unclear. Nevertheless, the fact that senile osteoporosis is primarily a disease of women, coupled with the known effect of estrogens in producing a positive calcium balance and reducing the incidence of fracture in these patients, has led to the use of these compounds in the treatment of this type of osteoporosis, along with other measures. The effectiveness of the prophylactic use of estrogens in the prevention or mitigation of postmenopausal osteoporosis is not clearly established, but they are used widely for this purpose.

Smoking and Disease

Although some of the relationships presently thought to exist between smoking and disease have been referred to, a brief recapitulation of current views is included here. Cigarette smoking may be the most common potentially lethal and at the same time potentially remedial condition met by physicians. As noted previously, over half the adult male population of the United States smoke cigarettes at the present time, four years after the Surgeon General's Advisory Committee issued its report. The proportion of women who smoke is smaller, but nevertheless considerable. The health impact of this habit is not confined to the smoker, but also makes a substantial contribution to the likelihood that his children will adopt the habit.

Recent studies have confirmed the associations noted earlier between cigarette smoking and death rates from coronary heart disease, which are higher in smokers than in nonsmokers; on the average this death rate may be 70 per cent higher, and in some patients 200 per cent higher or more, in the presence of other "risk" factors. Cessation of cigarette smoking is followed by a reduction in the risk of dying compared with the risk incurred by those who continue to smoke. The association between cigarette smoking and cerebral vascular disease has also been strengthened by recent studies.

The most recent (1967) Surgeon General's Report notes that cigarette smoking is the most important cause of chronic nonneoplastic bronchopulmonary disease in this country, outweighing the contributions of atmospheric pollution and occupational exposure. It greatly increases the risk of dying from chronic bronchitis and emphysema, in addition to being a common cause of cough, sputum production, and reduction in ventilatory function. Cessation of smoking is followed by a reduction in mortality from chronic bronchopulmonary disease relative to the mortality of those who continue to smoke.

The association between cigarette smoking, and to a much smaller extent, pipe and cigar smoking and lung cancer has been strengthened by recent studies. Duration, manner of smoking, and quantity of cigarettes smoked per day appear to be related to the risk of developing lung cancer. Male cigarette smokers of less than one pack a day have mortality ratios as high as 10, and smokers of more than one pack a day have mortality ratios as high as 30. Cessation of cigarette smoking reduces sharply the risk of dying of lung cancer relative to the risk of those who continue.

Associations also exist between cigarette smoking and cancers of the buccal cavity, pharynx, larynx, esophagus, and urinary bladder.

The bulk of evidence indicates that smoking is, in the main, conditioned by psychologic and social factors, whether or not underlying constitutional or hereditary influences are operative. The cessation of smoking can only be accomplished at present by the mobilization of psychosocial pressures, and this mobilization must be regarded as a significant responsibility of every physician. Smokers should be informed of the foregoing epidemiologic facts so they will have a sound basis upon which to make and reinforce decisions relative to cessation of the habit.

Obesity

Some of the health associations of obesity have been referred to previously. Because obesity is another exceedingly common, potentially correctable disorder with significant impact on health, it should be approached as an important pathological condition whenever it is encountered by the physician. Associated disorders include a higher incidence of arterial hypertension and diabetes as well as ischemic heart disease. The latter may be, at least in part, related to the former two factors. Other conditions bearing at least a partial clinical relationship to obesity include the hypoventilation syndrome, sometimes associated with cardiopulmonary failure, as well as an increased incidence of toxemia of pregnancy, increased risk in surgical procedures, various orthopedic difficulties, such as low back syndromes and osteoarthritis of the weight-bearing joints, and gall bladder disease.

The well-documented excessive mortality among the obese relates in part to some of the above associations. Therapy should be aggressive in the hope that at least part of the lethality of obesity may be reversible.

In the absence of specific psychologic or somatic contraindications, the effort to treat obesity should always be made when it is encountered. The patient should be educated in the concept that the disorder cannot be cured, but can only be rendered latent; that is, that it will surely recur if any terminable treatment program is adopted. Rather, therapy should aim toward a permanent alteration of the individual's eating habits, i.e., of his relationship with food. The writer has never seen long-sustained weight loss as the result of using appetite-suppressing drugs. It is sobering to reflect that with present techniques the five-year cure rate for obesity approaches zero. Efforts to prevent obesity through educational programs applied to populations or individuals may hold some promise, but the outlook in this regard seems gloomy in the setting of overalimentation that characterizes our society, and in the light of the frequent use of food for the purpose of assuaging anxiety.

Cancer Screening*

It seems likely that the most effective technique presently available for cancer screening consists of a careful history and physical examination by a competent physician. Many internal malignancies first make themselves manifest by inducing organ dysfunction, and the meticulous system review is the most sensitive method available for detecting these changes. Thus, anorexia, alteration of bowel habits, postmenopausal or excessive menstrual bleeding, pain, cough, rectal bleeding, and many other early indicators of possible cancer can only be elicited in this manner. The physical examination is probably somewhat less sensitive as a case-finding technique, but may reveal malignant lesions of the oral cavity or breast, abdominal masses, rectal tumors, lymph node enlargement, and a number of other findings, including the cutaneous lesions that may suggest visceral neoplasia.

The routine blood count, urinalysis, and stool guaiac afford simple laboratory screening techniques that should be available in every physician's office. The chest x-ray as a screening procedure for primary neoplasms of the lung appears to have a yield of about 2 per thousand (Lilienfeld *et al.*, 1966); this may be increased by combining chest x-rays with cytologic examination of sputum specimens for neoplastic cells.

Routine proctosigmoidoscopy, particularly in those over 40 years of age, is employed increasingly as a case-finding technique for carcinomas of the rectum and sigmoid. It should be noted that 35 per cent of all large bowel cancers are within reach of the examining finger on rectal examination, and an additional 30 per cent are within reach of the sigmoidoscope.

Smears for cytologic examination by the Papanicolaou technique should be taken from the cervix and the endocervical canal in all adult women at least once yearly. This technique reveals a large number of uterine malignancies, many of them early and presymptomatic. Cure rates are higher for endometrial and cervical carcinomas found in this manner than for those found when presenting flagrant symptoms, uterine enlargement, or other signs of advanced lesions.

Other screening techniques for the early identification of cancer are presently under study; for example, the widespread use of soft tissue x-rays of the breasts (mammography), in an effort to improve case-finding. Hopefully some of these will provide new

* See also Chapter 8.

methods of sufficient applicability, sensitivity, and specificity, so that many more patients with early disease may be identified and treated. Until these are established, the physician must rely on meticulous history-taking, physical examination, the ancillary procedures noted above, a high index of suspicion, and readiness to carry out further diagnostic procedures on the basis of any reasonable suggestion that a malignancy may be present.

PREVENTION OF INFECTIOUS AND OTHER DISEASES

Immunization

The principles of active and passive immunization are considered in Chapter 10. The potential impact of immunization procedures on individual and public health may be emphasized by considering the sharp reduction in the incidence of paralytic polio-myelitis that has occurred since the introduction of effective vaccines for this disease. Thus, in the early 1950's the incidence of the paralytic form of the disease in this country was 14.6 per 100,000. In 1965 there were only 61 cases, with 5 deaths. Similarly, the experience with smallpox vaccine has been associated with such a level of effectiveness that in the United States at the present time a single case may be considered an epidemic.

Although many vaccines do not approach the level of efficacy of these two, numerous opportunities for the prevention of infectious disease by active or passive immunization are available to the physician. A number of these will be considered.

Active Immunization.   Bacterial infections against which active immunization is feasible include diphtheria and pertussis, tetanus, typhoid fever, cholera, and tuberculosis. Immunization against diphtheria and pertussis is usually carried out simultaneously in infancy and childhood through the use of a combined preparation that often contains tetanus toxoid as well. Adverse reactions to pertussis and diphtheria vaccines may occur when these materials are administered to adults. Ordinarily 3 doses of the combined vaccine are administered a month apart, beginning at about 3 months of age. Booster injections are given at 2 and 5 years of age. Initial immunization against tetanus should be carried out in infancy and childhood. Effective circulating levels of antibody can probably be maintained thereafter with booster doses at intervals of 5 to 10 years. In patients previously immunized who have sustained wounds or injuries associated with tissue devitalization or soil contamination a booster dose should also be given, particularly if such has not been received in the past year. Nonimmunized persons who have sustained such injuries should be actively immunized as protection against future injuries. Typhoid vaccine should be administered to those living in or traveling to areas in which typhoid fever is hyperendemic. Three subcutaneous doses of 0.5 ml 7 to 10 days apart are given; annual booster doses of single injections of vaccine are often given, though at best the immunity conferred by this vaccine is not strong; even individuals who have received the full series of 3 doses a year before should perhaps have this repeated if heavy exposure to typhoid is likely. Cholera vaccine provides partial but incomplete protection against cholera. It is usually administered to those living or traveling in endemic areas in 2 doses 7 to 10 days apart. Active immunization against tuberculosis has been more widely used elsewhere than in the United States, and some controversy exists concerning the most appropriate circumstances for its application. The vaccine, an attenuated strain referred to as BCG (Bacillus Calmette-Guérin), may be given to tuberculin-negative individuals exposed to tubercle bacilli in the home, school, or laboratory, though some authorities prefer chemoprophylaxis with isoniazid under these circumstances.

Viral infections for which active immunizing procedures are available are several. Routine smallpox vaccination in infancy is practiced in this country, with revaccination at school entry and at risk of exposure to infection. The present extent of foreign travel makes the latter occasion a common one. Vaccination should be avoided in patients with dysgammaglobulinemias, systemic malignancies, such as lymphomas, eczema, and other dermatitides, and those receiving immunosuppressive therapy, radiation therapy, or adrenal cortical steroids, as well as in siblings of children with eczema. For immunization against poliomyelitis the weight of present evidence indicates that oral poliomyelitis vaccine is the preferred immunizing agent. Immunity of a very high order is conferred by this preparation; both effective levels of circulating neutralizing antibody and intestinal immunity are produced. Infants should receive oral poliomyelitis vaccine during the first year of life and again on entering school. Monovalent vaccines are preferred. Adults should also probably be immunized routinely. Immunization should generally be carried out in the cooler months of the year, when the prevalence of interfering enteroviruses is lowest. Type II vaccine is usually given first, Type I is given 8 weeks later, and Type III is given 6 or more weeks after that. Transient protection against influenza can be conferred with presently available vaccines. These contain inactivated, chick embryo-grown strains of influenza A and B viruses. Administration of the vaccine to all patients with chronic pulmonary disease and heart disease, as well as to the elderly, is strongly advised, as these are the groups with the highest case fatality rates from influenza. Such immunization should be carried out annually in the autumn by administration of 1.0 ml of vaccine subcutaenously. For immunization against measles effective live virus vaccines are now available. These consist of attenuated strains of measles virus, and probably confer immunity comparable in degree and duration to that following the natural infection. Ultimately, artificial immunization against measles will probably become routine in pediatric practice. Mumps immunization is indicated primarily in adult males who have not had the disease but who may be exposed—i.e., those with young children. Immunization is indicated in an effort to prevent orchitis, a painful and sometimes sterilizing complication. Live virus vaccine, is used. Because rabies is uniformly lethal, appropriate immunizing procedures afford the only known means of saving the life of an individual bitten by a rabid animal. Difficulties are introduced into the situation when the animal is not clearly rabid at the time of the bite, or when it escapes or is killed. The level of endemicity of rabies in the community is also a factor in deciding about prophylactic therapy, as is the fact that the vaccines themselves may induce neurological injury in addition to the serum sickness that may follow attempts to induce passive immunity with antirabies serum. The decision to initiate preventive treatment in the individual case should be made in consultation with local health authorities at the time of the bite or other contact. It is to be recalled that not only dogs, but wolves, foxes, bats, coyotes, jackals, ermines, and other species may transmit the infection. Avian embryo vaccines appear to be safer than the older preparations, and when administered together with antirabies serum or its globulin fractions, afford the best-known prophylactic treatment for severe bites. Yellow fever vaccine should be administered to those living or traveling in endemic areas. Effective immunization can be accomplished with the chick embryo-grown virus preparations used in this country, and may last for 10 years or more.

Of the Rickettsial infections, active immunization has been most effective in relation to epidemic typhus. Both the incidence and the severity of the disease are reduced; the mortality rate among vaccinated individuals who contract the disease is very low. Two doses of 1.0 ml each are given subcutaneously 10 days to 2 weeks apart; booster doses of 1.0 ml may be given at intervals of a few months if exposure is expected.

Passive Immunization. The relation of gamma globulin preparations to passive immunization against infectious hepatitis and perhaps against serum hepatitis has already been considered. For immunization against tetanus, human antitoxin (tetanus immune globulin) is now available, and should be used in preference to antitoxin of equine or bovine origin because it does not cause serum sickness or anaphylactic shock. This material is given intramuscularly to nonimmunized individuals who have sustained serious trauma or who are not seen until 48 hours or more after the injury. For lesser degrees of injury seen earlier a single injection of 1.2 million units of benzathine penicillin has been recommended as an adequate prophylactic measure. Passive protection against measles is afforded by intramuscular administration of gamma globulin. Given in appropriate doses (0.025 to 0.05 ml per pound of body weight, depending on age) in the first half of the incubation period, it attenuates the course of the disease. In larger doses the disease can be prevented altogether; this should be attempted in very young or debilitated children, pregnant women, and those with leukemia or lymphomas, or on immuno-suppressive or adrenal cortical steroid therapy who are exposed and susceptible.

Resistance to Infections: General Aspects

Several of the more specific physiologic processes involved in resistance to infections have achieved some clarification in recent years; and a number of correlations of an apparently less discrete nature exist. Some of the latter are well founded and others rest primarily on clinical suspicion. The group as a whole can, to varying degrees, be interfered with by the physician with resultant improvement in the patient's resistance. Among the more specific problems that can be approached are the effects of adrenal cortical steroids and immunosuppressive drugs on resistance to infections. These must be used cautiously, only on proper indications, with full awareness of this aspect of their impact on the patient. The various immunologic deficiency states, particularly the congenital and idiopathic varieties of hypogammaglobulinemia, may be approached through the intramuscular administration of gamma globulin in doses and at intervals appropriate to the maintenance of circulating levels above 150 to 200 mgm per 100 ml. The association of increased risk of infection with chronic lymphoid leukemia, lymphosarcoma, and widespread Hodgkin's disease is also related, at least in part, to hypogammaglobulinemia. Multiple myeloma and macroglobulinemia may be complicated by interference with normal immunoglobulin synthesis and an increased incidence of infection. The nephrotic syndrome may result in lowered concentrations of gamma globulin in body fluids because of urinary loss of the protein and dilution. Children who have been subjected to splenectomy have an increased incidence of bacteremias; the nature of this phenomenon is unclear. In the management of all these types of patients the increased susceptibility to infection must be borne in mind and appropriate preventive or therapeutic efforts directed accordingly.

Nutritional deficiency is also associated with an increased incidence of infections (see Chapter 11). The nature of this association is unclear, though the implications in the preventive aspects of medical care are not. Social and political factors are often important in the complex of forces behind marked malnutrition, and the physician's efforts may sometimes be appropriately directed to these as well as to the individual patient.

Alcohol, when used in substantial quantities, may contribute to a reduction in resistance to infections. Indeed, case fatality rates in some diseases are higher in alcoholics; pneumococcal lobar pneumonia is an example. This is undoubtedly a complex phenomenon, though recent studies have demonstrated interference with phagocytosis by cells of rats given large amounts of alcohol.

Exposure probably bears some relation to resistance to infections, though experimental corroboration is lacking. Nevertheless, clinical experience, as well as the cumulative experience of countless mothers, suggests a relationship, at least to viral respiratory disease.

Birth Defects and Genetic Counseling

Genetic counseling is discussed elsewhere in this volume (see Chapter 2) and is germane to understanding a large but as yet quantitatively ill-defined proportion of defects and disorders that become clinically apparent at any age from intrauterine life to late adulthood. The ability of the physician to prevent a significant number of these disorders has in large measure to do with eugenics, but a sound factual basis for genetic advice to patients is often lacking. On the other hand, the recent appearance of an epidemic of phocomelia traced to the ingestion of a drug, thalidomide, by women early in pregnancy points up environmental influences in the genesis of birth defects. The extent to which other drugs or additional adverse impacts on the fetus may be operative is unknown, but it is likely to be great. A well-recognized instance of birth defects clearly related to maternal disease during pregnancy is rubella; about 10 to 15 per cent of infants born to women who acquire the disease in the first trimester have evident congenital defects recognizable at birth or in the first year of life, including cataracts, glaucoma, congenital heart disease, thrombocytopenic purpura, and lesions of the long bones. The suggestion has been made that Down's syndrome (mongolism) may be related to viral hepatitis in the mother. A number of other associations have been suspected. That the physician must develop and retain a lively interest in this area is indicated by the fact that abnormal conditions of congenital origin are a leading cause of death and disability in the United States. It has been estimated that 500,000 fetal deaths and at least 62,000 deaths among the live-born are associated with birth defects each year, and that 15 million persons in this country alone have one or more congenital defects that affect their daily lives (Apgar and Stickle, 1968).

Case Finding*

An important preventive and epidemiologic responsibility of the physician relates to identification of diseased individuals whose existence in the community is revealed by the appearance of illness in their contacts. Many of these persons may be unaware of the presence of disease, and hence are untreated. Failure to identify them permits them to operate as continuing public health hazards. These problems relate chiefly to infectious and parasitic disease, including tuberculosis, venereal infections, and various parasitic infestations. The typhoid carrier is also in this category, as is the blood stream carrier of the agent of serum hepatitis. In addition to seeking the source of the patient's infection, the physician should, in certain circumstances, extend case-finding activities to those who may have acquired the disease from the patient. Thus, spread among the patient's contacts should be sought not only in the conditions noted above, but also in relation to infectious hepatitis, beta hemolytic streptococcal and meningococcal infections, and perhaps even such mundane afflictions as athlete's foot. The central point is the physician's responsibility to wonder, in relation to a number of conditions, from whom the disease came and to whom it may have gone. The corollary responsibility of notifying appropriate health authorities of diagnoses of reportable diseases is also to be noted, as such notification is the basis on which valid conclusions as to the nature and prevalence of various diseases in the community are to be drawn.

AVOIDANCE OF POTENTIALLY HARMFUL DIAGNOSTIC AND THERAPEUTIC MANEUVERS

There is virtually no diagnostic or therapeutic procedure that is not potentially harmful to some degree. In the evaluation and treatment of every patient the physician must continually balance these risks against the magnitude of the disease he is attempting to diagnose or treat. It has been said that no drug is as harmless as water, including water. It might be added that, therapeutically speaking, one should never hunt a mouse with a howitzer.

These accumulated risks have been formulated by Barr (1955) as the price we pay for modern management of disease. The bulk of information presently available concerns the acute toxic or other adverse side effects of diagnostic and treatment measures. The long-term untoward effects are largely unknown, though such risks as that deriving from the cumulative x-ray exposure experienced by the individual during his lifetime have been identified qualitatively, if not quantitatively (see Chapter 4). It would be naïve to assume that the acute adverse effects of drugs represent the totality of the risk they present to the patient. The physician must acknowledge our ignorance in this area, and use it to temper further his use of diagnostic and therapeutic agents,

* See also Chapter 10.

restricting them to those necessary for the proper care of the patient, and selecting whenever possible those associated with the least apparent risk.

So-called "iatrogenic disease" does not refer primarily to conditions produced by inappropriate therapy, quackery, or gross malpractice. Rather it has to do with the dangers inherent in diagnostic and treatment procedures themselves—even those selected with the greatest care, administered in appropriate dosages and with proper indications, and given with indicated precautions. Even under these circumstances there exists an irreducible minimum of risk; the physician's responsibility is to see to it that this is not inadvertently enhanced.

Among the diagnostic procedures that have been associated with substantial adverse effects are the intravenous administration of dyes for radiologic studies of the urinary tract or biliary tree (anaphylactic reactions), oral cholecystography (renal failure), sternal puncture for bone marrow examination (cardiac perforation and tamponade), thoracentesis and paracentesis (perforation of lung or bowel, infection), lumbar puncture (death from herniation of cerebellar tonsils, infection), cardiac catheterization and angiocardiography (cardiac puncture, death from arrhythmias, anaphylaxis), needle biopsy of the liver (bile peritonitis, hemorrhage), venepuncture (syncope with injury, infection), sigmoidoscopy (bowel perforation), and intravenous administration of dehydrocholic acid for determination of circulation time (anaphylactic reactions).

Adverse reactions to drugs include intoxications due to extension of the usual pharmacologic actions of the agent (e.g., digitalis intoxication, bleeding due to anti-coagulant therapy), difficulties due to modifications of the internal environment (e.g., due to diuretics, intravenous therapy, continuous gastric suction, sodium restriction, administration of potassium salts), and allergic reactions (cutaneous eruptions, drug fever, serum sickness, some blood dyscrasias). Potential interactions among the various types of adverse drug effects abound—for example, the potentiation of digitalis effect by hypokalemia due to diuretics.

An additional type of drug-induced disease is the precipitation of a clinical entity in an individual in whom it may or may not have been present in latent form; examples are the appearance of diabetes mellitus or hyperuricemia and gout in patients treated with thiazide derivatives, or the development of gastric ulcers in those on adrenal steroids. In some instances syndromes resembling naturally occurring disease have been produced, as in the lupus-like syndrome associated with the use of hydralazine.

Drug-induced liver injury is increasingly common. It has followed a wide variety of types of pharmacologic agents, including antimicrobial drugs (para-amino salicylic acid, some salts of erythromycin), tranquilizers (chlorpromazine, prochlorperazine), anti-inflammatory agents (phenylbutazone), and numerous general anesthetics. The pathogenesis of the lesions seen under these circumstances is poorly understood, but prolonged illness and death may result.

The introduction of infection by needles, indwelling venous or arterial catheters, and urinary tract instrumentation or catheterization is another type of injury that may be produced by treatment efforts. The use of blood and certain blood products is associated with the risk of infection with the agents of viral hepatitis and occasionally with other infections (see Chapter 10), as well as with the dangers of mismatched transfusions.

The occurrence of these risks is known to every physician. Their frequency is great; in Barr's experience they constituted, in the aggregate, one of the commonest conditions seen on the wards of a large general hospital, amounting to 5 per cent of those admitted. To some extent these disorders can be avoided or minimized; to that extent they represent preventable disease, and one of the physician's greatest challenges and opportunities. This responsibility will become even more important as time passes and the potency of therapeutic agents increases. The ancient admonition must be remembered always: *Primum non nocere*. First, be sure you do no harm.

PSYCHIATRIC AND SOCIAL PATHOLOGY

Suicide

In the United States suicide has ranked among the first ten causes of death in adults for most of the past 50 years. Approximately 20,000 individuals take their own lives annually in this country, and it has been estimated that a suicide attempt is made, on the average, once every minute. It is overwhelmingly likely that every physician at some time in his professional life will have a patient who makes a suicide attempt, successful or unsuccessful.

The person who is seriously contemplating suicide may be conceived of as one who is undergoing a crisis in which he is not his normal self, and who needs help during this crisis to protect him from himself (*Public Health Service Publication*, 1961). At the heart of suicide prevention lies the attempt to recognize the individual who represents a suicidal risk.

It is of importance in this regard that some 60 per cent of actual suicides have made prior attempts. In addition, studies of attempted suicides who survive have established that about 10 per cent eventually kill themselves.

It should be axiomatic that all suicide threats and attempts should be taken seriously. It is not true that those who talk about suicide don't actually do it; rather, about 80 per cent of those who conduct successful suicide attempts have given some sort of warning of their intent. Repeated talk of death may constitute such a warning, and should be evaluated carefully, though clearly many such individuals are not contemplating suicide. Overt references to intended suicide are not infrequent. In our culture, suicide attempts usually reflect some type of emotional disturbance. Although the gamut of psychiatric entities, from nonpsychotics to advanced schizophrenics, is run by suicidal patients, depression is a frequent emotional setting. It must be borne in mind that suicidal attempts are frequently made as the individual begins to improve and to emerge from his depression; special caution must be exercised during this period.

The triggering event may be one that elicits feelings of anger, disappointment, or frustration; or it may involve financial loss or severe loss of status. Among those at risk of suicide in a setting of some acute personal crisis, vigilance must be especially maintained for the three months or so afterward, because many suicides occur during this period.

In general, the physician must remember that no group in the population is immune to the risk of suicide. Appropriate care must be taken to identify and protect those at risk, in concert with the patient's family, and with the diagnostic and therapeutic help of the psychiatrist. Patients who have made suicide attempts, or those in whom the physician judges that such a risk is real, should have the benefit of psychiatric evaluation so that some expert treatment judgment may be made.

Alcohol

The extent to which alcoholism or its major complications can be prevented by the physician is small, and permanent cures among "addictive" types of chronic alcoholics are infrequent. The complex admixture of psychologic and social factors that are operative in this disorder contribute to the difficulties. Nevertheless, the physician is frequently consulted by the alcoholic or his family; efforts of a preventive nature can be addressed to several aspects of the problem. Attempts to persuade the patient to reduce his alcohol intake, if not to abstain completely, are sometimes effective, particularly in the earlier stages of the disorder. In some cases psychiatric evaluation and treatment are helpful. Protection of the patient against the hepatic, neurologic, pancreatic, and myocardial diseases associated with alcohol excess are dependent on reduction of intake, though describing or exploring the specters of these conditions with the patient is almost uniformly ineffective in inducing him to stop drinking, and often represents mobilization of hostile feelings in the physician by the alcoholic.

In patients with peripheral neuropathy or the Korsakoff-Wernicke syndrome, administration of thiamine may result in dramatic relief of symptoms and signs, but except for this, specific drug therapy has not been of striking use, either in the treatment of complications of alcoholism or in efforts to prevent the ingestion of alcohol.

The impact of alcoholism on those around the patient, particularly his family, may be severe. On some occasions the opportunity for sympathetic counseling with the physician may be helpful to the spouse or children of the alcoholic, and may aid in mitigating some of the adverse effects on the family that are likely to appear.

Counseling with the patient himself can be productive if he is able to recognize that alcohol is a problem for him, that he needs help in its management, and that he must be an active contributor to his own treatment. If this can be accomplished, psychiatric evaluation may then be sought, and a decision made in relation to some type of psychotherapy; referral to Alcoholics Anonymous may seem appropriate in some cases, with or without psychiatric consultation.

Despite the poor prognosis associated with alcoholism of severe degree, the physician must seek opportunities to reduce its impact on the patient, his family, and the community. The problem of alcoholism is so common that every physician will be confronted by it many times.

Drug Dependence and Addiction

The area of drug dependence is vast and complex. It is estimated that there are about 50,000 persons in the United States who are active narcotic addicts, and another

500,000 who are habituated to or dependent on hypnotic drugs. Both figures may be low, but they serve as indices of the dimensions of the problem.

The primary preventive responsibility of the physician is to minimize his contribution to the genesis of these addictions. Many patients acquire narcotic dependence in medical situations in which the drugs are given for appropriate medical reasons; the physician must be careful to keep dosage and duration of therapy with potentially addicting drugs to the minimum necessary for the proper care of the patient. Although certain personality types are more likely than others to become addicted, any individual is at risk, depending on the type of drug administered, the dose given, and the duration of therapy.

Similarly, the indiscriminate use of sedatives and hypnotics must be recognized as a procedure that not only fails to resolve anxieties, tensions, and insomnia over any long period of time, but that exposes patients to the risk of habituation and dependence, as well as to a variety of types of adverse drug reactions.

Efforts to treat the individual addict and thus protect him and society from the adverse effects of illicit use of narcotic drugs are better carried out in public or private institutions devoted to the management of this problem, rather than by the individual physician. Under these circumstances drug withdrawal can be accomplished, efforts at psychologic and social rehabilitation inaugurated, and plans for postinstitutional follow-up and therapy formulated. Prevention of relapse is uncommon, particularly in patients who must return to living conditions in urban slum areas; about 90 per cent of such individuals relapse within a year.

Other approaches, including maintenance therapy with methadone and organizations of ex-addicts analagous to Alcoholics Anonymous are presently being tried. Although varying degrees of effectiveness are reported, it is likely that neither represents the final answer to narcotic addiction; rather, it appears more likely that social advances and legislation attacking the root causes of poverty, slum living, and inequality of opportunity will be required to remove some of the pressures that appear to trigger narcotic use in susceptible individuals.

Other Problems

Numerous other factors potentially detrimental to health are operative in our culture, and are associated with opportunities for prevention of morbidity and mortality by the individual physician. Among these are to be mentioned such areas as physical abuse of children (the so-called "battered child syndrome"); malnutrition, with its potential for inducing permanent untoward effects on physical development and mental performance; traffic accidents, which are a major cause of death and disability in this country, and in relation to which important correlations exist with some types of personality structure and with alcoholism among drivers, as well as with automobile and highway design and construction; and the effects of noise, crowding, and living and working conditions, the results of which in terms of human misery, illness, and malfunctioning are almost certainly considerable, though largely unknown.

Many others could be identified, but the conditions and problems listed serve to indicate the scope of the social and environmental health problems that the physician should add to the responsibilities that are primarily clinical as he attempts to concern himself with the broad aspects of reduction of morbidity in his patient population.

THE PERIODIC HEALTH EXAMINATION— MULTIPHASIC SCREENING*

Periodic examinations of presumably healthy individuals have been gaining wide acceptance in recent years. They have been endorsed by many corporations, trade unions, subdivisions of government, medical centers, and practicing physicians, as well as by very large numbers of patients.

These health evaluations are based on three fundamental premises: (1) It is possible to construct an examination with sufficient sensitivity and specificity to separate out individuals with established disease, much of it presymptomatic, or with conditions or habits likely to lead to disease, from those lacking such trends, habits, or diseases. (2) A significant proportion of the pathology or the pre-pathologic conditions thus found will be remediable. (3) Altering or remedying such conditions or trends will result in reduced morbidity or mortality risk for the individual.

On balance, these examinations represent a worth-while effort to reduce morbidity and prolong life, but enthusiasm for them must be tempered with the realization that clear proof of their validity in accomplishing these ends is lacking. Thus, it is clear that significant and even life-threatening disease, such as some instances of severe coronary artery atherosclerosis, various malignancies, and some brain tumors, may be missed completely despite the careful application of all the clinical techniques used in such examinations; indeed, some instances of these or other conditions may not be detectable by any clinical diagnostic technique presently available. Further, it is clear that many of the conditions discovered are not remediable in any fundamental sense by any known therapeutic modality, and that, in relation to a number of those that can be approached therapeutically, we lack clear evidence of reversal, amelioration, or eradication as a result of such treatment. Thus, some reservations are indicated in evaluating the degree to which periodic health examinations accomplish their object.

A number of studies have given some indication of the diagnostic yield of these health evaluations. The figures obtained are based largely on the *first* examination of groups of asymptomatic adults; in populations examined repeatedly at intervals, e.g., annually, the yield of newly discovered conditions is considerably lower.

The commonest potentially remediable health threat uncovered is cigarette smoking. As indicated previously, this will be found in 40 to 50 per cent of adults examined. The impact on this incidence of a concerted effort to reduce it on the part of those conducting periodic examinations is unknown; the same is true in relation to a number of the disorders that may be found.

Other commonly discovered and potentially remediable conditions are obesity, noted in 10 to 30 per cent of examinations, and hypertension, found in 5 to 20 per cent in various series. Rectal or sigmoid adenomatous polyps have been reported in 5 to 15

* See also Chapter 8.

per cent, peptic ulcer in 5 to 10 per cent, inguinal hernia in 5 to 10 per cent, anemia in 5 to 10 per cent, cholelithiasis in 4 to 7 per cent, and glaucoma in 1 to 2 per cent.

Other commonly encountered conditions for which varying degrees of symptomatic relief can often be provided, though with less likelihood of reversal, include arthritis, found in 10 to 20 per cent; ischemic heart disease, 5 to 20 per cent; anxiety states, 5 to 20 per cent; diabetes mellitus, 1 to 3 per cent; and renal calculus, 1 to 2 per cent (Roberts, 1959).

Encountered less often are instances of congenital or rheumatic heart disease, active pulmonary tuberculosis, and a variety of malignancies. In relation to the latter, the value of discovery of presymptomatic neoplasms is based on the concept that cure rates are higher for malignancies that are found "early"—i.e., without associated regional or distant spread. Feinstein (1964) has emphasized some of the assumptions on which this idea is founded, and has pointed out the contribution made to the clinical pattern of tumor behavior by the intrinsic biologic properties of the neoplasm.

In recent years, coincident with the availability of automated techniques for performing multiple biochemical tests on blood, a number of such determinations have been added to health examinations. These have included measurement of blood urea nitrogen, fasting or postprandial blood sugar, serum cholesterol, serum calcium, serum protein-bound iodine, bilirubin, uric acid, and acid and alkaline phosphatase activities. The necessity for or usefulness of a number of these ancillary tests is not established at present.

If periodic health examinations are to be conducted, it would seem reasonable to center them about a careful history and physical examination. Various ancillary procedures should be added, including a complete blood count, urinalysis, stool guaiac, and chest x-ray. Electrocardiograms should probably be done on males over 40 or 45 years of age, and on females over 45 or 50; the yield of abnormalities approximates 10 per cent in this group, and abnormal findings may sometimes be used appropriately to reinforce advice concerning weight loss or cigarette smoking; in addition, it is often helpful to have base-line cardiograms available against which to compare tracings obtained later.

Cervical and endocervical smears should be obtained on females over the age of 30 to 35, and proctosigmoidoscopy should probably be included for individuals over 40 or 45 years of age.

Of the blood chemical determinations available, it is probably useful to obtain a measurement of total serum cholesterol concentration and the postprandial blood sugar or the blood sugar 2 hours after administration of a measured oral dose of glucose, usually 100 gm. The usefulness of determining blood urea nitrogen in those with no history of kidney disease or hypertension and with normal urinalyses has been debated, but occasionally unsuspected abnormalities are found. Serum uric acid may also be measured, in light of the frequency of gout and the correctability of hyperuricemia with probenecid or allopurinol; protection of the individual against tissue deposition of urate and urinary tract urate calculi may be accomplished in this way.

Other tests and procedures may be added on the basis of facts uncovered during the history or physical examination, or the initial laboratory work-up.

The further investigation of any abnormalities revealed by the periodic health evaluation must be considered and conducted by the physician in the hope that he can rule in a significant remediable condition at the least possible risk to the patient, and that the patient's health outlook will thereby be improved.

EDUCATION OF THE PUBLIC

Numerous opportunities to aid in the long-term reduction of disease morbidity and mortality are available to the physician in his potential role as an educator of his own patients, his social contacts, and the public at large.

For example, the dangers of self-medication are unknown or inadequately appreciated by many. Drugs remaining from prior prescriptions are self-administered by significant numbers of individuals for complaints similar to those for which the medication was originally given. This type of self-treatment involves the assumption of diagnostic responsibility by the patient, as does the ingestion of the host of proprietary, nonprescription preparations available in drug stores. In addition, the widespread use of such remedies exposes the patient to the risk of adverse drug reactions as well as the dangers of delay in appropriate therapy resulting from suppression of symptoms by analgesics, antinauseants, remedies for "indigestion," antipruritics, and so on.

Similarly, the inappropriateness to health maintenance or restoration of the galaxy of "tonics" and vitamin preparations that are so intensely marketed and so widely consumed should be clarified by physicians, and quack remedies should be exposed whenever possible.

Proper evaluation of proposed new public health measures, with education of lay persons concerning them, is an additional responsibility. The recent controversy concerning the fluoridation of public water supplies is an instance.

The physician should concern himself with and use his influence, where possible, to interfere with or modify advertising of proprietary remedies, cigarettes, and other health threats. This type of civic responsibility extends also to such diverse areas as advice concerning housing, noise control, and food inspection.

Of great long-term importance is the potential impact of the physician on the vivisection controversy. Continuing explanation of the necessity for and value of animal experimentation in human welfare is essential to combat the unreasoning and emotional appeals of antivivisectionists. There can be no doubt that the sum total of suffering in the world has been substantially reduced by thoughtful and properly conducted animal experimentation; the physician is in a uniquely advantageous position to formulate and explain this.

Of equal or greater importance is the opportunity available to every physician to clarify the nature of scientific medicine to the nonmedical world. It is essential for patients and potential patients to develop a clearer understanding of the nature and limitations of the diagnostic and therapeutic processes as well as efforts to prevent disease or morbidity. A more realistic appraisal by the population generally of the capacities and limitations of the physician, and of the systems of probabilities on which much of medical practice rests, will serve to improve the quality of the dialogue between the individual physician and his patient as well as that between the medical and nonmedical worlds.

OPPORTUNITIES FOR EPIDEMIOLOGIC AND OTHER INVESTIGATIVE EFFORTS

Some aspects of individual practice provide unique opportunities for studies of the incidence or prevalence of disease, or of its modifiability. In several respects these opportunities cannot be matched in institutional practice. Thus, the advantages of long-term study by a single observer obviate many of the errors introduced by variations in diagnostic criteria and other judgments when multiple observers are involved. Further, the practitioner is likely to deal with a patient population significantly different from that which comprises a hospital's practice; this is true whether one considers in-patients or out-patients. Finally, the practicing physician is likely to have a greater opportunity to make extended observations, often over a period of years, on a patient population that is likely to be a good deal more stable than that available to a hospital. Thus, long-term prospective studies may be more feasible, observations on the incidence and prevalence of nonhospitalizing illness may be more accurate, evaluations of familial occurrence of disease may be facilitated, and study of groups other than those that compose ward populations of patients in hospitals may be accomplished by the practitioner.

Other types of investigations may also be conducted effectively by the practitioner. Opportunities for significant studies should be sought and exploited by the physician as such efforts tend to make him more critical and more knowledgable. They are likely to improve the quality of care received by his patients, and to supplement the types of studies more readily carried out in hospitals, medical schools, and research institutes.

REFERENCES

ABELSON, P. H.: Changing attitudes toward smoking. Editorial, *Science*, **161**, July 26, 1968.

AHRENS, E. H., JR., HIRSCH, J., OETTE, K., FARQUHAR, J. W., and STEIN, Y.: Carbohydrate-induced and fat-induced lipemia. *Trans Ass Amer Physicians*, **74**:134–46, 1961.

APGAR, V., and STICKLE, G.: Birth defects; their significance as a public health problem. *JAMA*, **204**:371–74, 1968.

BARR, D. P.: Hazards of modern diagnosis and therapy—the price we pay. Frank Billings Memorial Lecture. *JAMA*, **159**:1452–56, 1955.

BURROWS, B., NIDEN, A. H., BARCLAY, W. R., and KASIK, J. E.: Chronic obstructive lung disease. I. Clinical and physiologic findings in 175 patients and their relationship to age and sex. *Amer Rev Resp Dis*, **91**:521–40, 1965.

CASTLEMAN, B., and KRICKSTEIN, H. I.: Do adenomatous polyps of the colon become malignant? *New Eng J Med*, **267**:469–75, 1962.

COCHRANE, A. L.: A medical scientist's view of screening. *Public Health*, **81**:207–13, 1967.

DOYLE, J. T., *et al.*: The relationship of cigarette smoking to coronary heart disease; the second report of the combined experience of the Albany, N.Y., and Framingham, Mass., studies. *JAMA*, **190**:886–90, 1964.

FEINSTEIN, A. R.: Symptomatic patterns, biologic behavior and prognosis in cancer of the lung. Practical application of Boolean algebra and clinical taxonomy. *Ann Intern Med*, **61**:27–43, 1964.

FREDERICKSON, D. S., and LEES, R. S.: Familial hyperlipoproteinemia. In Stanbury, J. B. Wyngaarden, J. B., and Frederickson, D. S. (eds.): *The Metabolic Basis of Inherited Disease*, 2nd ed. McGraw-Hill Book Co., New York, 1965.

GRAHAM, J. H., and HELWIG, E. B.: Precancerous skin lesions and systemic cancer. In Cumley, R. W., *et al.* (eds.): *Tumors of the Skin*. Year Book Publishers, Chicago, 1964.

GRAHAM, P. A.: Screening for chronic glaucoma. *Proc Roy Soc Med*, **59**:1215–19, 1966.

KANNEL, W. B., DAWBER, T. R., COHEN, M. E., and McNAMARA, P. M.: Vascular disease of the brain—epidemiologic aspects: The Framingham Study. *Amer J Public Health*, **55**:1355–66, 1965.

KUO, P. T.: Hyperglyceridemia in coronary artery disease and its management. *JAMA*, **201**:87–94, 1967.

LARAGH, J. H., SEALEY, J. E., LEDINGHAM, J. G. G., and NEWTON, M. A.: Oral contraceptives. Renin, aldosterone and high blood pressure. *JAMA*, **201**:918–22, 1967.

LEISHMAN, A. W. D.: Merits of reducing high blood pressure. *Lancet*, **1**:1284–88, 1963.

LILIENFELD, A., *et al.*: An evaluation of radiologic and cytologic screening for the early detection of lung cancer: a cooperative pilot study of the American Cancer Society and the Veterans Administration. *Cancer Res*, **26**:2083–2121, 1966.

MAYER, J.: Some aspects of the problem of regulation of food intake and obesity. *New Eng J Med*, **274**:722–31, 1966.

OLIVER, M. F.: Presymptomatic diagnosis of ischaemic heart disease. *Proc Roy Soc Med*, **59**:1180–84, 1966.

OLIVER, W. L.: Multiple screening tests for chronic diseases. *New York J Med*, **67**:302–8, 1967.

REID, D. D., HOLLAND, W. W., and ROSE, G. A.: An Anglo-American cardiovascular comparison. *J Lancet*, **2**:1375–78, 1967.

ROBERTS, N. J.: The values and limitations of periodic health examinations. *J Chronic Dis*, **9**:95–116, 1959.

SCHREINER, G. E.: The nephrotoxicity of analgesic abuse. *Ann Intern Med*, **57**:1047–52, 1962.

THOMAS, C. B., and ROSS, D. C.: Precursors of hypertension and coronary disease among healthy medical students: discriminant function analysis. IV. Using certain habits of daily life (sleeping, eating, drinking, studying and exercise) as the criteria. *Johns Hopkins Med J*, **122**:196–217, 1968.

TRUETT, J., CORNFIELD, J., and KANNEL, W.: A multivariate analysis of the risk of coronary heart disease in Framingham. *J Chronic Dis*, **20**:511–24, 1967.

U.S. PUBLIC HEALTH SERVICE: *The Health Consequences of Smoking: 1968 Supplement to the 1967 Public Health Service Review*.

————: *Smoking and Health: Report of the Advisory Committee to the Surgeon General of the Public Health Service*. 1964.

————: *Some Facts About Suicide: Causes and Prevention*. PHS Pub. no. 852. U.S. Government Printing Office, 1961.

WOOD, F. H., FEINSTEIN, A. R., TARANTA, A., EPSTEIN, J. S., and SIMPSON, R.: Rheumatic fever in children and adolescents. III. Comparative effectiveness of three prophylaxis regimens in preventing streptococcal infections and rheumatic recurrences. *Ann Intern Med* (Suppl. no. 5), **60**:31–46, 1964.

INDEX